Frontiers in Antimicrobial Biomaterials

Frontiers in Antimicrobial Biomaterials

Editor

Helena Felgueiras

MDPI • Basel • Beijing • Wuhan • Barcelona • Belgrade • Manchester • Tokyo • Cluj • Tianjin

Editor
Helena Felgueiras
Centro de Ciência e
Tecnologia Têxtil
Universidade do Minho
Guimarães
Portugal

Editorial Office
MDPI
St. Alban-Anlage 66
4052 Basel, Switzerland

This is a reprint of articles from the Special Issue published online in the open access journal *International Journal of Molecular Sciences* (ISSN 1422-0067) (available at: www.mdpi.com/journal/ijms/special_issues/antimicro_biomaterials).

For citation purposes, cite each article independently as indicated on the article page online and as indicated below:

LastName, A.A.; LastName, B.B.; LastName, C.C. Article Title. *Journal Name* **Year**, *Volume Number*, Page Range.

ISBN 978-3-0365-5218-7 (Hbk)
ISBN 978-3-0365-5217-0 (PDF)

Contents

Helena P. Felgueiras
Frontiers in Antimicrobial Biomaterials
Reprinted from: *Int. J. Mol. Sci.* **2022**, *23*, 9377, doi:10.3390/ijms23169377 1

Jakub Spałek, Przemysław Ociepa, Piotr Deptuła, Ewelina Piktel, Tamara Daniluk and Grzegorz Król et al.
Biocompatible Materials in Otorhinolaryngology and Their Antibacterial Properties
Reprinted from: *Int. J. Mol. Sci.* **2022**, *23*, 2575, doi:10.3390/ijms23052575 5

Maria Minodora Marin, Raluca Ianchis, Rebeca Leu Alexa, Ioana Catalina Gifu, Madalina Georgiana Albu Kaya and Diana Iulia Savu et al.
Development of New Collagen/Clay Composite Biomaterials
Reprinted from: *Int. J. Mol. Sci.* **2021**, *23*, 401, doi:10.3390/ijms23010401 29

Adewale O. Fadaka, Samantha Meyer, Omnia Ahmed, Greta Geerts, Madimabe A. Madiehe and Mervin Meyer et al.
Broad Spectrum Anti-Bacterial Activity and Non-Selective Toxicity of Gum Arabic Silver Nanoparticles
Reprinted from: *Int. J. Mol. Sci.* **2022**, *23*, 1799, doi:10.3390/ijms23031799 49

Rūta Minickaitė, Birutė Grybaitė, Rita Vaickelionienė, Povilas Kavaliauskas, Vidmantas Petraitis and Rūta Petraitienė et al.
Synthesis of Novel Aminothiazole Derivatives as Promising Antiviral, Antioxidant and Antibacterial Candidates
Reprinted from: *Int. J. Mol. Sci.* **2022**, *23*, 7688, doi:10.3390/ijms23147688 67

Ayuni Yussof, Brian Cammalleri, Oluwanifemi Fayemiwo, Sabrina Lopez and Tinchun Chu
Antibacterial and Sporicidal Activity Evaluation of Theaflavin-3,3′-digallate
Reprinted from: *Int. J. Mol. Sci.* **2022**, *23*, 2153, doi:10.3390/ijms23042153 87

Yoshie Umehara, Miho Takahashi, Hainan Yue, Juan Valentin Trujillo-Paez, Ge Peng and Hai Le Thanh Nguyen et al.
The Antimicrobial Peptides Human -Defensins Induce the Secretion of Angiogenin in Human Dermal Fibroblasts
Reprinted from: *Int. J. Mol. Sci.* **2022**, *23*, 8800, doi:10.3390/ijms23158800 109

Xuewu Zhu, Fangyi Chen, Shuang Li, Hui Peng and Ke-Jian Wang
A Novel Antimicrobial Peptide Sparanegtin Identified in *Scylla paramamosain* Showing Antimicrobial Activity and Immunoprotective Role In Vitro and Vivo
Reprinted from: *Int. J. Mol. Sci.* **2021**, *23*, 15, doi:10.3390/ijms23010015 121

Ying Yang, Fangyi Chen, Kun Qiao, Hua Zhang, Hui-Yun Chen and Ke-Jian Wang
Two Male-Specific Antimicrobial Peptides SCY2 and Scyreprocin as Crucial Molecules Participated in the Sperm Acrosome Reaction of Mud Crab *Scylla paramamosain*
Reprinted from: *Int. J. Mol. Sci.* **2022**, *23*, 3373, doi:10.3390/ijms23063373 139

Wan Yang, Vijay Singh Gondil, Dehua Luo, Jin He, Hongping Wei and Hang Yang
Optimized Silica-Binding Peptide-Mediated Delivery of Bactericidal Lysin Efficiently Prevents *Staphylococcus aureus* from Adhering to Device Surfaces
Reprinted from: *Int. J. Mol. Sci.* **2021**, *22*, 12544, doi:10.3390/ijms222212544 161

Karina Egle, Ingus Skadins, Andra Grava, Lana Micko, Viktors Dubniks and Ilze Salma et al.
Injectable Platelet-Rich Fibrin as a Drug Carrier Increases the Antibacterial Susceptibility of Antibiotic—Clindamycin Phosphate
Reprinted from: *Int. J. Mol. Sci.* **2022**, *23*, 7407, doi:10.3390/ijms23137407 . . . . **177**

Do Nam Lee, Yeong Rim Kim, Sohyeon Yang, Ngoc Minh Tran, Bong Joo Park and Su Jung Lee et al.
Controllable Nitric Oxide Storage and Release in Cu-BTC: Crystallographic Insights and Bioactivity
Reprinted from: *Int. J. Mol. Sci.* **2022**, *23*, 9098, doi:10.3390/ijms23169098 . . . . **195**

International Journal of
Molecular Sciences

MDPI

Editorial

Frontiers in Antimicrobial Biomaterials

Helena P. Felgueiras

Centre for Textile Science and Technology (2C2T), University of Minho, Campus de Azurém, 4800-058 Guimarães, Portugal; helena.felgueiras@2c2t.uminho.pt

Biomaterials can be used as implantable devices or drug delivery platforms, which have significant impacts on the patient's quality of life. Indeed, every year, a substantial number of new biomaterials and scaffolding systems are engineered and introduced in the biomedical field, with increased health benefits observed, as reported by Spalek et al. [1]. However, their long-term use can be threatened by the adhesion and proliferation of microorganisms, which can interact and form biofilms, or by the formation of fibrosis and consequent triggered cytotoxic responses. Pathogenic microorganisms may cause local infections and lead to implant failures. Additionally, they can hinder the delivery of therapeutic molecules by specialized carriers, rendering them ineffective. Many alternatives have been proposed over the years to prevent such events, including the use of antiseptics and antibiotics or the physical modification of the biomaterial surface, with the incorporation of biomolecules having developed into an area of interest. From specialized polymers and functional groups to silver and, more recently, antimicrobial peptides and natural extracts, different functionalization and modification techniques have been employed in this fight against pathogenic agents [1–7]. Marin et al., for instance, introduced a new generation of collagen-based biomaterials embedded with nanoclay for skin regeneration, demonstrating an improved antimicrobial potential. They reported that, depending on the nanoclay type used, both the cellular viability and antimicrobial activity (potentiated by gentamicin) could be controlled for a prolonged action over time [8]. This Special Issue aims at furthering our understanding of the antimicrobial actions of specialized biomaterials and introducing new surface modification strategies, original polymeric chemical structures, and new antimicrobial agent–material combinations, from which infection control or microbial eradication can be achieved.

Citation: Felgueiras, H.P. Frontiers in Antimicrobial Biomaterials. *Int. J. Mol. Sci.* **2022**, *23*, 9377. https://doi.org/10.3390/ijms23169377

Received: 16 August 2022
Accepted: 18 August 2022
Published: 19 August 2022

In this collection of research, many important findings can be highlighted, namely the engineering and synthesis of novel antimicrobial agents. Fadaka et al. took a well-known nanomaterial, the silver nanoparticles, and modified its synthesis to improve its physical-chemical properties. They used gum arabic, sodium borohydride, and their combination as reducing agents and evaluated the particles' antimicrobial and cytotoxic profiles. Gum arabic was deemed to be the most effective reducing agent in improving the bactericidal efficiency of the synthesized silver nanoparticles. However, the authors concluded that the nanoparticle toxicity could not be completely overcome, even by using a greener synthesis methodology, which is required in order to establish ranges of effectiveness for human safety [9]. Novel aminothiazoles with superior antiviral, antioxidant, and antibacterial activities were also synthesized by Minickaitė et al. They demonstrated that, by using substitutes in the thiazole ring, optimized antimicrobial structures could be generated with target specificity [10]. Yussof et al. revealed similar outcomes when exploring the antibacterial and sporicidal effectiveness of theaflavin-3,3′-digallate. They determined the potential of this polyphenol, derived from the leaves of *Camellia sinensis*, to fight against a range of bacteria, including the spore-forming *Bacillus* spp., and established its promising broad-spectrum antibacterial and anti-spore activities [11].

Antimicrobial peptides are considered a new generation of antimicrobial agents. Indeed, in recent years, they have been explored as potential alternatives to antibiotics and other immunomodulatory drugs [12]. Umehara et al. studied the well-characterized skin-derived human β-defensins antimicrobial peptides and demonstrated their influence on the secretion of angiogenin, a potent angiogenic factor. They revealed that various human β-defensins can stimulate the production of angiogenin while maintaining their antimicrobial activities and other immunomodulatory properties [13]. Zhu et al. identified a new antimicrobial peptide gene, the Sparanegtin gene from the mud crab *Scylla paramamosain*, whose transcripts were particularly abundant in the testis of that species. The recombinant Sparanegtin was found to be effective against both Gram-positive and Gram-negative bacteria, including *Pseudomonas aeruginosa*, and its immunomodulatory effects on specific bacteria were also revealed [14]. Yang et al. also identified two male-specific antimicrobial peptides, SCY2 and Scyreprocin from the mud crab *Scylla paramamosain*, and established their dual role in reproductive immunity and sperm acrosome reactions while maintaining their antimicrobial profiles [15].

In light of the size and sensitivity to physiological conditions of most bioactive agents, including antimicrobial peptides, optimizing their localized and target deliveries are essential. With this in mind, Yang et al. proposed the incorporation of ClyF, an anti-staphylococcal lysin, into constructs of silica-binding peptide for application as device coatings for the prevention of *Staphylococcal*-related infections. The ClyF-immobilized surfaces supported the normal attachment and growth of mammalian cells and displayed significant bactericidal features, being deemed potentially effective in preventing the growth of antibiotic-resistant microorganisms [16]. In turn, Egle et al. studied the influence of an engineered platelet-rich fibrin, used as a carrier matrix in the antibacterial properties of clindamycin phosphate, on Gram-positive bacteria. The carrier was observed to induce structural changes in the clindamycin, giving rise to a more active compound that significantly decreased the minimal bactericidal concentrations required to eliminate *Staphylococcal* strains. The researchers attested to the safety of the engineered carrier for human cells in vitro, thus evidencing the system's potential to reduce the risk of postoperative infection [17]. Finally, Lee et al. proposed the controlled storage and release of nitric oxide from metal organic nanosized frameworks formed from Cu-BTC for prospective uses in drug delivery systems. The nitric oxide release was maintained as constant for 12 h, meeting the requirements for clinical applications. Most importantly, the authors verified the structures' antibacterial potential by their significant elimination of six bacteria strains, highlighting the synergistic effects between the payload and carrier [18].

Funding: This research was funded by the Portuguese Foundation for Science and Technology (FCT) via grants PTDC/CTMTEX/28074/2017 and UID/CTM/00264/2021.

Conflicts of Interest: The author declares no conflict of interest.

References

1. Spałek, J.; Ociepa, P.; Deptuła, P.; Piktel, E.; Daniluk, T.; Król, G.; Góźdź, S.; Bucki, R.; Okła, S. Biocompatible Materials in Otorhinolaryngology and Their Antibacterial Properties. *Int. J. Mol. Sci.* **2022**, *23*, 2575. [CrossRef] [PubMed]
2. Teixeira, M.A.; Antunes, J.C.; Seabra, C.L.; Tohidi, S.D.; Reis, S.; Amorim, M.T.P.; Felgueiras, H.P. Tiger 17 and pexiganan as antimicrobial and hemostatic boosters of cellulose acetate-containing poly (vinyl alcohol) electrospun mats for potential wound care purposes. *Int. J. Biol. Macromol.* **2022**, *209*, 1526–1541. [CrossRef] [PubMed]
3. Felgueiras, H.P. An insight into biomolecules for the treatment of skin infectious diseases. *Pharmaceutics* **2021**, *13*, 1012. [CrossRef] [PubMed]
4. Antunes, J.C.; Domingues, J.M.; Miranda, C.S.; Silva, A.F.G.; Homem, N.C.; Amorim, M.T.P.; Felgueiras, H.P. Bioactivity of chitosan-based particles loaded with plant-derived extracts for biomedical applications: Emphasis on antimicrobial fiber-based systems. *Mar. Drugs* **2021**, *19*, 359. [CrossRef] [PubMed]
5. Felgueiras, H.P.; Homem, N.C.; Teixeira, M.; Ribeiro, A.; Teixeira, M.O.; Antunes, J.; Amorim, M. Biodegradable wet-spun fibers modified with antimicrobial agents for potential applications in biomedical engineering. *J. Phys. Conf. Ser.* **2021**, *1765*, 012007. [CrossRef]
6. Teixeira, M.O.; Antunes, J.C.; Felgueiras, H.P. Recent advances in fiber–hydrogel composites for wound healing and drug delivery systems. *Antibiotics* **2021**, *10*, 248. [CrossRef] [PubMed]
7. Miranda, C.S.; Ribeiro, A.R.; Homem, N.C.; Felgueiras, H.P. Spun biotextiles in tissue engineering and biomolecules delivery systems. *Antibiotics* **2020**, *9*, 174. [CrossRef] [PubMed]

8. Marin, M.M.; Ianchis, R.; Leu Alexa, R.; Gifu, I.C.; Kaya, M.G.A.; Savu, D.I.; Popescu, R.C.; Alexandrescu, E.; Ninciuleanu, C.M.; Preda, S.; et al. Development of New Collagen/Clay Composite Biomaterials. *Int. J. Mol. Sci.* **2022**, *23*, 401. [CrossRef] [PubMed]
9. Fadaka, A.O.; Meyer, S.; Ahmed, O.; Geerts, G.; Madiehe, M.A.; Meyer, M.; Sibuyi, N.R.S. Broad Spectrum Anti-Bacterial Activity and Non-Selective Toxicity of Gum Arabic Silver Nanoparticles. *Int. J. Mol. Sci.* **2022**, *23*, 1799. [CrossRef] [PubMed]
10. Minickaitė, R.; Grybaitė, B.; Vaickelionienė, R.; Kavaliauskas, P.; Petraitis, V.; Petraitienė, R.; Tumosienė, I.; Jonuškienė, I.; Mickevičius, V. Synthesis of Novel Aminothiazole Derivatives as Promising Antiviral, Antioxidant and Antibacterial Candidates. *Int. J. Mol. Sci.* **2022**, *23*, 7688. [CrossRef] [PubMed]
11. Yussof, A.; Cammalleri, B.; Fayemiwo, O.; Lopez, S.; Chu, T. Antibacterial and Sporicidal Activity Evaluation of Theaflavin-3,3′-digallate. *Int. J. Mol. Sci.* **2022**, *23*, 2153. [CrossRef] [PubMed]
12. Felgueiras, H.P.; Amorim, M.T.P. Functionalization of electrospun polymeric wound dressings with antimicrobial peptides. *Colloids Surf. B Biointerfaces* **2017**, *156*, 133–148. [CrossRef] [PubMed]
13. Umehara, Y.; Takahashi, M.; Yue, H.; Trujillo-Paez, J.V.; Peng, G.; Nguyen, H.L.T.; Okumura, K.; Ogawa, H.; Niyonsaba, F. The Antimicrobial Peptides Human β-Defensins Induce the Secretion of Angiogenin in Human Dermal Fibroblasts. *Int. J. Mol. Sci.* **2022**, *23*, 8800. [CrossRef] [PubMed]
14. Zhu, X.; Chen, F.; Li, S.; Peng, H.; Wang, K.-J. A Novel Antimicrobial Peptide Sparanegtin Identified in Scylla paramamosain Showing Antimicrobial Activity and Immunoprotective Role In Vitro and Vivo. *Int. J. Mol. Sci.* **2022**, *23*, 15. [CrossRef] [PubMed]
15. Yang, Y.; Chen, F.; Qiao, K.; Zhang, H.; Chen, H.-Y.; Wang, K.-J. Two Male-Specific Antimicrobial Peptides SCY2 and Scyreprocin as Crucial Molecules Participated in the Sperm Acrosome Reaction of Mud Crab Scylla paramamosain. *Int. J. Mol. Sci.* **2022**, *23*, 3373. [CrossRef] [PubMed]
16. Yang, W.; Gondil, V.S.; Luo, D.; He, J.; Wei, H.; Yang, H. Optimized Silica-Binding Peptide-Mediated Delivery of Bactericidal Lysin Efficiently Prevents Staphylococcus aureus from Adhering to Device Surfaces. *Int. J. Mol. Sci.* **2021**, *22*, 12544. [CrossRef] [PubMed]
17. Egle, K.; Skadins, I.; Grava, A.; Micko, L.; Dubniks, V.; Salma, I.; Dubnika, A. Injectable Platelet-Rich Fibrin as a Drug Carrier Increases the Antibacterial Susceptibility of Antibiotic—Clindamycin Phosphate. *Int. J. Mol. Sci.* **2022**, *23*, 7407. [CrossRef] [PubMed]
18. Lee, D.N.; Kim, Y.R.; Yang, S.; Tran, N.M.; Park, B.J.; Lee, S.J.; Kim, Y.; Yoo, H.; Kim, S.-J.; Shin, J.H. Controllable Nitric Oxide Storage and Release in Cu-BTC: Crystallographic Insights and Bioactivity. *Int. J. Mol. Sci.* **2022**, *23*, 9098. [CrossRef]

International Journal of
Molecular Sciences

Review

Biocompatible Materials in Otorhinolaryngology and Their Antibacterial Properties

Jakub Spałek [1,2,*], Przemysław Ociepa [2], Piotr Deptuła [3], Ewelina Piktel [4], Tamara Daniluk [3], Grzegorz Król [1], Stanisław Góźdź [1], Robert Bucki [1,3] and Sławomir Okła [1,2,*]

1 Institute of Medical Science, Collegium Medicum, Jan Kochanowski University of Kielce, IX Wieków Kielc 19A, 25-317 Kielce, Poland; g.krol@op.pl (G.K.); stanislaw.gozdz@onkol.kielce.pl (S.G.); buckirobert@gmail.com (R.B.)
2 Department of Otolaryngology, Head and Neck Surgery, Holy-Cross Cancer Center, Artwińskiego 3, 25-734 Kielce, Poland; pr.ociepa@gmail.com
3 Department of Medical Microbiology and Nanobiomedical Engineering, Medical University of Bialystok, Mickiewicza 2C, 15-222 Bialystok, Poland; piotr.deptula@umb.edu.pl (P.D.); tamara.daniluk@umb.edu.pl (T.D.)
4 Independent Laboratory of Nanomedicine, Medical University of Bialystok, Mickiewicza 2B, 15-222 Bialystok, Poland; ewelina.piktel@wp.pl
* Correspondence: jspalek@ujk.edu.pl (J.S.); slawomir.okla@gmail.com (S.O.)

Abstract: For decades, biomaterials have been commonly used in medicine for the replacement of human body tissue, precise drug-delivery systems, or as parts of medical devices that are essential for some treatment methods. Due to rapid progress in the field of new materials, updates on the state of knowledge about biomaterials are frequently needed. This article describes the clinical application of different types of biomaterials in the field of otorhinolaryngology, i.e., head and neck surgery, focusing on their antimicrobial properties. The variety of their applications includes cochlear implants, middle ear prostheses, voice prostheses, materials for osteosynthesis, and nasal packing after nasal/paranasal sinuses surgery. Ceramics, such as as hydroxyapatite, zirconia, or metals and metal alloys, still have applications in the head and neck region. Tissue engineering scaffolds and drug-eluting materials, such as polymers and polymer-based composites, are becoming more common. The restoration of life tissue and the ability to prevent microbial colonization should be taken into consideration when designing the materials to be used for implant production. The authors of this paper have reviewed publications available in PubMed from the last five years about the recent progress in this topic but also establish the state of knowledge of the most common application of biomaterials over the last few decades.

Keywords: biomaterials; nanomaterials; antimicrobial action; osteosynthesis; tissue engineering; voice prosthesis

Citation: Spałek, J.; Ociepa, P.; Deptuła, P.; Piktel, E.; Daniluk, T.; Król, G.; Góźdź, S.; Bucki, R.; Okła, S. Biocompatible Materials in Otorhinolaryngology and Their Antibacterial Properties. *Int. J. Mol. Sci.* **2022**, *23*, 2575. https://doi.org/10.3390/ijms23052575

Academic Editor: Helena Felgueiras

Received: 15 January 2022
Accepted: 20 February 2022
Published: 25 February 2022

1. Introduction

Biomaterial is any substance (other than a drug) or combination of substances, natural or synthetic, that can be used for a period of time, independently or as part of a system which treats, augments, or replaces any tissue, organ, or function of the body [1]. The first application of biomaterial in history is most likely a case that was reported a few centuries after the Common Era of ancient medicine for wound closure. Romans have described urologic catheters, and Aztecs used gold dental fillings [2]. Nowadays, technological progress allows the development of implants that are based on innovative biomaterials. We can classify biomaterials by their applications, material physicochemical properties, or their interactions with the patient's tissue. The application of biomaterials in modern medicine is very wide, for example, artificial joints, bone grafts, dental implants, cardiovascular stents, artificial lenses, plastic surgery implants, trauma and reconstructive surgery materials, and surgical tools. Due to the variety of biomaterials' functions, their mechanical properties varied from very hard and stiff to very soft and flexible. According to the biomaterials' nature, we distinguish the builds of polymers, metals, composites, and ceramics materials. We can also classify biomaterials from their level of interaction with the host tissue as bioinert, bioactive, and bioresorbable [3–5]. One of the greatest risks associated with placing an implant within the living tissue of a patient is related to the colonization of the material by opportunistic/pathogenic microorganisms and the formation of a bacterial/fungal or mixed biofilm on an implant's surface. There are some methods to prevent this process, which are described in Section 4.

1.1. Polymers

Most common polymers used for the design and fabrication of biomaterials include natural polymers, such as collagen, alginate, or chitosan, and synthetic ones, such as polyethylene, polyethylene terephthalate, and polytetrafluorethylene. Polymers are classified by their permanent (biostable) or temporary (biodegradable) applications. Biostable polymers are used for long-term exploitation. When working with biostable polymers, the main challenge is to prevent the material degradation of the polymer by physiological tissue processes as oxidation of polyether segments in polyurethane at the α-position to the ether-oxygen [6], or the long-term hydrolysis of polyamides [7] or polyethylene terephthalate [7,8]. In most situations, biofilm growth is also a destructive factor for the polymers [9,10]. Biodegradable polymers are used as a base for local drug delivery or as a temporary support for tissue regeneration. These polymers are degraded non-enzymatically by hydrolysis or by specific enzymes [11]. The good biocompatibility makes them a good material for many medical applications [12–15]. Among the few polymers approved by the FDA, there are poly(glycolic acid) or poly(glycolide) (PGA), poly(lactic acid) or poly(lactide) (PLA), as well as poly(lactic-co-glycolic acid) or poly(lactide-co-glycolide) (PLGA) (Figure 1).

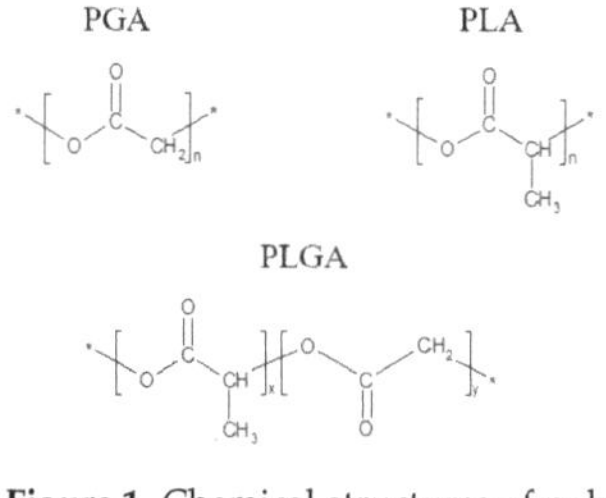

Figure 1. Chemical structures of poly(glycolic acid) (PGA), poly(lactic acid) (PLA), and poly(lactide-co-glycolide) (PLGA). (n: number of repeat units in PLA and PGA; x and y: number of lactic and glycolic units in PLGA, respectively). * another unit of PGA/PLA.

In 1970, the US Food and Drug Administration approved these materials for bioresorbable surgical sutures, then, in 1986, the first bioresorbable drug delivery PLGA microspheres were approved [16]. PLGA co-polymers undergo degradation in the way of hydrolysis. The ester bonds are cleaved by the hydrolytic degradation that occurs throughout the whole PLGA microparticle matrix. PLGA degradation into monomers can be divided into three phases. In this process of random chain scission, the polymer divides into the oligomers and finally into soluble monomers. In the first phase, the weight loss and soluble monomer formed are not appreciable, and, in the second phase, there is rapid loss of mass. Once the monomers are formed, they are eliminated by physiological pathways. Lactic acid enters the tricarboxylic acid cycle and is metabolized and eliminated in carbon dioxide and water, while glycolic acid is excreted unchanged by the kidneys or metabolized by the tricarboxylic acid cycle [16–18] (Figure 2). So far, 15 products based on PLA/PLGA microparticles have been approved and marketed, and more than 35 products have been successfully developed for medical use [19].

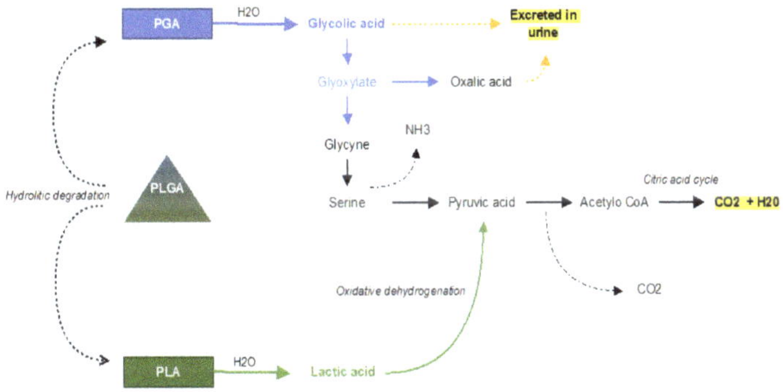

Figure 2. Schematic illustration showing the degradation of PLGA co-polymer and the PGA and PLA monomers. As a result, carbon dioxide and water are finally produced.

1.2. Metals and Metals Alloys

Titanium and its alloys, as well as iron-based alloys and cobalt-based alloys, are commonly used in medicine as materials for all kinds of implants and biomedical constructions, such as orthopedic and bone fracture surgical treatment or as a scaffold of cardiologic self-expanded stents [20,21]. These materials are the most popular metallic biomaterials applied in the broad field of medicine. Stainless steel was applied in the 1920s as a biomaterial, and the first cobalt-based alloy was introduced into dental practice in 1907 [22]. Titanium alloys since the eighties have been model metallic materials used in various types of biomedical constructions [20], unfortunately this material has significant flaws. For many years, toxic alloying agents in titanium alloys, such as aluminum and vanadium, have raised doubts. Studies prove the toxicity of these elements and induction of many diseases after long-term periods of use [23,24]. The main disadvantage of some of these materials is also a very common local inflammatory host reaction or toxicity, which can be decreased by coating them by other biocompatible materials as for example polymers. However, sometimes the local tissue reaction to the material is beneficial, such as stimulating new bones through the use of magnesium alloys in the healing of bone fractures [25]. In recent years, new titanium-based materials with non-toxic additives, such as molybdenum and niobium, which are austenitic steels without the addition of toxic nickel, have been investigated [26–28].

1.3. Ceramics

Ceramics are a group of biomaterials with very good biocompatibility features. This group generally does not cause an allergic reaction and a cytotoxic effect [29]. But on the other hand these materials are brittle and low impact resistance [30]. Ceramics biomaterials are commonly use in bone replacement, dental and maxillo-facial reconstructions. Aluminum trioxide is still used for dental implants but zirconia, which was introduced as a dental implants material in 1970s is nowadays commonly used because of its similar color to human teeth [31,32].

1.4. Composites

Composite materials are made of at least two constituents to decrease their disadvantages. Composite materials are used for bulk soft tissues replacements, space fillers, catheters, ureter prostheses, tendons and ligaments, and vascular grafts. Fiber-reinforced polymer composites are the most commonly used composites in orthopedics [33].

2. Methods

Innovative biomaterials for otolaryngology have already been developed. This article aims to review recent publications in this area. Available bibliographies in PubMed were searched, and the latest or the most significant papers, in the authors' opinions, were quoted. Publications from the last five years (2015–2020) were reviewed in PubMed. Some publications included in this review were published more than five years ago or not found by the queries mentioned below but, in the authors' opinions, these publications were significant and important. There were 163 articles quoted in this review, following the authors' research. The following amounts of articles (January 2022) were found after typing some keywords in PubMed: polymers + otolaryngology (828), polymers + head and neck cancers (476), polymers + sinus surgery (263), polymers + head and neck tissue engineering (149), polymers + head and neck implants (125), polymers + cochlear implants (38), and polymers + nasal packing (37).

3. Biomaterials Used in Otorhinolaryngology

3.1. Cochlear Implants

Cochlear implants are commonly used for the successful treatment of deaf-born children and deafened adults. The idea of this technically advanced method is to implant a cochlear implant's electrode into the cochlea to allow the electrical stimulation of the auditory nerve [34]. The interaction between the electrode and the auditory neurons is essential for long and effective treatment. The cochlear implant–electrode array consists of platinum–iridium and silicone. Despite its materials' good biocompatibility, cochlear implants are recognized as foreign bodies. The efficiency of cochlear implants is affected by postoperative connective tissue growth around the electrode array. This results in tissue fibrosis around the electrode, which happens due to fibrocyte migration after the electrode implantation. This process is undesirable because of the increase in impedance that it results in. Glucocorticoids—mainly dexamethasone—are locally applied to decrease fibrosis. One of the methods of its application is drug depot accommodation in the silicon carrier of the electrode [35] (Figure 3). This approach has a more continuous and longer profile of drug release, which is more effective than other methods of dexamethasone application [2,36]. It is desirable to minimize the space between electrodes and auditory neuronal dendrites. For this reason, neurotrophic factors, such as the glial cell-derived neurotrophic factor (GDNF) and the brain-derived neurotrophic factor (BDNF), are also used. Local application of these factors to the cochlear implant electrodes is one of the methods that have a proven positive effect on the anti-fibrosis process, the regeneration of auditory neuron dendrites, and the in vivo preservation of neurons in animals [36–39]. Lehner et al. have tested a new type of Poly-(D,L-lactic-co-glycolic acid) (PLGA)-based biodegradable implant for intracochlear delivery of drugs on animals to find the appropriate size and mechanical properties, as well as to prove the general feasibility of its administration. They found that the use of Polyethylene glycol (PEG) as an additional excipient was beneficial in two aspects. PEG softens the extrudates and prevents cracking during bending, and PEG accelerates the initial drug release rate so that it matches the desired profile [37]. The release of dexamethasone from the PLGA without PEG was measured at 6.5% within the first week, this then accelerated to reach almost 50% after two weeks and 80% after three weeks. It is connected to initial slow water penetration and the autocatalytic degradation of the polymer [38].

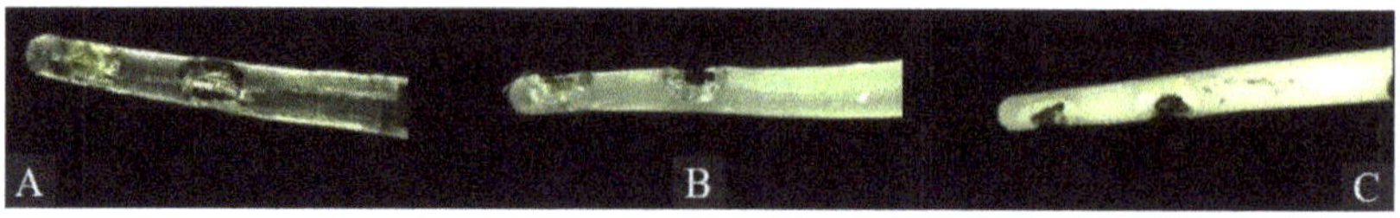

Figure 3. (**A**): pure silicone electrode array without DEX (0%); (**B**): electrode array containing 1% DEX (16 ng/day delivery rate); (**C**): electrode array containing 10% DEX (49 ng/day delivery rate). Adapted from an open-access source: [36].

The developed intracochlear drug-loaded implant can be administrated with or without a neuroprosthetic cochlear implant. Some experimental studies also showed the positive application of biodegradable drug delivery systems as a salvage therapy for idiopathic sudden sensorial hearing loss (ISSHL) [37,39]. A carrier of dexamethasone was used along with a PLGA polymer matrix containing a mixture of polymer chains with free and esterified carboxylic end groups without a preservative. The PLGA matrix slowly degrades to lactic acid and glycolic acid.

3.2. Tympanostomy Tube

The implantation of a tympanostomy tube in the eardrum allows the drainage of fluid from the middle ear. This procedure is usually performed in patients with otitis media. Biofilm formation on this device is the main factor of post-tympanostomy complications, such as otorrhea, tube occlusion, and discomfort. There are some studies where authors have faced this problem. In some in vitro studies, the use of a vancomycin coating or a piperacillin-tazobactam coating of the tympanostomy tube were tested with positive promising results [40,41].

Another approach is to change the tube-surface properties of resisting bacterial colonization and biofilm formation. The model implemented by Saidi et. al suggests that the adherence properties of the tube may be more important than antibacterial coatings in terms of the prevention of persistent otorrhea [42]. Jang et al. suggest that the surface modification by an ion bombardment is not enough on its own to resist ciprofloxacin-resistant *Pseudomonas aeruginosa* biofilm formation [43]. Joe et. al designed a novel tympanostomy tube type, i.e., a tympanostomy stent (TS), which had a smooth and minimized surface area to prevent the adherence of biofilm by preserving its own function of drainage. Furthermore, it was coated with TiO_2. The authors reported the promising outcomes of their study [44].

3.3. Middle-Ear Prosthesis

The ossicular chain reconstruction of the middle ear may be carried out with either a partial ossicular replacement prosthesis or a total ossicular replacement prosthesis. Implantable middle-ear hearing aids are used in the treatment of mild–moderate, mixed or conductive hearing loss and, in some cases, to treat sensorineural hearing loss [45]. There is a variety of materials used by surgeons for ossicular reconstruction. Some studies indicate that titanium ossicular prostheses are the most popular among surgeons, because of their efficiency in sound transmission and the fact that they are delicate and easy to handle. Titanium is the most lightweight and biocompatible material among all allogenic materials used for ossicular reconstruction [46,47]. Moreover, titanium clip prostheses have proven long-term results in ossiculoplasty [48]. A ceramic (hydroxyapatite) prosthesis commonly used for ossicular reconstruction also exists; however, it has high incidence of extrusion when it is placed in contact with the tympanic membrane [49,50]. A retrospective study comparing hearing and anatomical outcomes after ossicular chain reconstruction with titanium or hydroxyapatite prostheses concluded that both types of prosthesis had satisfactory functional and anatomical results, and no preponderance could be stated, except for the hearing results of partial titanium prostheses [51]. One of the materials used for middle ear surgery is a composite HAPEX (Smith and Nephew). It is composed of 40% synthetic hydroxyapatite (HAp) and 60% high-density polyethylene (HDPE). In a clinical study, HAPEX has proven to be a stable implant/bone bonding material. It was observed that middle-ear prostheses became overgrown by fibrous tissue inside a thin epithelial layer [52]. Problems with extrusion, migration, and reactivity occur with some alloplastic materials, such as Polyethylene, high-density polyethylene sponge (HDPS), polytetrafluoroethylene (PTFE), and Proplast (PTFE–carbon composite), which are also regarded as ossicular prostheses [53]. There are many reports of different artificial materials used in ossicular surgery, but the histocompatibility and long-term outcomes still remain uncertain. Moreover, none of the materials mentioned above possess bactericidal properties [54]. Such activity is looked for as it indicates the same information as the detection of biocompatibility or physical properties. There are some studies about new antimicrobial system, which are fully described in Section 4.

3.4. Nasal Packing Materials

Endoscopic sinus surgery (ESS), conchotomy, or septoplasty procedures are currently very common surgical treatments. They are often associated with such postoperative complications as nasal bleeding, adhesions, and stenosis, which could be prevented by nasal packing [55]. The efficiency of and the patient's tolerance for nasal packing products vary [56]. The currently used packing materials can be classified into nonbiodegradable (e.g., vaselinized gauze, Telfapads, cotton-stuffed latex finger cots, Silastic sheeting, Merocel sponges) and biodegradable types (e.g., gel film, MeroGel, hyaluronic acid gels, FloSeal, cellulose gels, Nasopore, NASASTENT) (Figure 4). Nasopore is a fully synthetic biodegradable, fragmenting foam that absorbs water while supporting the surrounding tissue. This process provides local hemostasis by compressing bleeding vessels in the nasal cavity. After several days, it dissolves and can be suctioned from the nasal cavity. Research indicates that biodegradable packing is more comfortable because it results in less pain, bleeding, nasal blockage, and facial edema in the early postoperative period. However, there is no significant difference in the long-term post-operative outcomes of ESS [57]. Wang et al. performed the meta-analysis of 459 articles and concluded that Nasopore (absorbable) is superior to Merocel (non-absorbable), with regard to pain upon removal, bleeding, in situ pain, pressure, and general satisfaction, and equal to Merocel, with regard to nasal obstruction, tissue adhesion, and mucosal healing [58].

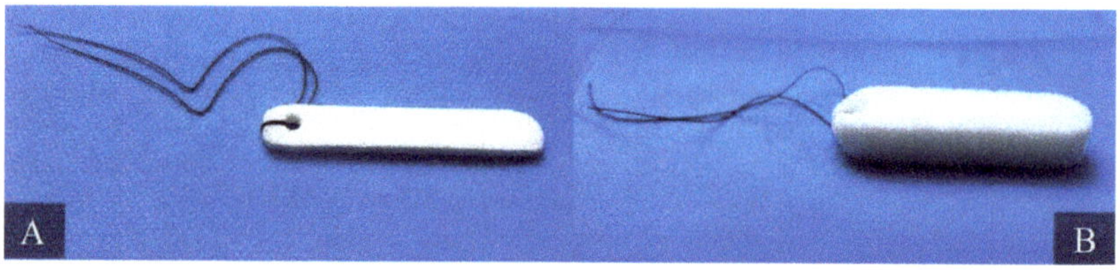

Figure 4. Nonabsorbable nasal packing Merocel (Medtronic Inc., Minneapolis, MN, USA). Panel (**A**) presents compressed, dehydrated sponge. Panel (**B**) shows the sponge decompressed, 30 s after hydration with saline. Material from the authors' collection.

3.5. Corticosteroid-Eluting Sinus Stents

As nasal packing materials have a positive impact on short-term postoperative outcomes, corticosteroid-eluting sinus stents could increase long-term outcomes. The European Position Paper on Rhinosinusitis and Nasal Polyps (EPOS 2020) guidelines recommend Corticoid-Eluting Sinus Stents as a therapeutic option in patients who have undergone surgical treatment of chronic rhinosinusitis (CRS) to decrease the percentage of re-operations in the future [59]. Recent advancements in bioabsorbable and drug-eluting stents provide an option for improving the long-term outcomes of postoperative endoscopic sinus surgery (ESS). Some patients had sinus neo-ostium stenosis or synechiae formation, middle turbinate (MT) lateralization, after surgery. To prevent this situation and to improve longer-term outcomes, surgeons have used nonabsorbable frontal stents that were typically placed immediately after surgery and removed in the clinic between four and six weeks later because of significant crusting and/or symptomatic pressure. For these reasons, sinus stents have been used sparingly [60]. In 2011, the first corticosteroid-eluting sinus stent (Inter- sect ENT) was approved by the FDA for patients after ethmoid sinus surgery. Then, in 2016 and 2017, the FDA approved similar devices for frontal and maxillary sinus surgeries. [61] Nowadays, there are plenty of bioresorbable stents releasing mainly mometasone for patients with CRS after ESS. There are two models of steroid-eluting sinus implants that have been U.S. Food and Drug Administration (FDA)-approved for use in CRS patients: short-duration Propel family devices (Propel, Propel Mini, Propel Contour; Intersect ENT, Menlo Park, CA, USA) and long-duration Sinuva devices (Intersect ENT, Menlo Park, CA, USA). (Figure 5).

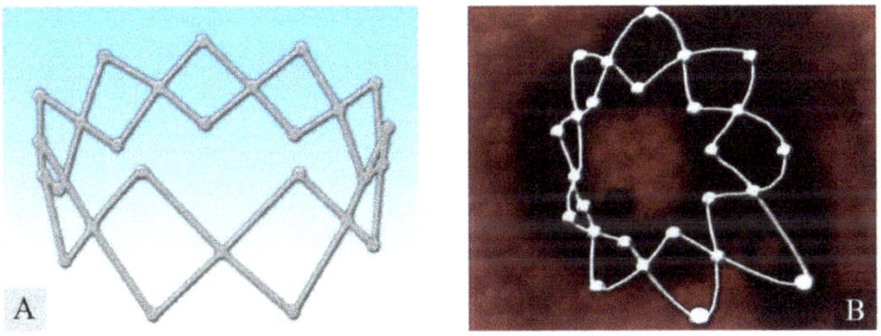

Figure 5. Mometasone-loaded (**A**) spring-like Propel™ sinus implant expands when placed into the sinus mucosa (**B**), thus keeping the middle meatus open and, hence, promoting mucous drainage and wound healing. Adapted from an open-access source: [15].

These novel devices have had promising outcomes in some clinical trials [62–65]. Drug-eluting nasal implants ensure continuous drug release over longer periods of time to the nasal mucosa, in contrast to the nasal sprays (Figure 6). The corticosteroid was encapsulated in a biodegradable polymer matrix in the form of micro- and nano-particles, and then attached to the biodegradable scaffolds of implants to achieve longer periods of drug release. The most commonly used materials for these implants are biodegradable polymers such as polylactic acid (PLA) and polylactic-co-glycolic acid (PLGA). These materials have good biocompatibility and good tolerance and have been biodegraded by the hydrolysis of their ester linkages. [66,67]. This feature results in the main advantage of these materials, i.e., bioresorption, which means that these products do not require additional surgery to remove.

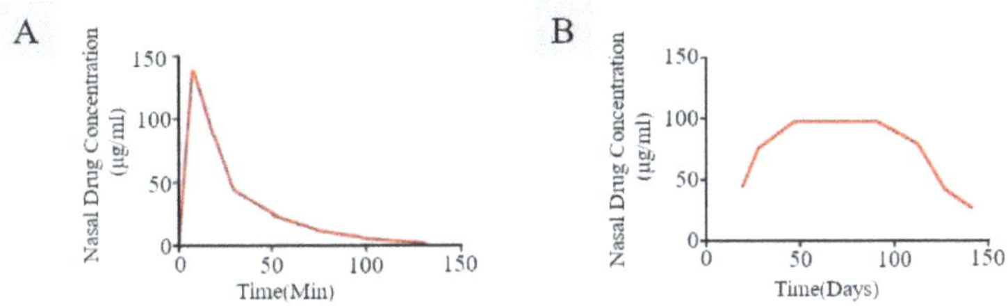

Figure 6. Nasal drug concentration versus time, obtained after administration of nasal sprays and drug-eluting implants. Nasal sprays show rapid clearance of the drug from the nasal mucosa (panel (**A**)) as compared to locally acting implants (panel (**B**)). Adapted from an open-access source: [15].

3.6. Materials for Osteosynthesis

Plate osteosyntheses allow three dimensional reconstructions of complex face fractures and the skull base. The general standard treatment uses a titanium plate system because of its resistance to corrosion, strength, ease of handling, lack of dimensional changes, mechanical properties closest to the bone compared with the other metallic bioinert biomaterials, minimal scatter on computed tomography (CT) scanning, and compatibility with radiography and magnetic resonance imaging [68,69]. Titanium screws marketed in the internal fixation systems are commonly produced from a titanium alloy, Ti–6Al–4V alloy, which is the most widely used alloy. On the other hand, osteosynthesis plates are generally produced from CP-Ti (commercially pure titanium, usually grade 2) [70,71]. These materials have some disadvantages, such as poor resistance to wear, which results in the deposition of friction in the surrounding tissue, infections, and sensitivity perturbations [72]. The other issue is the secondary surgery needed for implant removal in 5–40% of cases [68], because of its translocation thermal sensitivity, interference with diagnostic imaging, osteopenia of cortical bone induced by stress, and corrosion [73,74]. Moreover, titanium particles, as products of wear, have been found in scar tissue covering these plates, as well as in locoregional lymph nodes [68]. Therefore, in some cases, titanium osteofixation implant materials should be removed after fulfilling their functions. Pinto et al. do not see the need for routine removal of these osteosynthesis implants after installation, except when there is a clinical indication that this should be done. There is, however, no consensus in the oral and maxillofacial surgery literature regarding the removal of bone plate in asymptomatic cases [71]. To minimize the above limitations, biodegradable bone fixation materials based on polyhydroxy acids (polyglycolide acid (PGA), polylactide (PLLA and PDLA)) have been developed [72,75–79] (Table 1).

Table 1. Characteristics of bioresorbable materials and commercially available systems for maxillofacial osteosynthesis.

Material	**PGA Polyglycolic Acid**	**PLA Polylactic Acid**		**Copolymers of PGA, PLLA, PDLA**	**uHA/PLLA Composites of Unsintered Hydroxyapatite and Poly-L-Lactide**
		PLLA Poly-L-Lactide	**PDLA Poly-D-Lactide**		
	1st Generation			**2nd Generation**	**3rd Generation**
	High molecular weight; highly crystalline; rapidly degradable; radiotransparency; first bioresorbable polymer clinically used.	High molecular weight due to its crystallinity and hydrophobicity; resistant to hydrolysis; radiotransparency.	High molecular weight; lower crystallinity; less resistant to hydrolysis; highly biocompatible compared to PLLA radiotransparency.	Their properties can be controlled by varying the ratio of glycolide to lactide for different compositions. Radiotransparency.	Contains 30–40% weight fractions of raw hydroxyapatite, neither calcined nor sintered material. Osteoconductive capacity (can be complete replacement by bone tissue); radiopacity.
Application	Early loss of mechanical strength after 4–7 weeks, clearance time is 6–12 months [79]	Total resorption is over 3.5 years in vivo, in vitro about 2 years [79]	-	Resorption time of 12–18 months. In general, a higher glycolide content leads to a faster rate of degradation.	The PLLA matrix is completely absent from the composites after 4 years and almost all u-HA particles are replaced after 5.5 years [77]
	Pure PGA, due to its durability, which is insufficient to allow for complete bone healing, has rather minimal usefulness in maxillofacial surgery [68]. Biofix® SR-PGA (self-reinforced PGA).	GrandFix® FixSorb-MX®	There is no study using pure PDLA for osteofixation in the maxillofacial surgery.	SonicWeld Rx® (PDDLA 100%) LactoSorb® (PLLA (82%) + PGA (18%)) RapidSorb® (PLLA 85% + PGA 15%) Delta® PLLA (85%) + PGA (10%) + PDLA (5%) PolyMax® (PLLA70% + PLDLA (30%)	Osteotrans MX® (plate: PLLA 60 wt% + u-HA 40 wt%; screw: PLLA (70 wt%) + u-HA (30 wt%))

The idea of biodegradable plates may have emerged from absorbable sutures [75]. The use of biodegradable materials to stabilize fractured facial skeletons was first reported in 1971 [74]. Since then, resorbable polymeric plates and screws have been used widely in pediatric patients with maxillofacial traumas, so as to reduce any interference with craniofacial growth in children [69,76]. The biodegradation process depends on many factors, such as: contact with body fluids, temperature, motion, molecular weight, the crystal form and geometry of the material, and the nature of the tissue where the implant is implanted. The ideal biodegradable osteofixation material provides appropriate strength while degrading in a predictable fashion throughout the healing process without causing adverse reactions. Recently, the concept has changed from simply "resorbable materials" to "bioabsorbable materials", which means the materials have the characteristics of biodegradation plus stimulation of osteoconduction [75]. Unfortunately, they are weaker than conventional titanium plates and can provoke an inflammatory, bacterial foreign-body reaction [1,72,80]. However, Cural et al. found that resorbable (PDLLA) and titanium plates and screws did not differ in terms of biomechanical behaviors after stabilization of the fracture of the mandible angle [77], but the thickness of conventional bioresorbable plates is, on average, two to three times that of metal plates of comparable flexural strength [69]. Larger and thicker plates can lead to greater patient discomfort, as they may be palpable through the skin [78]. Furthermore, the thickness of the plates causes limitations in use—this can be a factor that influences the complication of plate exposure and wound dehiscence, especially in regions with very thin oral mucosa.

The mechanical properties of bioresorbable materials are close to that of the human bone, thereby preventing stress-shielding atrophy and weakening of the fixed bone caused by rigid metallic fixation [79]. Sukegawa et al. did not observe a border between the bone and u-HA/PLLA screws during their histological examination, indicating that the material directly bonded with the human bone [80]. Poly-L/D lactide plates and u-HA/PLLA composite plates are easily bendable with fingers at room temperature, combining waveforms with angles and torsion, and can be maintained in the desired position without heating if slower bending and less force are applied [75]. However, long-term stability and relapse frequency in bioabsorbable osteofixation are still insufficiently studied, especially in cases concerning segmental movements of great magnitude or segmental movements to a position where bony resistance exists.

In contrast to metallic osteosynthesis, bioresorbable implants cannot be sterilized in the operating room through autoclaving. Manufacturers thus use either γ-irradiation or ethylene oxide gas (EtO) for sterilization of implants [81].

Magnesium has also been highlighted as a new material to replace polymer-based osteofixation material in maxillofacial bone surgery. The use of magnesium for bone implants was first described by Lambotte in 1932 [82]. The rapid corrosion of Mg and Mg alloys is a significant limitation regarding the use of these materials. Magnesium alloys possess good mechanical stability, which provides total degradability, but their biocompatibility is still questionable [81]. There is only one case report using Mg-based osteofixative materials in the maxillofacial area in humans [83]. Further research will be necessary to eliminate potential risk and to exclude the risk of non-biocompatibility.

3.7. Bone Substitution Materials

Bone is the second most transplanted tissue after blood [84]. Each bone defect within the maxillofacial skeleton resulting from trauma, disease (i.e., tumors, cysts), or congenital malformation is a significant health problem. Biomaterials used as bone grafts must meet specific requirements to achieve new, healthy, well-vascularized bone tissue formation. Autologous, allogenic, alloplastic, or xenogenic materials are used in bone regeneration [85]. Although autologous bone is still the gold-standard graft material and is not a biomaterial per se, other grafts are used very often (alone or in combination) [86]. A large variability exists between the bone-forming capabilities of various bone grafts, and the osteoinductive potential remains one of the key features to improve the integration of implanted bone grafts. For the regeneration of small osseous defects, bone-substitute biomaterials covered by a membrane are commonly used.

DBBM (deproteinized bovine bone mineral) is the biomaterial with the most documentation in the scientific literature for bone grafting [87]. Deproteinized bone matrix of cortical or cancellous xenogenic bone used as a bone graft material shows biocompatibility, provides a supportive osteoconductive structure, and releases calcium and phosphate ions, thus stimulating osteogenesis. However, when the proteins in its structure are not fully eliminated prior to use, it may provoke foreign body reactions. In addition, there is a potential for cross-infection [88,89]. Although the authors have not found a case of infection from xenotransplantation in maxillofacial surgery, despite them having been reported, there is a potential risk and certain precautions must be taken.

Commercially available xenogenic osteoconductive biomaterials are made of bovine bone (e.g., Bio-Oss®, Gen-Ox®, Cerabone), porcine bone (e.g., Gen-Os), or horse bone (e.g., Bio-Gen). The deproteinization processes for xenogenic grafts can be performed by chemical or heat treatments. Uklejowski et al. showed that the thermal deproteinization process leads to numerous cracks on the surface of the trabeculae of cancellous bone but is much shorter, while bone specimens after the deproteinization process with the chemical agents are generally smooth [90]. According to their study, the most complete and most effective chemical deproteinization process is obtained when using 7 wt% H_2O_2 solution —bone specimens are deproteinized by 90% after 14 days of process. Due to the mechano-structural properties and effectiveness, the chemical deproteinization processes are more suitable for bone tissue replacements [90].

Synthetic materials are not as widely accepted as the allograft materials, despite their obvious benefits; they still lack a significant amount of documented clinical studies supporting their effectiveness. The most investigated calcium phosphate (CaP) bone graft substitutes are hydroxyapatite (HA), B-tricalcium phosphate (B-TCP), and their combination, also called biphasic calcium phosphate (BCF) [71,90]. Their bioactivity and degradation time can be controlled by changing their chemical compositions and sintering temperatures. When compared to synthetic polymers, synthetic bioceramics are superior for bone repairs due to their improved biocompatibility, bioactivity, and strength [71,91]. Yahav et al. show that biphasic calcium sulfate sets hard, acting like a "bone cement", no membrane is required, and primary closure is not mandatory. The material has a complete conversion to bone over a period of four to six months. They achieved similar clinical results as with other grafting products [92]. Miron et al., in a study of the osteoinductive potential of bone grafting material, showed that the xenograft (DBBM) has no potential to form ectopic bone formations, but BCP (biphasic calcium phosphate fabricated from a 10:90 ratio of hydroxyapatite and β-tricalcium phosphate) was able to stimulate ectopic bone formation [93]. Donos et al. obtained similar results in relation to DBBM [94]. Guillaume obtained satisfactory results for bone regeneration with B-TCP for pre-implant surgery, sinus floor elevation, and lateralization of the inferior alveolar nerve (IAN) [95].

Besides the "traditional" use for osseous defect repair, a variety of innovative applications are emerging; for instance, recent studies have interestingly highlighted the suitability of bioactive glasses and glass–ceramics for wound healing applications and soft tissue engineering.

Even though the ideal properties of bone grafts were defined in the literature three decades ago, the market still has no ideal biomaterial which has all of these properties [71]. In a consensus report of Group 2 of the 15 h European Workshop on Periodontology on Bone Regeneration we can read that the future of craniomaxillofacial bone regeneration will probably entail the manufacturing of personalized biomaterial from 3D digital data obtained from patients [90]. Manufacturing customized scaffolds or bones with 3D printing that will perfectly fit to the bone defect shape is a dream of many scientists and surgeons. So far, surgical templates printed using a 3D printer have been increasingly used to facilitate and speed up the surgical procedure (Figure 7).

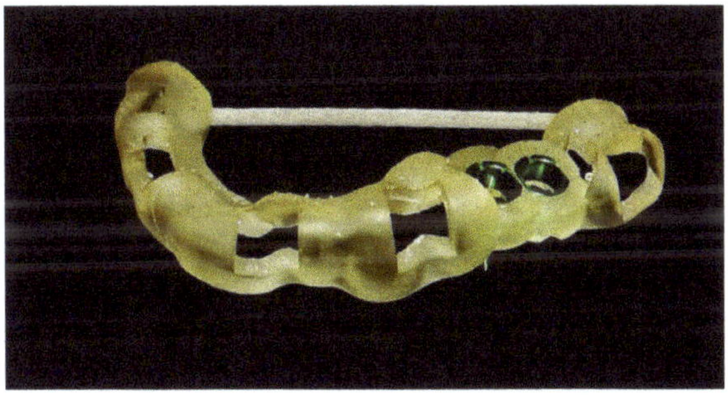

Figure 7. Surgical templates printed using a 3D printer personalized to the patient's anatomical features, fitted on CT scan and oral scanner. Used to facilitate and speed up the surgical procedure of dental implants. Material from the authors' collection.

Bone regeneration techniques need resorbable or non-resorbable membranes as well. The barrier membranes prevent the invasion of surrounding soft tissue, provide stability to the bone graft, prevent soft tissue from collapsing into the defect, accumulate growth factors, and permit osteogenic cells to repopulate bone defects. [96–98]. At present, resorbable materials of xenogeneic origin, such as collagen, are the most commonly used option in guided bone regeneration [98]. However, PTFE membranes also have many uses. Compared with biodegradable membranes, they have a superior space-making capability, mainly when they have titanium reinforcement, which makes them the ideal membranes for vertical bone regeneration [90]. Garcia et al. systematically reviewed the available literature to ascertain the clinical outcomes of two different resorbable collagen membranes and concluded that GBR procedures, through resorbable collagen membranes, achieve volumetric bone gains with no statistical significance between the cross-link and the non-cross-link membranes. However, in terms of biocompatibility, tissue integration, and postoperative complications, the results suggest that non-cross-link membranes present better results [99]. Sbricoli et al. reached a similar conclusion, i.e., that collagen membranes show advantageous biological and clinical features compared to both non-resorbable and other resorbable membranes, but they are not free from possible complications [100].

Martin-Thomé et al. undertook a case series study of a bi-layered synthetic resorbable PLGA membrane (Tisseos®, Biomedical Tissues SAS, 129 Nantes, France). This membrane is made of poly-D,L-lactic/glycolic acid 85/15 (PLGA) and completely degrades by hydrolysis after 4–6 months without signs of inflammation and has a bi-layered structure with a dense film to prevent gingival epithelial cell invasion and a micro-fibrous layer to support osteogenic cells and bone healing. Re-epithelialisation and normal wound closure were observed in patients, where the membrane was exposed after surgery [101].

3.8. Voice Prosthesis

The most common and effective method of voice rehabilitation among post-laryngectomy patients is a tracheoesophageal puncture with voice prosthesis (VP) implantation [102]. The most serious disadvantage of silicone-polymer-based voice prosthesis devices is their colonization and damage by fungi and bacterial biofilm [9,10] (Figure 8). The most common yeasts isolated from VPs' biofilms are *Candida* spp., which forms a tridimensional network leading to device malfunction [103]. There are few voice prostheses manufacturers in the market, but, beyond the prosthesis shape and insertion procedure technique, the polymer material is generally still the same as it has been for years. The new polymeric material should be improved to prevent or slow down the VP degradation process. A modification that will result in antimicrobial properties would be highly desirable. To achieve such a goal, commonly used polymers should be modified with antimicrobial nanosystems or chemical compounds [104–108] that might reduce the ability of microorganisms to adhere to and develop biofilms on the prosthesis' surface. Another approach is to find materials that will have relatively better physical and/or antimicrobial features and/or bacterial and fungal anti-attachment properties. Among popular polymers, some authors selected nine because of their relatively good features, such as the polymers' costs, chemistries, and toxicities. They have found that AODMBA [(R) α acryloyloxy β,β dimethyl γ butyrolactone] was demonstrated to be 3D printable and exhibited strong anti attachment properties, which were retained in its AODMBA printed forms. These tests showed that anti attachment by AODMBA is just as effective against the drug-resistant isolates as against a standard *C. albicans* strain [109]. Further investigations should be performed in this area. Looking for methods that will prevent the initial adherence of hyphae (an essential step in biofilm formation) should be considered essential in the development of future VP material.

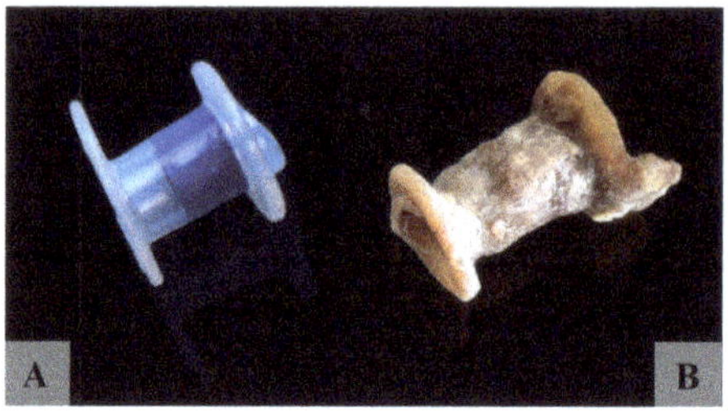

Figure 8. Figure presents Provox voice prostheses. Panel (**A**) shows a completely new prosthesis. Panel (**B**) shows the voice prosthesis after 26 months of use. Its surface is covered with microbial biofilm. Material from the authors' collection.

3.9. Tissue Engineering

Tissue engineering (TE) has the potential for reconstruction with autologous tissue that is not limited by availability of patient donor-site tissue. TE is applicable in otolaryngology in nose, external ear, laryngo-tracheal, and facial skeleton reconstruction [110]. Otolaryngology has a symbolic association with TE because of the memorable picture of the Vacanti mouse bearing a human ear on its back from 1996 [111]. Nowadays, for nasal reconstruction, tissue-engineered cartilaginous constructs are alternatives for synthetic or allogenic materials. The method is based on the implantation of biodegradable collagen scaffolds with seeded chondrocytes and progenitor cells instead of nasal cartilages. The literature reports cases of reconstructions of the two-layer alar lobule or the nasal dorsum in patients after tumor resections or cleft lip–nose deformities. They have achieved good aesthetic and functional outcomes using autologous nasal septal chondrocytes seeded on utilized collagen membranes or scaffolds [112,113]. As with the nasal TE, the otologic appliance has focused on auricular reconstructions. Investigators expanded harvested microtia chondrocytes, seeded these on a 3D-printed biodegradable scaffold, and cultured the construct in vitro. They reported satisfactory post-implantation aesthetic outcomes [114]. On the other hand, bacterial nanocellulose (BNC), which is non-degradable biocompatible material that promotes chondrocyte adhesion and proliferation, also exists. Nimeskern et al. presented BNC as having the capability to reach mechanical properties of relevance for ear cartilage replacement; it can be produced in patient-specific ear shapes [115].

There are also investigations into the regeneration of inner- and middle-ear structures. Chitosan patches (E-CPs) that release epidermal growth factor (EGF) as a patch therapy to replace surgical methods of the perforated tympanic membrane reconstructions have also been developed [116]. The inner-ear treatment by TE is focused on in vitro models of decellularized cochleae and the establishment of pluripotent stem cell lines with the goal of generating functional inner-ear hair cells [117]. Regenerative medicine for laryngotracheal replacements has, in recent years, focused on investigations concerning ideal scaffold materials for tracheal reconstruction [110]. Commonly used scaffold materials include decellularized tissue, poly-lactic-co-glycolic acid (PLGA), poly-ϵ-caprolactone (PCL), polyethylene terephthalate (PET), and polyurethane (PU). There is still no answer as to which material is optimal for this procedure [118–121]. Simultaneously, investigators are examining the ideal cellular source for graft seeding. Moreover, some in vivo animal model studies with stem cell-seeded constructs were performed with positive outcomes in restoring larynx phonation function [122,123].

4. Improving the Safety of Biomaterials by Preventing Their Microbial Colonization and Host Immune Response

Despite the extremely important role of newly formed biomaterials in improving the health and quality of the lives of patients with dysfunctions within the head and neck region, not all safety issues related to their functions within the patients' bodies have been resolved. One of the greatest risks associated with placing an implant within the living tissue of a patient is related to the colonization of the material by opportunistic/pathogenic microorganisms and the formation of a bacterial/fungal biofilm on the implant's surface. This is an important issue, because the presence of microorganisms on the surface of the implant not only changes its mechanical properties, accelerates its wear [10], and increases the risk of explanation [124], but also, above all, can be a source of life-threatening infections leading to the development of sepsis [125,126]. Under the conditions of the human body, excessive colonization of tissue surfaces by pathogenic microorganisms is limited due to specific, mucilaginous barriers, the presence of natural microflora, and the synthesis of a number of endogenous substances characterized by antibacterial and immunomodulatory activity. In the case of implanted biomaterials, such protection does not occur, which forces the search for protective methods limiting the formation of biofilm on their surface to take place. In other words, the restoration of the live tissue's ability to prevent microbial colonization should be taken into consideration within the design of materials for implant production.

The group of methods limiting microorganism growth and hampering microbial adherence includes the fabrication of materials with anti-fouling features [127], covering the surface of implants with anti-adhesive substances [128], surface charge modifications [129], coating with antibiotics and antimicrobial peptides [130], or the use of nanoparticles as antimicrobial covering. Particularly, the use of nanotechnological methods has recently attracted more interest due to their lower potential to induce microbial drug resistance and both potent, broad-spectrum antimicrobial activity and immunomodulatory features. The above-mentioned methods and their applications are presented in Table 2.

Table 2. Various methods to synthetize materials with antimicrobial properties and their uses.

Method of Material Antimicrobial Functionalization	Application
anti-fouling	cochlear implants [127,131]
anti-adhesive	dental resin and polydi-methylsiloxane elastomer (PDMS) [128]
surface–charge modification	titanium micro-screws [129]
coating with antibiotics	bone implants [132], tympanostomy tubes [41], paranasal sinus stents [133],
coating with antimicrobial agent such as nanoparticles	nasal mucosa splints [134], inner ear implants [135], middle ear implants [54], bone tissue scaffolds [86,90,91]

4.1. *Methods of Biomaterial Modifications to Increase Their Antimicrobial Properties*

Antibacterial coating. There are three main methods for fixing antibacterial agents on the material surface: (i) covalent grafting, (ii) material blending, and (iii) layer-by-layer (LBL) assembly. Covalent grafting is more stable than other methods, such as non-covalent bonding (electrostatic attraction and hydrogen bonding). There are some very detailed publications describing two categories of covalent grafting—'grafting to' and 'grafting from' [136–139]. Moreover, the technology of photo-initiation of some monomers or polymers by UV also exists. This technique can be very efficient to prevent the formation of bacterial biofilms on medical devices [140].

The LBL assembly is considered to be a universal technique for making antimicrobial coatings on medical devices. It relies on the adsorption of electrolytes or complementary compounds on the substrate surface [141]. The applications of this method are very wide-ranging, there are some works that report the modification of different materials by LBL assembly as: polyacrylic acid (PAA, as the polyanion) and polyetherimide (PEI, as the polycation) used to obtain a multilayer PAA/PEI assembled film [142], chitosan and heparin [143], chitosan and collagen [144], polydimethylaminoethyl methacrylate (polycation) and cellobiose dehydrogenase (CDH, polyanion), and polybenzenesulfonic salt (polyanion) [145].

Material blending is a method of mixing different types of polymers. The final antimicrobial effects depend on the features of the used substrates and their proportions. This technology was used in polyhexamethyleneguanidine dodecylbenzenesulfonate (PHMG-DBS)-coated tracheal intubation tubes (good antimicrobial outcomes were reported) [146]. Indeed, a polyurethane (PU) catheter modified with poly(diallyldimethylammonium chloride) (pDADMAC) demonstrated good bactericidal features [147].

Antibiotic delivery systems. In some cases, polymers could serve as an antibiotic-controlled release systems. Rossi et al. described their method of incubation of poly(hydroxybutyric-co-hydroxyvalerate) (PHBV) in a solution of chloroform and gentamicin in a shaking water bath at 55 °C for 24 h. The authors reported a good profile of drug release and good bactericidal effect [148]. Another study reported that the release of antibiotics from different material formats of silk (films, microspheres, hydrogels, coatings) and biodegradable chitosan had good functional profiles and the potential to achieve the needed local concentrations while also minimizing systemic exposure [149,150].

Polymers with nanoparticles. Silver nanoparticles alone have a proven bactericidal effect in the treatment of local infections. The mechanism of their action is based on the ability to damage the bacterial cell membrane. There are some studies that report the method of silver nanoparticles' incorporation into polymer materials to achieve antifungal and bactericidal features. Polymer systems containing silver nanoparticles can be synthesized in situ using the polymer matrix as a reaction medium or ex situ when silver nanoparticles are incorporated into the polymeric matrix already synthetized [151,152]. The latest studies report the use of silver nanoparticles modified with zwitterionic poly (carboxybetaine-co-dopamine methacrylamide) copolymer (PCBDA@AgNPs), which was firmly fixed onto soft contact lenses through the mussel-inspired surface chemistry [153] or hybrid nanocoatings [154]. Ye et al. described the method of connection between antimicrobial peptides, GL13K and AgNP, to create a hybrid nanocoating on a Ti implant. Due to the combined application of these two antimicrobial agents with different antimicrobial mechanisms, they achieved more potent synergistic effects.

4.2. Selected Biomaterials with Antimicrobial Modifications for Use in Otorhinolaryngology

In one of the more interesting studies, Duda et al. presented the possibility of coating Bioverit® II middle ear prostheses using silver containing silica. In their study, rabbits were implanted with silver-functionalized middle-ear prostheses, and this group was compared with pure silica coatings and 1% silver sulfadiazine cream applied on a silica coating. The authors demonstrated the clinical justification of the study, and the usefulness of the developed implants for reconstructive middle-ear surgery and reduced fibrosis was observed. Nevertheless, some signs of acute toxicity of the silver coatings on the mucosal ear tissue (particularly single necrotic and apoptotic cells) were observed, which prompted further studies into the safety of such an approach [155]. Another problem is the formation of bacterial biofilm on medical devices, such as cochlear implants (CI), that can lead to chronic infections. In response to this, a vancomycin-releasing PCL/polyethylene oxide (PEO) nanofiber mat was proposed to prevent MRSA biofilm formation on the surface of ossicular prostheses and in the environment of otitis media, due to effective delivery of vancomycin for prolonged time [156].

Kirchhoff et al. found in vitro that bioactive glass (BAG of type S53P4) consisting of silicon dioxide, sodium oxide, calcium oxide, and phosphorus pentoxide induces significant changes in the biofilm morphology of the most common bacterial strains responsible for biofilm-related implant infections. Its antibacterial activity was tested with three types of materials commonly used in cochlear implants: silicone, titanium, and platinum. In each case, significant alterations in biofilm morphology could be detected via SEM. Höing et al. also found that bioactive glass S53P4 can reduce biofilm formation on CI materials in vitro [131].

The formation of fungal biofilm can be seen as a separate problem in the implementation of medical devices. Filastatin inhibits the adhesion of multiple pathogenic *Candida* species. Vargas-Blanco et al. report that treatment with Filastatin significantly inhibited the ability of *C. albicans* to adhere to bioactive glass (by 99.06%), silicone (by 77.27%), and dental resin (by 60.43%) in vivo.

The first middle-ear implant that has the bactericidal activity and hearing improvement confirmed in the clinical trial conducted by Ziąbka and Malec [157] (Figure 9).

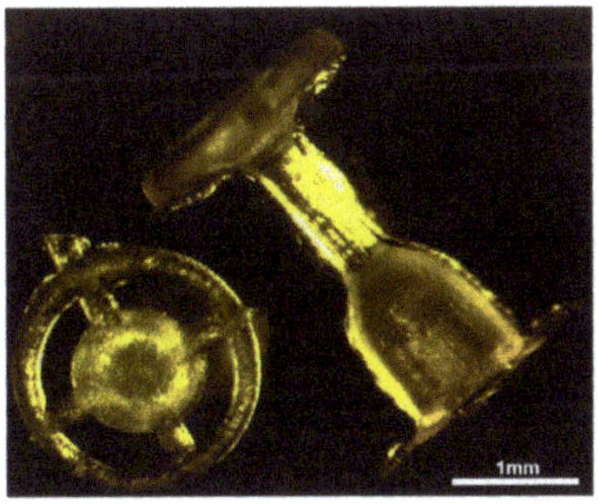

Figure 9. Middle-ear prosthesis for ossicular reconstruction made of ABS polymer. Adapted from an open-access source: [158].

Recent experimental ossicular chain implants made of ABS polymer material (poly)acrylonitrile butadiene styrene (INEOS SyrolutionEurope GmbH, Frankfurt, Germany) and modified with silver nanoparticles, AgNPs 45T, have shown promising antimicrobial efficacy [57,159,160]. Such activity is regarded as being the same as biocompatibility or physical properties.

Silver nanoparticles, used to provide antimicrobial activity, were also used as coatings for nasal tampons [134]. Research carried out using rats to test such tampons when applied for 48 h demonstrated that silver nanoparticle-embedded tampons were far more efficient in limiting *Haemophilus parainfluenzae* colonization when compared to silicone- or PEG-based nasal splints. A decreased inflammatory response was also noted, which suggest the utility of AgNPs in the prevention of secondary infections [134]. A nanotechnology approach was also used for the preparation of ciprofloxacin and azithromycin nanoparticle suspension for the coating of sinus stents with anti-*Pseudomonas aeruginosa* properties [133].

In the context of bone substitution materials, nanohydroxyapatite can be loaded with chlorhexidine digluconate using electrostatic interactions between the cationic group of CHX and the phosphate group of nanoHA in order to prevent surface bacterial accumulation [159]. Nevertheless, in the case of bone infections, poor bone/plasma ratios of parenterally administrated antibiotics, along with the ability of bacteria to form biofilm inside the bone, considerably hampers the fighting of bacterial infections. To increase the amount and efficiency of antibiotics against bone infection-causing pathogens, Parent et al. proposed the incorporation of vancomycin in tri-dimensional hydroxyapatite-based scaffolds for local, prophylactic delivery of antibiotics [132]. Similarly, Weng et al. demonstrated recently that a local three-dimensional scaffold strategy strongly contributes to the improvement of anti-MRSA therapies, as a result of coating the bone biomaterial with a significant amount of silver nanoparticles [160].

Another promising approach for decreasing bacterial adherence to the implants is surface–charge modification. Kao et al. found in in vivo models, that charge modification decreased the colonization by *P. aeruginosa* of titanium screw implants.

Another method to improve the function of biomaterials and protect implants from microbial exposure is to modulate the inflammatory response of the host. Nevertheless, this effect should be balanced between a beneficial, antimicrobial effect and a redundant, toxic effect that damages tissues and increases the risk of inflammation.

Although the number of studies examining the immunomodulatory activity of biomaterials coatings has decreased when compared to studies examining antimicrobial ones, some interesting studies have been undertaken recently. In one of the newer studies, lithium niobate nanoparticles were proven to exert an immunomodulatory effect, possess the ability to stimulate beta-defensin in epithelial cells, and shown to be effective against *Pseudomonas aeruginosa* bacteria, which supports their utility for inner-ear-device fabrication [135]. In another study, magnetic hexagonal ferrite nanoparticles were incorporated into bone hydroxyapatite/chitosan scaffolds to recruit endogenous stem cells [161]. The promising results were also obtained using a mouse soft-tissue implant-associated infection model, where anti-biofilm and the immunomodulatory activities of zinc oxide nanoparticle (ZnO NPs) were investigated. According to Wang et al., this effect was achieved by a combination of factors, including (i) the antimicrobial efficiency of ZnO NPs, (ii) the nanoparticle-mediated induction of inflammatory cytokines release, and (iii) promoting phagocytosis [162]. Although the results of these studies are not application specific, they can certainly be thought of in terms of their subsequent use in the production of implants in otorhinolaryngology. Zinc-incorporated titanium oxide nanotubes were also noted to accelerate bone formation when fabricated on titanium implant materials [163].

The above research confirms that the development of implantable biomaterials with an appropriate safety–effectiveness ratio is extremely important and worthy of further research.

5. Conclusions

In general, the most widely used materials in the field of otorhinolaryngology are polymer-based synthetics. They have the potential to be an ideal material in this case, if it is possible to achieve modification of their properties, such as the ability to prevent the growth of microorganisms. As we currently face the challenge of an increasing number of infections caused by antibiotic-resistant strains of bacteria, there is an urgent need to find a new class of antibacterial agents. AMPs, their synthetic mimics, and nanosystems containing metallic nanoparticles have a promising potential as a more efficient alternative to conventional antibiotics, due to their microbiocidal properties that cover large spectrum of microorganisms, as well as their low ability to induce drug resistance. There is no doubt that the development of these molecules for the antibacterial modification of materials used in medical devices in otorhinolaryngology will be beneficial. At the same time, we should look for new materials that will have better biocompatibility and mechanical properties. The ability to customize the shapes of this biomaterial with 3D printers will also be of benefit to patients in need.

Author Contributions: Conceptualization, J.S. and R.B.; methodology, J.S.; software, J.S. and P.D.; validation, J.S., P.D., E.P. and R.B.; formal analysis, R.B. and S.O.; investigation, J.S. and P.O.; resources, J.S., P.O. and E.P.; data curation, J.S.; writing—original draft preparation, J.S., P.O. and E.P.; writing—review and editing, P.D., T.D., G.K. and R.B.; visualization, J.S., G.K. and P.O.; supervision, S.G., S.O. and R.B.; All authors have read and agreed to the published version of the manuscript.

Funding: This work was supported by the National Science Center, Poland under Grant UMO-2018/31/B/NZ6/02476 (to RB), Medical University of Bialystok (SUB/1/NN/21/002/1122 to

T.D.), and by a program of the Minister of Science and Higher Education under the name "Regional Initiative of Excellence in 2019–2022", project number: 024/RID/2018/19, financing amount: 11.999.000,00 PLN.

Institutional Review Board Statement: Not applicable.

Informed Consent Statement: Not applicable.

Data Availability Statement: Publicly available datasets were analyzed in this study. This data can be found in PubMed.

Conflicts of Interest: The authors declare no conflict of interest.

References

1. Bergman, C.P.; Aisha, S. *Dental Ceramics: Microstructure, Properties and Degradation*; Springer: Berlin/Heidelberg, Germany, 2013; 84p.
2. Sternberg, K. Current requirements for polymeric biomaterials in otolaryngology. *GMS Curr. Top. Otorhinolaryngol. Head Neck Surg.* **2009**, *8*, Doc11. [CrossRef]
3. Jones, J.R.; Hench, L.L. Biomedical materials for new millennium: Perspective on the future. *Mater. Sci. Technol.* **2001**, *17*, 891–900. [CrossRef]
4. Hermawan, H.; Mantovani, D. Degradable metallic biomaterials: The concept, current developments and future directions. *Minerva Biotecnol.* **2009**, *21*, 207–216.
5. Bohner, M. Resorbable biomaterials as bone graft substitutes. *Mater. Today* **2010**, *13*, 24–30. [CrossRef]
6. Mathur, A.B.; Collier, T.O.; Kao, W.J.; Wiggins, M.; Schubert, M.A.; Hiltner, A.; Anderson, J.M. In vivo biocompatibility and biostability of modified polyurethanes. *J. Biomed. Mater. Res.* **1997**, *36*, 246–257. [CrossRef]
7. Heumann, S.; Eberl, A.; Pobeheim, H.; Liebminger, S.; Fischer-Colbrie, G.; Almansa, E.; Cavaco-Paulo, A.; Gubitz, G.M. New model substrates for enzymes hydrolysing polyethyleneterephthalate and polyamide fibres. *J. Biochem. Biophys. Methods* **2006**, *69*, 89–99. [CrossRef] [PubMed]
8. King, R.N.; Lyman, D.J. Polymers in contact with the body. *Environ. Health Perspect.* **1975**, *11*, 71–74. [CrossRef]
9. Galli, J.; Calo, L.; Meucci, D.; Giuliani, M.; Lucidi, D.; Paludetti, G.; Torelli, R.; Sanguinetti, M.; Parrilla, C. Biofilm in voice prosthesis: A prospective cohort study and laboratory tests using sonication and SEM analysis. *Clin. Otolaryngol.* **2018**, *10*, 1260–1265. [CrossRef]
10. Spałek, J.; Deptuła, P.; Cieśluk, M.; Strzelecka, A.; Łysik, D.; Mystkowska, J.; Daniluk, T.; Król, G.; Góźdź, S.; Bucki, R.; et al. Biofilm Growth Causes Damage to Silicone Voice Prostheses in Patients after Surgical Treatment of Locally Advanced Laryngeal Cancer. *Pathogens* **2020**, *9*, 793. [CrossRef]
11. Lendlein, A. Polymere als Implantatwerkstoffe. *Chem. Unserer Zeit* **1999**, *33*, 279–295. [CrossRef]
12. Unverdorben, M.; Spielberger, A.; Schywalsky, M.; Labahn, D.; Hartwig, S.; Schneider, M.; Lootz, D.; Behrend, D.; Schmitz, K.; Degenhardt, R.; et al. A polyhydroxybutyrate biodegradable stent: Preliminary experience in the rabbit. *Cardiovasc. Interv. Radiol.* **2002**, *25*, 127–132. [CrossRef] [PubMed]
13. Sodian, R.; Hoerstrup, S.P.; Sperling, J.S.; Martin, D.P.; Daebritz, S.; Mayer, J.E., Jr.; Vacanti, J.P. Evaluation of biodegradable, three-dimensional matrices for tissue engineering of heart valves. *ASAIO J.* **2000**, *46*, 107–110. [CrossRef] [PubMed]
14. Ray, S.; Kalia, V.C. Biomedical Applications of Polyhydroxyalkanoates. *Indian J. Microbiol.* **2017**, *57*, 261–269. [CrossRef]
15. Parikh, A.; Anand, U.; Ugwu, M.C.; Feridooni, T.; Massoud, E.; Agu, R.U. Drug-eluting nasal implants: Formulation, characterization, clinical applications and challenges. *Pharmaceutics* **2014**, *6*, 249–267. [CrossRef] [PubMed]
16. Blasi, P. Poly(lactic acid)/poly(lactic-co-glycolic acid)-based microparticles: An overview. *J. Pharm. Investig.* **2019**, *49*, 337–346. [CrossRef]
17. Elmowafy, E.M.; Tiboni, M.; Soliman, M.E. Biocompatibility, biodegradation and biomedical applications of poly(lactic acid)/poly(lactic-co-glycolic acid) micro and nanoparticles. *J. Pharm. Investig.* **2019**, *49*, 347–380. [CrossRef]
18. Schoubben, A.; Ricci, M.; Giovagnoli, S. Meeting the unmet: From traditional to cutting-edge techniques for poly lactide and poly lactide-co-glycolide microparticle manufacturing. *J. Pharm. Investig.* **2019**, *49*, 381–404. [CrossRef]
19. Zhong, H.; Chan, G.; Hu, Y.; Hu, H.; Ouyang, D. A Comprehensive Map of FDA-Approved Pharmaceutical Products. *Pharmaceutics* **2018**, *10*, 263. [CrossRef]
20. Long, M.; Rack, H.J. Titanium alloys in total joint replacement—A materials science perspective. *Biomaterials* **1998**, *19*, 1621–1639. [CrossRef]
21. Yazdimamaghani, M.; Razavi, M.; Vashaee, D.; Moharamzadeh, K.; Boccaccini, A.R.; Tayebi, L. Porous magnesium-based scaffolds for tissue engineering. *Mater. Sci. Eng. C Mater. Biol. Appl.* **2017**, *71*, 1253–1266. [CrossRef]
22. Marti, A. Cobalt-base alloys used in bone surgery. *Injury* **2000**, *31*, D18–D21. [CrossRef]
23. Ortiz, A.J.; Fernandez, E.; Vicente, A.; Calvo, J.L.; Ortiz, C. Metallic ions released from stainless steel, nickel-free, and titanium orthodontic alloys: Toxicity and DNA damage. *Am. J. Orthod. Dentofac. Orthop.* **2011**, *140*, e115–e122. [CrossRef] [PubMed]
24. Gomes, C.C.; Moreira, L.M.; Santos, V.J.; Ramos, A.S.; Lyon, J.P.; Soares, C.P.; Santos, F.V. Assessment of the genetic risks of a metallic alloy used in medical implants. *Genet. Mol. Biol.* **2011**, *34*, 116–121. [CrossRef] [PubMed]

25. Zhao, D.; Witte, F.; Lu, F.; Wang, J.; Li, J.; Qin, L. Current status on clinical applications of magnesium-based orthopaedic implants: A review from clinical translational perspective. *Biomaterials* **2017**, *112*, 287–302. [CrossRef]
26. Lourenço, M.L.; Cardoso, G.C.; dos Santos Jorge Sousa, K.; Donato, T.A.G.; Pontes, F.M.L.; Grandini, C.R. Development of novel Ti-Mo-Mn alloys for biomedical applications. *Sci. Rep.* **2020**, *10*, 6298. [CrossRef]
27. Jakubowicz, J. Special Issue: Ti-Based Biomaterials: Synthesis, Properties and Applications. *Materials* **2020**, *13*, 1696. [CrossRef]
28. Yang, K.; Ren, Y. Nickel-free austenitic stainless steels for medical applications. *Sci. Technol. Adv. Mater.* **2010**, *11*, 014105. [CrossRef]
29. Aldini, N.N.; Fini, M.; Giavaresi, G.; Torricelli, P.; Martini, L.; Giardino, R.; Ravaglioli, A.; Krajewski, A.; Mazzocchi, M.; Dubini, B.; et al. Improvement in zirconia osseointegration by means of a biological glass coating: An in vitro and in vivo investigation. *J. Biomed. Mater. Res.* **2002**, *61*, 282–289. [CrossRef]
30. Saenz, A.; Brostow, W.; Rivera-Muñoz, E. Ceramic biomaterials: An introductory overview. *J. Mater. Educ.* **1999**, *21*, 297–306.
31. Cranin, A.N.; Schnitman, P.A.; Rabkin, S.M.; Onesto, E.J. Alumina and zirconia coated vitallium oral endosteal implants in beagles. *J. Biomed. Mater. Res.* **1975**, *9*, 257–262. [CrossRef]
32. Depprich, R.; Zipprich, H.; Ommerborn, M.; Naujoks, C.; Wiesmann, H.P.; Kiattavorncharoen, S.; Lauer, H.C.; Meyer, U.; Kübler, N.R.; Handschel, J. Osseointegration of zirconia implants compared with titanium: An in vivo study. *Head Face Med.* **2008**, *4*, 30. [CrossRef]
33. Scholz, M.S.; Blanchfield, J.P.; Bloom, L.D.; Coburn, B.H.; Elkington, M.; Fuller, J.D.; Gilbert, M.E.; Muflahi, S.A.; Pernice, M.F.; Rae, S.I.; et al. The use of composite materials in modern orthopaedic medicine and prosthetic devices: A review. *Compos. Sci. Technol.* **2011**, *71*, 1791–1803. [CrossRef]
34. Lenarz, T.; Lesinski-Schiedat, A.; Weber, B.P.; Frohne, C.; Buchner, A.; Battmer, R.D.; Parker, J.; von Wallenberg, E. The Nucleus Double Array Cochlear Implant: A new concept in obliterated cochlea. *Laryngorhinootologie* **1999**, *78*, 421–428. [CrossRef] [PubMed]
35. Scheper, V.; Hessler, R.; Hutten, M.; Wilk, M.; Jolly, C.; Lenarz, T.; Paasche, G. Local inner ear application of dexamethasone in cochlear implant models is safe for auditory neurons and increases the neuroprotective effect of chronic electrical stimulation. *PLoS ONE* **2017**, *12*, e0183820. [CrossRef] [PubMed]
36. Wilk, M.; Hessler, R.; Mugridge, K.; Jolly, C.; Fehr, M.; Lenarz, T.; Scheper, V. Impedance Changes and Fibrous Tissue Growth after Cochlear Implantation Are Correlated and Can Be Reduced Using a Dexamethasone Eluting Electrode. *PLoS ONE* **2016**, *11*, e0147552. [CrossRef] [PubMed]
37. Lehner, E.; Gundel, D.; Liebau, A.; Plontke, S.; Mader, K. Intracochlear PLGA based implants for dexamethasone release: Challenges and solutions. *Int. J. Pharm. X* **2019**, *1*, 100015. [CrossRef]
38. Fredenberg, S.; Wahlgren, M.; Reslow, M.; Axelsson, A. The mechanisms of drug release in poly(lactic-co-glycolic acid)-based drug delivery systems—A review. *Int. J. Pharm.* **2011**, *415*, 34–52. [CrossRef]
39. Plontke, S.K.; Glien, A.; Rahne, T.; Mader, K.; Salt, A.N. Controlled release dexamethasone implants in the round window niche for salvage treatment of idiopathic sudden sensorineural hearing loss. *Otol. Neurotol.* **2014**, *35*, 1168–1171. [CrossRef]
40. Jang, C.H.; Park, H.; Cho, Y.B.; Choi, C.H.; Park, I.Y. The use of piperacillin-tazobactam coated tympanostomy tubes against ciprofloxacin-resistant *Pseudomonas* biofilm formation: An in vitro study. *Int. J. Pediatr. Otorhinolaryngol.* **2009**, *73*, 295–299. [CrossRef]
41. Jang, C.H.; Park, H.; Cho, Y.B.; Choi, C.H. Effect of vancomycin-coated tympanostomy tubes on methicillin-resistant *Staphylococcus aureus* biofilm formation: In vitro study. *J. Laryngol. Otol.* **2010**, *124*, 594–598. [CrossRef]
42. Saidi, I.S.; Biedlingmaier, J.F.; Whelan, P. In vivo resistance to bacterial biofilm formation on tympanostomy tubes as a function of tube material. *Otolaryngol. Head Neck Surg.* **1999**, *120*, 621–627. [CrossRef]
43. Jang, C.H.; Cho, Y.B.; Choi, C.H. Effect of ion-bombarded silicone tympanostomy tube on ciprofloxacin-resistant *Pseudomonas aeruginosa* biofilm formation. *Int. J. Pediatr. Otorhinolaryngol.* **2012**, *76*, 1471–1473. [CrossRef]
44. Joe, H.; Seo, Y.J. A newly designed tympanostomy stent with TiO_2 coating to reduce *Pseudomonas aeruginosa* biofilm formation. *J. Biomater. Appl.* **2018**, *33*, 599–605. [CrossRef]
45. de Abajo, J.; Sanhueza, I.; Giron, L.; Manrique, M. Experience with the active middle ear implant in patients with moderate-to-severe mixed hearing loss: Indications and results. *Otol. Neurotol.* **2013**, *34*, 1373–1379. [CrossRef]
46. Stupp, C.H.; Stupp, H.F.; Grün, D. Replacement of ear ossicles with titanium prostheses. *Laryngorhinootologie* **1996**, *75*, 335–337. [CrossRef]
47. Maassen, M.M.; Löwenheim, H.; Pfister, M.; Herberhold, S.; Jorge, J.R.; Baumann, I.; Nüsser, A.; Zimmermann, R.; Brosch, S.; Zenner, H.P. Surgical-handling properties of the titanium prosthesis in ossiculoplasty. *Ear Nose Throat J.* **2005**, *84*, 142–144. [CrossRef]
48. Gostian, A.O.; Kouame, J.M.; Bremke, M.; Ortmann, M.; Hüttenbrink, K.B.; Beutner, D. Long term results of the titanium clip prosthesis. *Eur. Arch. Otorhinolaryngol.* **2016**, *273*, 4257–4266. [CrossRef]
49. Wongwiwat, P.; Boonma, A.; Lee, Y.S.; Narayan, R.J. Bioceramics in ossicular replacement prostheses: A review. *J. Long Term. Eff. Med. Implant.* **2011**, *21*, 169–183. [CrossRef]
50. Shinohara, T.; Gyo, K.; Saiki, T.; Yanagihara, N. Ossiculoplasty using hydroxyapatite prostheses: Long-term results. *Clin. Otolaryngol. Allied Sci.* **2000**, *25*, 287–292. [CrossRef]

51. Ocak, E.; Beton, S.; Meço, C.; Dursun, G. Titanium versus Hydroxyapatite Prostheses: Comparison of Hearing and Anatomical Outcomes after Ossicular Chain Reconstruction. *Turk. Arch. Otorhinolaryngol.* **2015**, *53*, 15–18. [CrossRef]
52. Meijer, A.G.; Segenhout, H.M.; Albers, F.W.; van de Want, H.J. Histopathology of biocompatible hydroxylapatite-polyethylene composite in ossiculoplasty. *ORL J. Otorhinolaryngol. Relat. Spec.* **2002**, *64*, 173–179. [CrossRef]
53. Ovsianikov, A.; Chichkov, B.; Adunka, O.; Pillsbury, H.; Doraiswamy, A.; Narayan, R.J. Rapid prototyping of ossicular replacement prostheses. *Appl. Surf. Sci.* **2007**, *253*, 6603–6607. [CrossRef]
54. Ziabka, M.; Menaszek, E.; Tarasiuk, J.; Wronski, S. Biocompatible Nanocomposite Implant with Silver Nanoparticles for Otology-In Vivo Evaluation. *Nanomaterials* **2018**, *8*, 764. [CrossRef]
55. Krings, J.G.; Kallogjeri, D.; Wineland, A.; Nepple, K.G.; Piccirillo, J.F.; Getz, A.E. Complications of primary and revision functional endoscopic sinus surgery for chronic rhinosinusitis. *Laryngoscope* **2014**, *124*, 838–845. [CrossRef]
56. Okushi, T.; Yoshikawa, M.; Otori, N.; Matsuwaki, Y.; Asaka, D.; Nakayama, T.; Morimoto, T.; Moriyama, H. Evaluation of symptoms and QOL with calcium alginate versus chitin-coated gauze for middle meatus packing after endoscopic sinus surgery. *Auris Nasus Larynx* **2012**, *39*, 31–37. [CrossRef]
57. Verim, A.; Seneldir, L.; Naiboglu, B.; Karaca, C.T.; Kulekci, S.; Toros, S.Z.; Oysu, C. Role of nasal packing in surgical outcome for chronic rhinosinusitis with polyposis. *Laryngoscope* **2014**, *124*, 1529–1535. [CrossRef]
58. Wang, J.; Cai, C.; Wang, S. Merocel versus Nasopore for nasal packing: A meta-analysis of randomized controlled trials. *PLoS ONE* **2014**, *9*, e93959. [CrossRef]
59. Fokkens, W.J.; Lund, V.J.; Hopkins, C.; Hellings, P.W.; Kern, R.; Reitsma, S.; Toppila-Salmi, S.; Bernal-Sprekelsen, M.; Mullol, J. Executive summary of EPOS 2020 including integrated care pathways. *Rhinology* **2020**, *58*, 82–111. [CrossRef]
60. Luong, A.; Ow, R.A.; Singh, A.; Weiss, R.L.; Han, J.K.; Gerencer, R.; Stolovitzky, J.P.; Stambaugh, J.W.; Raman, A. Safety and Effectiveness of a Bioabsorbable Steroid-Releasing Implant for the Paranasal Sinus Ostia: A Randomized Clinical Trial. *JAMA Otolaryngol. Head Neck Surg* **2018**, *144*, 28–35. [CrossRef]
61. US Food and Drug Administration (FDA). Premarket Approval (PMA). 2018. Available online: https://www.accessdata.fda.gov/scripts/cdrh/cfdocs/cfpma/pma.cfm (accessed on 10 January 2022).
62. Han, J.K.; Kern, R.C. Topical therapies for management of chronic rhinosinusitis: Steroid implants. *Int. Forum Allergy Rhinol.* **2019**, *9*, S22–S26. [CrossRef]
63. Smith, T.L.; Singh, A.; Luong, A.; Ow, R.A.; Shotts, S.D.; Sautter, N.B.; Han, J.K.; Stambaugh, J.; Raman, A. Randomized controlled trial of a bioabsorbable steroid-releasing implant in the frontal sinus opening. *Laryngoscope* **2016**, *126*, 2659–2664. [CrossRef]
64. Forwith, K.D.; Han, J.K.; Stolovitzky, J.P.; Yen, D.M.; Chandra, R.K.; Karanfilov, B.; Matheny, K.E.; Stambaugh, J.W.; Gawlicka, A.K. RESOLVE: Bioabsorbable steroid-eluting sinus implants for in-office treatment of recurrent sinonasal polyposis after sinus surgery: 6-month outcomes from a randomized, controlled, blinded study. *Int. Forum Allergy Rhinol.* **2016**, *6*, 573–581. [CrossRef]
65. Adriaensen, G.; Lim, K.H.; Fokkens, W.J. Safety and efficacy of a bioabsorbable fluticasone propionate-eluting sinus dressing in postoperative management of endoscopic sinus surgery: A randomized clinical trial. *Int. Forum Allergy Rhinol.* **2017**, *7*, 813–820. [CrossRef]
66. Makadia, H.K.; Siegel, S.J. Poly Lactic-co-Glycolic Acid (PLGA) as Biodegradable Controlled Drug Delivery Carrier. *Polymers* **2011**, *3*, 1377–1397. [CrossRef]
67. Margolis, J.R. The excel stent: A good DES, but can we really stop clopidogrel after 6 months? *JACC Cardiovasc. Interv.* **2009**, *2*, 310–311. [CrossRef]
68. Kanno, T.; Sukegawa, S.; Furuki, Y.; Nariai, Y.; Sekine, J. Overview of innovative advances in bioresorbable plate systems for oral and maxillofacial surgery. *Jpn. Dent. Sci. Rev.* **2018**, *54*, 127–138. [CrossRef]
69. Sukegawa, S.; Kanno, T.; Nagano, D.; Shibata, A.; Sukegawa-Takahashi, Y.; Furuki, Y. The Clinical Feasibility of Newly Developed Thin Flat-Type Bioresorbable Osteosynthesis Devices for the Internal Fixation of Zygomatic Fractures: Is There a Difference in Healing Between Bioresorbable Materials and Titanium Osteosynthesis? *J. Craniofac. Surg.* **2016**, *27*, 2124–2129. [CrossRef]
70. Haugen, H.J.; Lyngstadaas, S.P.; Rossi, F.; Perale, G. Bone grafts: Which is the ideal biomaterial? *J. Clin. Periodontol.* **2019**, *46*, 92–102. [CrossRef]
71. Pinto, C.M.; Asprino, L.; de Moraes, M. Chemical and structural analyses of titanium plates retrieved from patients. *Int. J. Oral Maxillofac. Surg.* **2015**, *44*, 1005–1009. [CrossRef]
72. Acero, J.; Calderon, J.; Salmeron, J.I.; Verdaguer, J.J.; Concejo, C.; Somacarrera, M.L. The behaviour of titanium as a biomaterial: Microscopy study of plates and surrounding tissues in facial osteosynthesis. *J. Cranio-Maxillofac. Surg.* **1999**, *27*, 117–123. [CrossRef]
73. Lin, K.Y.; Bartlett, S.P.; Yaremchuk, M.J.; Grossman, R.F.; Udupa, J.K.; Whitaker, L.A. An experimental study on the effect of rigid fixation on the developing craniofacial skeleton. *Plast. Reconstr. Surg.* **1991**, *87*, 229–235. [CrossRef]
74. Cutright, D.E.; Hunsuck, E.E.; Beasley, J.D. Fracture reduction using a biodegradable material, polylactic acid. *J. Oral Surg.* **1971**, *29*, 393–397.
75. Park, Y.-W. Bioabsorbable osteofixation for orthognathic surgery. *Maxillofac. Plast. Reconstr. Surg.* **2015**, *37*, 6. [CrossRef]
76. Suuronen, R.; Kallela, I.; Lindqvist, C. Bioabsorbable plates and screws: Current state of the art in facial fracture repair. *J. Craniomaxillofac. Trauma* **2000**, *6*, 19–27.
77. Cural, Ü.; Atalay, B.; Yildirim, M.S. Comparison of Mechanical Stabilization of the Mandibular Angulus Fracture Fixation, With Titanium Plates and Screws, Resorbable Plates and Screws, and Bone Adhesives. *J. Craniofac. Surg.* **2018**, *29*, 1780–1787. [CrossRef]

78. Sukegawa, S.; Kanno, T.; Matsumoto, K.; Sukegawa-Takahashi, Y.; Masui, M.; Furuki, Y. Complications of a poly-L-lactic acid and polyglycolic acid osteosynthesis device for internal fixation in maxillofacial surgery. *Odontology* **2018**, *106*, 360–368. [CrossRef]
79. On, S.-W.; Cho, S.-W.; Byun, S.-H.; Yang, B.-E. Bioabsorbable Osteofixation Materials for Maxillofacial Bone Surgery: A Review on Polymers and Magnesium-Based Materials. *Biomedicines* **2020**, *8*, 300. [CrossRef]
80. Sukegawa, S.; Kawai, H.; Nakano, K.; Kanno, T.; Takabatake, K.; Nagatsuka, H.; Furuki, Y. Feasible Advantage of Bioactive/Bioresorbable Devices Made of Forged Composites of Hydroxyapatite Particles and Poly-L-lactide in Alveolar Bone Augmentation: A Preliminary Study. *Int. J. Med. Sci.* **2019**, *16*, 311–317. [CrossRef]
81. Schumann, P.; Lindhorst, D.; Wagner, M.E.H.; Schramm, A.; Gellrich, N.C.; Rücker, M. Perspectives on Resorbable Osteosynthesis Materials in Craniomaxillofacial Surgery. *Pathobiology* **2013**, *80*, 211–217. [CrossRef]
82. Lambotte, A. L'utilisation du magnesium comme materiel perdu dans l'osteosynthèse. *Bull. Mem. Soc. Nat. Chir.* **1932**, *28*, 1325–1334.
83. Leonhardt, H.; Franke, A.; McLeod, N.M.H.; Lauer, G.; Nowak, A. Fixation of fractures of the condylar head of the mandible with a new magnesium-alloy biodegradable cannulated headless bone screw. *Br. J. Oral Maxillofac. Surg.* **2017**, *55*, 623–625. [CrossRef]
84. Shegarfi, H.; Reikeras, O. Review article: Bone transplantation and immune response. *J. Orthop. Surg.* **2009**, *17*, 206–211. [CrossRef]
85. Kloss, F.R.; Offermanns, V.; Kloss-Brandstätter, A. Comparison of allogeneic and autogenous bone grafts for augmentation of alveolar ridge defects-A 12-month retrospective radiographic evaluation. *Clin. Oral Implant. Res.* **2018**, *29*, 1163–1175. [CrossRef]
86. Sohn, H.S.; Oh, J.K. Review of bone graft and bone substitutes with an emphasis on fracture surgeries. *Biomater. Res.* **2019**, *23*, 9. [CrossRef]
87. Caballé-Serrano, J.; Fujioka-Kobayashi, M.; Bosshardt, D.D.; Gruber, R.; Buser, D.; Miron, R.J. Pre-coating deproteinized bovine bone mineral (DBBM) with bone-conditioned medium (BCM) improves osteoblast migration, adhesion, and differentiation in vitro. *Clin. Oral Investig.* **2016**, *20*, 2507–2513. [CrossRef]
88. Katz, J.; Mukherjee, N.; Cobb, R.R.; Bursac, P.; York-Ely, A. Incorporation and immunogenicity of cleaned bovine bone in a sheep model. *J. Biomater Appl.* **2009**, *24*, 159–174. [CrossRef]
89. Cho, J.S.; Kim, H.-S.; Um, S.-H.; Rhee, S.-H. Preparation of a novel anorganic bovine bone xenograft with enhanced bioactivity and osteoconductivity. *J. Biomed. Mater. Res. Part. B Appl. Biomater.* **2013**, *101B*, 855–869. [CrossRef]
90. Sanz, M.; Dahlin, C.; Apatzidou, D.; Artzi, Z.; Bozic, D.; Calciolari, E.; De Bruyn, H.; Dommisch, H.; Donos, N.; Eickholz, P.; et al. Biomaterials and regenerative technologies used in bone regeneration in the craniomaxillofacial region: Consensus report of group 2 of the 15th European Workshop on Periodontology on Bone Regeneration. *J. Clin. Periodontol.* **2019**, *46* (Suppl. S21), 82–91. [CrossRef]
91. Baino, F.; Novajra, G.; Vitale-Brovarone, C. Bioceramics and Scaffolds: A Winning Combination for Tissue Engineering. *Front. Bioeng Biotechnol.* **2015**, *3*, 202. [CrossRef]
92. Yahav, A.; Kurtzman, G.M.; Katzap, M.; Dudek, D.; Baranes, D. Bone Regeneration: Properties and Clinical Applications of Biphasic Calcium Sulfate. *Dent. Clin. N. Am.* **2020**, *64*, 453–472. [CrossRef]
93. Miron, R.J.; Zhang, Q.; Sculean, A.; Buser, D.; Pippenger, B.E.; Dard, M.; Shirakata, Y.; Chandad, F.; Zhang, Y. Osteoinductive potential of 4 commonly employed bone grafts. *Clin. Oral Investig.* **2016**, *20*, 2259–2265. [CrossRef]
94. Donos, N.; Kostopoulos, L.; Tonetti, M.; Karring, T.; Lang, N.P. The effect of enamel matrix proteins and deproteinized bovine bone mineral on heterotopic bone formation. *Clin. Oral Implant. Res.* **2006**, *17*, 434–438. [CrossRef]
95. Guillaume, B. Filling bone defects with beta-TCP in maxillofacial surgery: A review. *Morphologie* **2017**, *101*, 113–119. [CrossRef]
96. Friedmann, A.; Dehnhardt, J.; Kleber, B.M.; Bernimoulin, J.P. Cytobiocompatibility of collagen and ePTFE membranes on osteoblast-like cells in vitro. *J. Biomed. Mater. Res. A* **2008**, *86*, 935–941. [CrossRef]
97. Rodella, L.F.; Favero, G.; Labanca, M. Biomaterials in maxillofacial surgery: Membranes and grafts. *Int J. Biomed. Sci* **2011**, *7*, 81–88.
98. Urban, I.A.; Monje, A. Guided Bone Regeneration in Alveolar Bone Reconstruction. *Oral Maxillofac. Surg. Clin. N. Am.* **2019**, *31*, 331–338. [CrossRef]
99. Jiménez Garcia, J.; Berghezan, S.; Caramês, J.M.M.; Dard, M.M.; Marques, D.N.S. Effect of cross-linked vs non-cross-linked collagen membranes on bone: A systematic review. *J. Periodontal. Res.* **2017**, *52*, 955–964. [CrossRef]
100. Sbricoli, L.; Guazzo, R.; Annunziata, M.; Gobbato, L.; Bressan, E.; Nastri, L. Selection of Collagen Membranes for Bone Regeneration: A Literature Review. *Materials* **2020**, *13*, 786. [CrossRef]
101. Martin-Thomé, H.; Bourdin, D.; Strube, N.; Saffarzadeh, A.; Morlock, J.F.; Campard, G.; Evanno, C.; Hoornaert, A.; Layrolle, P. Clinical Safety of a New Synthetic Resorbable Dental Membrane: A Case Series Study. *J. Oral Implant.* **2018**, *44*, 138–145. [CrossRef]
102. Souza, F.G.R.; Santos, I.C.; Bergmann, A.; Thuler, L.C.S.; Freitas, A.S.; Freitas, E.Q.; Dias, F.L. Quality of life after total laryngectomy: Impact of different vocal rehabilitation methods in a middle income country. *Health Qual. Life Outcomes* **2020**, *18*, 92. [CrossRef]
103. Bertl, K.; Zatorska, B.; Leonhard, M.; Matejka, M.; Schneider-Stickler, B. Anaerobic and microaerophilic pathogens in the biofilm formation on voice prostheses: A pilot study. *Laryngoscope* **2012**, *122*, 1035–1039. [CrossRef]
104. Bucki, R.; Niemirowicz-Laskowska, K.; Deptuła, P.; Wilczewska, A.Z.; Misiak, P.; Durnaś, B.; Fiedoruk, K.; Piktel, E.; Mystkowska, J.; Janmey, P.A. Susceptibility of microbial cells to the modified PIP(2)-binding sequence of gelsolin anchored on the surface of magnetic nanoparticles. *J. Nanobiotechnol.* **2019**, *17*, 81. [CrossRef]

105. Durnaś, B.; Wnorowska, U.; Pogoda, K.; Deptuła, P.; Wątek, M.; Piktel, E.; Głuszek, S.; Gu, X.; Savage, P.B.; Niemirowicz, K.; et al. Candidacidal Activity of Selected Ceragenins and Human Cathelicidin LL-37 in Experimental Settings Mimicking Infection Sites. *PLoS ONE* **2016**, *11*, e0157242. [CrossRef]
106. Durnaś, B.; Piktel, E.; Wątek, M.; Wollny, T.; Góźdź, S.; Smok-Kalwat, J.; Niemirowicz, K.; Savage, P.B.; Bucki, R. Anaerobic bacteria growth in the presence of cathelicidin LL-37 and selected ceragenins delivered as magnetic nanoparticles cargo. *BMC Microbiol.* **2017**, *17*, 167. [CrossRef]
107. Niemirowicz, K.; Durnaś, B.; Tokajuk, G.; Piktel, E.; Michalak, G.; Gu, X.; Kułakowska, A.; Savage, P.B.; Bucki, R. Formulation and candidacidal activity of magnetic nanoparticles coated with cathelicidin LL-37 and ceragenin CSA-13. *Sci. Rep.* **2017**, *7*, 4610. [CrossRef]
108. Niemirowicz-Laskowska, K.; Mystkowska, J.; Łysik, D.; Chmielewska, S.; Tokajuk, G.; Misztalewska-Turkowicz, I.; Wilczewska, A.Z.; Bucki, R. Antimicrobial and Physicochemical Properties of Artificial Saliva Formulations Supplemented with Core-Shell Magnetic Nanoparticles. *Int. J. Mol. Sci.* **2020**, *21*, 1979. [CrossRef]
109. Vallieres, C.; Hook, A.L.; He, Y.; Crucitti, V.C.; Figueredo, G.; Davies, C.R.; Burroughs, L.; Winkler, D.A.; Wildman, R.D.; Irvine, D.J.; et al. Discovery of (meth)acrylate polymers that resist colonization by fungi associated with pathogenesis and biodeterioration. *Sci. Adv.* **2020**, *6*, eaba6574. [CrossRef]
110. Niermeyer, W.L.; Rodman, C.; Li, M.M.; Chiang, T. Tissue engineering applications in otolaryngology-The state of translation. *Laryngoscope Investig. Otolaryngol.* **2020**, *5*, 630–648. [CrossRef]
111. Cao, Y.; Vacanti, J.P.; Paige, K.T.; Upton, J.; Vacanti, C.A. Transplantation of Chondrocytes Utilizing a Polymer-Cell Construct to Produce Tissue-Engineered Cartilage in the Shape of a Human Ear. *Plast. Reconstr. Surg.* **1997**, *100*, 297–302. [CrossRef]
112. Fulco, I.; Miot, S.; Haug, M.D.; Barbero, A.; Wixmerten, A.; Feliciano, S.; Wolf, F.; Jundt, G.; Marsano, A.; Farhadi, J.; et al. Engineered autologous cartilage tissue for nasal reconstruction after tumour resection: An observational first-in-human trial. *Lancet* **2014**, *384*, 337–346. [CrossRef]
113. Hoshi, K.; Fujihara, Y.; Saijo, H.; Kurabayashi, K.; Suenaga, H.; Asawa, Y.; Nishizawa, S.; Kanazawa, S.; Uto, S.; Inaki, R.; et al. Three-dimensional changes of noses after transplantation of implant-type tissue-engineered cartilage for secondary correction of cleft lip–nose patients. *Regen. Ther.* **2017**, *7*, 72–79. [CrossRef] [PubMed]
114. Zhou, G.; Jiang, H.; Yin, Z.; Liu, Y.; Zhang, Q.; Zhang, C.; Pan, B.; Zhou, J.; Zhou, X.; Sun, H.; et al. In Vitro Regeneration of Patient-specific Ear-shaped Cartilage and Its First Clinical Application for Auricular Reconstruction. *EBioMedicine* **2018**, *28*, 287–302. [CrossRef] [PubMed]
115. Nimeskern, L.; Martínez Ávila, H.; Sundberg, J.; Gatenholm, P.; Müller, R.; Stok, K.S. Mechanical evaluation of bacterial nanocellulose as an implant material for ear cartilage replacement. *J. Mech. Behav. Biomed. Mater.* **2013**, *22*, 12–21. [CrossRef]
116. Lee, M.C.; Seonwoo, H.; Garg, P.; Jang, K.J.; Pandey, S.; Park, S.B.; Kim, H.B.; Lim, J.; Choung, Y.H.; Chung, J.H. Chitosan/PEI patch releasing EGF and the EGFR gene for the regeneration of the tympanic membrane after perforation. *Biomater. Sci.* **2018**, *6*, 364–371. [CrossRef] [PubMed]
117. Mellott, A.J.; Shinogle, H.E.; Nelson-Brantley, J.G.; Detamore, M.S.; Staecker, H. Exploiting decellularized cochleae as scaffolds for inner ear tissue engineering. *Stem Cell Res. Ther.* **2017**, *8*, 41. [CrossRef]
118. Maughan, E.F.; Butler, C.R.; Crowley, C.; Teoh, G.Z.; den Hondt, M.; Hamilton, N.J.; Hynds, R.E.; Lange, P.; Ansari, T.; Urbani, L.; et al. A comparison of tracheal scaffold strategies for pediatric transplantation in a rabbit model. *Laryngoscope* **2017**, *127*, E449–E457. [CrossRef]
119. Zhao, L.; Sundaram, S.; Le, A.V.; Huang, A.H.; Zhang, J.; Hatachi, G.; Beloiartsev, A.; Caty, M.G.; Yi, T.; Leiby, K.; et al. Engineered Tissue-Stent Biocomposites as Tracheal Replacements. *Tissue Eng. Part A* **2016**, *22*, 1086–1097. [CrossRef]
120. Dharmadhikari, S.; Liu, L.; Shontz, K.; Wiet, M.; White, A.; Goins, A.; Akula, H.; Johnson, J.; Reynolds, S.D.; Breuer, C.K.; et al. Deconstructing tissue engineered trachea: Assessing the role of synthetic scaffolds, segmental replacement and cell seeding on graft performance. *Acta Biomate.r* **2020**, *102*, 181–191. [CrossRef]
121. Best, C.A.; Pepper, V.K.; Ohst, D.; Bodnyk, K.; Heuer, E.; Onwuka, E.A.; King, N.; Strouse, R.; Grischkan, J.; Breuer, C.K.; et al. Designing a tissue-engineered tracheal scaffold for preclinical evaluation. *Int. J. Pediatr. Otorhinolaryngol.* **2018**, *104*, 155–160. [CrossRef]
122. Brookes, S.; Voytik-Harbin, S.; Zhang, H.; Zhang, L.; Halum, S. Motor endplate-expressing cartilage-muscle implants for reconstruction of a denervated hemilarynx. *Laryngoscope* **2019**, *129*, 1293–1300. [CrossRef]
123. Herrmann, P.; Ansari, T.; Southgate, A.; Varanou Jenkins, A.; Partington, L.; Carvalho, C.; Janes, S.; Lowdell, M.; Sibbons, P.D.; Birchall, M.A. In vivo implantation of a tissue engineered stem cell seeded hemi-laryngeal replacement maintains airway, phonation, and swallowing in pigs. *J. Tissue Eng. Regen. Med.* **2019**, *13*, 1943–1954. [CrossRef] [PubMed]
124. Olsen, L.B.; Larsen, S.; Wanscher, J.H.; Faber, C.E.; Jeppesen, J. Postoperative infections following cochlear implant surgery. *Acta Otolaryngol.* **2018**, *138*, 956–960. [CrossRef] [PubMed]
125. Mikulskis, P.; Hook, A.; Dundas, A.A.; Irvine, D.; Sanni, O.; Anderson, D.; Langer, R.; Alexander, M.R.; Williams, P.; Winkler, D.A. Prediction of Broad-Spectrum Pathogen Attachment to Coating Materials for Biomedical Devices. *ACS Appl. Mater. Interfaces* **2018**, *10*, 139–149. [CrossRef] [PubMed]
126. Wei, B.P.; Shepherd, R.K.; Robins-Browne, R.M.; Clark, G.M.; O'Leary, S.J. Pneumococcal meningitis post-cochlear implantation: Potential routes of infection and pathophysiology. *Otolaryngol. Head Neck Surg.* **2010**, *143*, S15–S23. [CrossRef]

127. Kirchhoff, L.; Arweiler-Harbeck, D.; Arnolds, J.; Hussain, T.; Hansen, S.; Bertram, R.; Buer, J.; Lang, S.; Steinmann, J.; Höing, B. Imaging studies of bacterial biofilms on cochlear implants-Bioactive glass (BAG) inhibits mature biofilm. *PLoS ONE* **2020**, *15*, e0229198. [CrossRef]
128. Vargas-Blanco, D.; Lynn, A.; Rosch, J.; Noreldin, R.; Salerni, A.; Lambert, C.; Rao, R.P. A pre-therapeutic coating for medical devices that prevents the attachment of Candida albicans. *Ann. Clin. Microbiol. Antimicrob.* **2017**, *16*, 41. [CrossRef]
129. Kao, W.K.; Gagnon, P.M.; Vogel, J.P.; Chole, R.A. Surface charge modification decreases *Pseudomonas aeruginosa* adherence in vitro and bacterial persistence in an in vivo implant model. *Laryngoscope* **2017**, *127*, 1655–1661. [CrossRef]
130. Chen, R.; Willcox, M.D.; Ho, K.K.; Smyth, D.; Kumar, N. Antimicrobial peptide melimine coating for titanium and its in vivo antibacterial activity in rodent subcutaneous infection models. *Biomaterials* **2016**, *85*, 142–151. [CrossRef]
131. Höing, B.; Kirchhoff, L.; Arnolds, J.; Hussain, T.; Buer, J.; Lang, S.; Arweiler-Harbeck, D.; Steinmann, J. Bioactive Glass Granules Inhibit Mature Bacterial Biofilms on the Surfaces of Cochlear Implants. *Otol. Neurotol.* **2018**, *39*, e985–e991. [CrossRef]
132. Parent, M.; Magnaudeix, A.; Delebassée, S.; Sarre, E.; Champion, E.; Viana Trecant, M.; Damia, C. Hydroxyapatite microporous bioceramics as vancomycin reservoir: Antibacterial efficiency and biocompatibility investigation. *J. Biomater. Appl.* **2016**, *31*, 488–498. [CrossRef]
133. Lim, D.J.; Skinner, D.; Mclemore, J.; Rivers, N.; Elder, J.B.; Allen, M.; Koch, C.; West, J.; Zhang, S.; Thompson, H.M.; et al. In-vitro evaluation of a ciprofloxacin and azithromycin sinus stent for *Pseudomonas aeruginosa* biofilms. *Int Forum Allergy Rhinol.* **2020**, *10*, 121–127. [CrossRef] [PubMed]
134. Şevik Eliçora, S.; Erdem, D.; Dinç, A.E.; Altunordu Kalaycı, Ö.; Hazer, B.; Yurdakan, G.; Külah, C. Effects of polymer-based, silver nanoparticle-coated silicone splints on the nasal mucosa of rats. *Eur. Arch. Otorhinolaryngol.* **2017**, *274*, 1535–1541. [CrossRef] [PubMed]
135. Danti, S.; Azimi, B.; Candito, M.; Fusco, A.; Sorayani Bafqi, M.S.; Ricci, C.; Milazzo, M.; Cristallini, C.; Latifi, M.; Donnarumma, G.; et al. Lithium niobate nanoparticles as biofunctional interface material for inner ear devices. *Biointerphases* **2020**, *15*, 031004. [CrossRef]
136. Edmondson, S.; Osborne, V.L.; Huck, W.T.S. Polymer brushes via surface-initiated polymerizations. *Chem. Soc. Rev.* **2004**, *33*, 14–22. [CrossRef]
137. Kabirian, F.; Ditkowski, B.; Zamanian, A.; Hoylaerts, M.F.; Mozafari, M.; Heying, R. Controlled NO-Release from 3D-Printed Small-Diameter Vascular Grafts Prevents Platelet Activation and Bacterial Infectivity. *ACS Biomater. Sci. Eng.* **2019**, *5*, 2284–2296. [CrossRef]
138. Gao, Q.; Yu, M.; Su, Y.; Xie, M.; Zhao, X.; Li, P.; Ma, P.X. Rationally designed dual functional block copolymers for bottlebrush-like coatings: In vitro and in vivo antimicrobial, antibiofilm, and antifouling properties. *Acta Biomater.* **2017**, *51*, 112–124. [CrossRef]
139. Cheng, Q.; Asha, A.B.; Liu, Y.; Peng, Y.-Y.; Diaz-Dussan, D.; Shi, Z.; Cui, Z.; Narain, R. Antifouling and Antibacterial Polymer-Coated Surfaces Based on the Combined Effect of Zwitterions and the Natural Borneol. *ACS Appl. Mater. Interfaces* **2021**, *13*, 9006–9014. [CrossRef]
140. Kurowska, M.; Eickenscheidt, A.; Guevara-Solarte, D.-L.; Widyaya, V.T.; Marx, F.; Al-Ahmad, A.; Lienkamp, K. A Simultaneously Antimicrobial, Protein-Repellent, and Cell-Compatible Polyzwitterion Network. *Biomacromolecules* **2017**, *18*, 1373–1386. [CrossRef]
141. Qiu, H.; Si, Z.; Luo, Y.; Feng, P.; Wu, X.; Hou, W.; Zhu, Y.; Chan-Park, M.B.; Xu, L.; Huang, D. The Mechanisms and the Applications of Antibacterial Polymers in Surface Modification on Medical Devices. *Front. Bioeng. Biotechnol.* **2020**, *8*. [CrossRef]
142. Wong, S.Y.; Han, L.; Timachova, K.; Veselinovic, J.; Hyder, M.N.; Ortiz, C.; Klibanov, A.M.; Hammond, P.T. Drastically Lowered Protein Adsorption on Microbicidal Hydrophobic/Hydrophilic Polyelectrolyte Multilayers. *Biomacromolecules* **2012**, *13*, 719–726. [CrossRef]
143. Meng, S.; Liu, Z.; Shen, L.; Guo, Z.; Chou, L.L.; Zhong, W.; Du, Q.; Ge, J. The effect of a layer-by-layer chitosan–heparin coating on the endothelialization and coagulation properties of a coronary stent system. *Biomaterials* **2009**, *30*, 2276–2283. [CrossRef] [PubMed]
144. Li, D.; Dai, F.; Li, H.; Wang, C.; Shi, X.; Cheng, Y.; Deng, H. Chitosan and collagen layer-by-layer assembly modified oriented nanofibers and their biological properties. *Carbohydr. Polym.* **2021**, *254*, 117438. [CrossRef] [PubMed]
145. Vaterrodt, A.; Thallinger, B.; Daumann, K.; Koch, D.; Guebitz, G.M.; Ulbricht, M. Antifouling and Antibacterial Multifunctional Polyzwitterion/Enzyme Coating on Silicone Catheter Material Prepared by Electrostatic Layer-by-Layer Assembly. *Langmuir* **2016**, *32*, 1347–1359. [CrossRef]
146. Ghamrawi, S.; Bouchara, J.-P.; Tarasyuk, O.; Rogalsky, S.; Lyoshina, L.; Bulko, O.; Bardeau, J.-F. Promising silicones modified with cationic biocides for the development of antimicrobial medical devices. *Mater. Sci. Eng. C* **2017**, *75*, 969–979. [CrossRef]
147. Dirain, C.O.; Silva, R.C.; Antonelli, P.J. Prevention of biofilm formation by polyquaternary polymer. *Int. J. Pediatric Otorhinolaryngol.* **2016**, *88*, 157–162. [CrossRef] [PubMed]
148. Rossi, S.; Azghani, A.O.; Omri, A. Antimicrobial efficacy of a new antibiotic-loaded poly(hydroxybutyric-co-hydroxyvaleric acid) controlled release system. *J. Antimicrob. Chemother.* **2004**, *54*, 1013–1018. [CrossRef] [PubMed]
149. Pritchard, E.M.; Valentin, T.; Panilaitis, B.; Omenetto, F.; Kaplan, D.L. Antibiotic-Releasing Silk Biomaterials for Infection Prevention and Treatment. *Adv. Funct. Mater.* **2013**, *23*, 854–861. [CrossRef]
150. Marsili, L.; Dal Bo, M.; Berti, F.; Toffoli, G. Chitosan-Based Biocompatible Copolymers for Thermoresponsive Drug Delivery Systems: On the Development of a Standardization System. *Pharmaceutics* **2021**, *13*, 1876. [CrossRef]

151. Divya, K.P.; Miroshnikov, M.; Dutta, D.; Vemula, P.K.; Ajayan, P.M.; John, G. In Situ Synthesis of Metal Nanoparticle Embedded Hybrid Soft Nanomaterials. *Acc. Chem. Res.* **2016**, *49*, 1671–1680. [CrossRef]
152. Sharma, V.K.; Yngard, R.A.; Lin, Y. Silver nanoparticles: Green synthesis and their antimicrobial activities. *Adv. Colloid Interface Sci.* **2009**, *145*, 83–96. [CrossRef]
153. Ma, L.; Li, K.; Xia, J.; Chen, C.; Liu, Y.; Lang, S.; Yu, L.; Liu, G. Commercial soft contact lenses engineered with zwitterionic silver nanoparticles for effectively treating microbial keratitis. *J. Colloid Interface Sci.* **2022**, *610*, 923–933. [CrossRef] [PubMed]
154. Ye, Z.; Sang, T.; Li, K.; Fischer, N.G.; Mutreja, I.; Echeverría, C.; Kumar, D.; Tang, Z.; Aparicio, C. Hybrid nanocoatings of self-assembled organic-inorganic amphiphiles for prevention of implant infections. *Acta Biomater.* **2022**, *140*, 338–349. [CrossRef] [PubMed]
155. Duda, F.; Bradel, S.; Bleich, A.; Abendroth, P.; Heemeier, T.; Ehlert, N.; Behrens, P.; Esser, K.H.; Lenarz, T.; Brandes, G.; et al. Biocompatibility of silver containing silica films on Bioverit®II middle ear prostheses in rabbits. *J. Biomater. Appl.* **2015**, *30*, 17–29. [CrossRef]
156. Jang, C.H.; Cho, Y.B.; Jang, Y.S.; Kim, M.S.; Kim, G.H. Antibacterial effect of electrospun polycaprolactone/polyethylene oxide/vancomycin nanofiber mat for prevention of periprosthetic infection and biofilm formation. *Int. J. Pediatr. Otorhinolaryngol.* **2015**, *79*, 1299–1305. [CrossRef] [PubMed]
157. Ziabka, M.; Dziadek, M.; Krolicka, A. Biological and Physicochemical Assessment of Middle Ear Prosthesis. *Polymers* **2019**, *11*, 79. [CrossRef] [PubMed]
158. Ziabka, M.; Dziadek, M.; Menaszek, E.; Banasiuk, R.; Krolicka, A. Middle Ear Prosthesis with Bactericidal Efficacy-In Vitro Investigation. *Molecules* **2017**, *22*, 681. [CrossRef]
159. Barros, J.; Grenho, L.; Fernandes, M.H.; Manuel, C.M.; Melo, L.F.; Nunes, O.C.; Monteiro, F.J.; Ferraz, M.P. Anti-sessile bacterial and cytocompatibility properties of CHX-loaded nanohydroxyapatite. *Colloids Surf. B Biointerfaces* **2015**, *130*, 305–314. [CrossRef]
160. Weng, W.; Li, X.; Nie, W.; Liu, H.; Liu, S.; Huang, J.; Zhou, Q.; He, J.; Su, J.; Dong, Z.; et al. One-Step Preparation of an AgNP-nHA@RGO Three-Dimensional Porous Scaffold and Its Application in Infected Bone Defect Treatment. *Int. J. Nanomed.* **2020**, *15*, 5027–5042. [CrossRef]
161. Wang, Q.; Tang, Y.; Ke, Q.; Yin, W.; Zhang, C.; Guo, Y.; Guan, J. Magnetic lanthanum-doped hydroxyapatite/chitosan scaffolds with endogenous stem cell-recruiting and immunomodulatory properties for bone regeneration. *J. Mater. Chem. B* **2020**, *8*, 5280–5292. [CrossRef]
162. Wang, J.; Zhou, H.; Guo, G.; Tan, J.; Wang, Q.; Tang, J.; Liu, W.; Shen, H.; Li, J.; Zhang, X. Enhanced Anti-Infective Efficacy of ZnO Nanoreservoirs through a Combination of Intrinsic Anti-Biofilm Activity and Reinforced Innate Defense. *ACS Appl. Mater. Interfaces* **2017**, *9*, 33609–33623. [CrossRef]
163. Chen, B.; You, Y.; Ma, A.; Song, Y.; Jiao, J.; Song, L.; Shi, E.; Zhong, X.; Li, Y.; Li, C. Zn-Incorporated TiO. *Int. J. Nanomed.* **2020**, *15*, 2095–2118. [CrossRef] [PubMed]

International Journal of
Molecular Sciences

MDPI

Article

Development of New Collagen/Clay Composite Biomaterials

Maria Minodora Marin [1,2,*], Raluca Ianchis [3,*], Rebeca Leu Alexa [1], Ioana Catalina Gifu [3], Madalina Georgiana Albu Kaya [2], Diana Iulia Savu [4], Roxana Cristina Popescu [4], Elvira Alexandrescu [3], Claudia Mihaela Ninciuleanu [3], Silviu Preda [5], Madalina Ignat [2], Roxana Constantinescu [2] and Horia Iovu [1,6,*]

1 Advanced Polymer Materials Group, Politehnica University of Bucharest, 1-7 Polizu Street, 011061 Bucharest, Romania; rebeca.leu@upb.ro
2 Collagen Department, Leather and Footwear Research Institute, 93 Ion Minulescu Street, 031215 Bucharest, Romania; albu_mada@yahoo.com (M.G.A.K.); madalina.fleancu@yahoo.com (M.I.); rodica.roxana@yahoo.com (R.C.)
3 National Research & Development Institute for Chemistry and Petrochemistry, ICECHIM, Spl. Independentei Nr. 202, 6th District, 060021 Bucharest, Romania; catalina.gifu@icechim-pd.ro (I.C.G.); elviraalexandrescu@yahoo.com (E.A.); claudia.ninciuleanu@icechim-pd.ro (C.M.N.)
4 Department of Life and Environmental Physics, Horia Hulubei National Institute of Physics and Nuclear Engineering, 077125 Magurele, Romania; savu_diana@yahoo.com (D.I.S.); Roxana.popescu@nipne.ro (R.C.P.)
5 Institute of Physical Chemistry "Ilie Murgulescu", Romanian Academy, Spl. Independentei 202, 6th District, 060021 Bucharest, Romania; predas01@yahoo.co.uk
6 Chemical Sciences Section, Academy of Romanian Scientists, 54 Splaiul Independentei, 50085 Bucharest, Romania
* Correspondence: maria_minodora.marin@upb.ro (M.M.M.); raluca.ianchis@icechim-pd.ro (R.I.); horia.iovu@upb.ro (H.I.)

Citation: Marin, M.M.; Ianchis, R.; Leu Alexa, R.; Gifu, I.C.; Kaya, M.G.A.; Savu, D.I.; Popescu, R.C.; Alexandrescu, E.; Ninciuleanu, C.M.; Preda, S.; et al. Development of New Collagen/Clay Composite Biomaterials. *Int. J. Mol. Sci.* **2022**, *23*, 401. https://doi.org/10.3390/ijms23010401

Academic Editor: Helena Felgueiras

Received: 5 December 2021
Accepted: 27 December 2021
Published: 30 December 2021

Abstract: The fabrication of collagen-based biomaterials for skin regeneration offers various challenges for tissue engineers. The purpose of this study was to obtain a novel series of composite biomaterials based on collagen and several types of clays. In order to investigate the influence of clay type on drug release behavior, the obtained collagen-based composite materials were further loaded with gentamicin. Physiochemical and biological analyses were performed to analyze the obtained nanocomposite materials after nanoclay embedding. Infrared spectra confirmed the inclusion of clay in the collagen polymeric matrix without any denaturation of triple helical conformation. All the composite samples revealed a slight change in the 2-theta values pointing toward a homogenous distribution of clay layers inside the collagen matrix with the obtaining of mainly intercalated collagen-clay structures, according X-ray diffraction analyses. The porosity of collagen/clay composite biomaterials varied depending on clay nanoparticles sort. Thermo-mechanical analyses indicated enhanced thermal and mechanical features for collagen composites as compared with neat type II collagen matrix. Biodegradation findings were supported by swelling studies, which indicated a more crosslinked structure due additional H bonding brought on by nanoclays. The biology tests demonstrated the influence of clay type on cellular viability but also on the antimicrobial behavior of composite scaffolds. All nanocomposite samples presented a delayed gentamicin release when compared with the collagen-gentamicin sample. The obtained results highlighted the importance of clay type selection as this affects the performances of the collagen-based composites as promising biomaterials for future applications in the biomedical field.

Keywords: clay; type II collagen; biomaterials

1. Introduction

The design of collagen biomaterials for use as implants poses various challenges for tissue engineers [1]. Biomaterials offer great advantages for medical therapies, facilitating a good response for clinical problems [2,3]. Biopolymers represent an important resource for biomedical applications because of their characteristics, for example, in cell adhesion, proliferation and compatibility with diverse categories of drugs, and of different chemical structure [4–6]. The forms of mixed biopolymers commonly used are hydrogels, membranes, spheres, fibers, and sponges.

Hydrogels are 3D crosslinked polymers structures with high capacity to absorb and retain important water amounts without the degradation of their tridimensional network. Hydrogels can be synthesized from natural, synthetic, or combined polymer chains. Hydrogels can serve as matrices for the obtaining of composite biomaterials, targeting adequate structures and morphologies beneficial for biomedical application [7–10]. Because of their availability and versatility, natural polymers such as collagen, alginate, chitosan, hyaluronic acid, and cellulose are mostly preferred for their use in various formulations and mixtures. These are regularly used for a series of remedies in regenerative medicine and drug delivery systems [11,12].

Collagen represents the foremost component of extracellular matrix with a unique triple helical structure, and it is renowned for its low antigenicity, abundance in vertebrate organism, exceptional biocompatibility, and desired biodegradability, unique features that recommend it as an exceptional biomaterial for medical application [13,14]. All these properties promote collagen for use in various biomaterials as wound dressings, bone substitutes, antithrombogenic surfaces, and ophthalmologic collagen shields. Moreover, collagen found application in tissue engineering, for skin replacement and artificial blood vessels and valves [15]. Type II collagen can be found in the extracellular matrix of the articular cartilage as the most important structural element alongside proteoglycans and others specific collagens [16]. Moreover, type II collagen is produced in vitreous, embryonic cornea, and retinal nerve membrane [17]. It is extensively used in food industry, cosmetics, and biomedical and pharmaceuticals applications. Nowadays, the requirement for type II collagen in biomaterials field is progressively growing [18,19]. However, collagen-based biomaterials applications are frequently limited by inadequate thermal stability and mechanical strength. Nevertheless, these drawbacks can be mitigated through the use of cross-linking agents, interpenetration with synthetic polymers, or through the addition of inorganic fillers [20,21].

Currently, several clays are being utilized in medicine and pharmaceuticals as active components or excipients, as well as in cosmetics for creams and emulsion preparation [22]. The majority of clays is obtained from alkaline volcanic sediments using a hydrothermal process. Clays are composed of very fine particles with mixed metal ions. Mostly, they include phyllosilicates such as hydrous silicates of aluminum (Al), zinc (Zn), magnesium (Mg), iron (Fe), and smaller amounts of other metal ions [23]. The structure of clays can be viewed in a platelet form having less than 2 μm in diameter and less than 10 nm in thickness. Furthermore, every level includes minimum one silica (SiO_2) tetrahedron (T) succeeded by one alumina (Al_2O_3) octahedron (O). Clays are divided into three large groups: serpentine-kaolin composed by the halloysite species with chemical formula $Al_2Si_2O_5(OH)_4{\cdot}2H_2O$; smectites that comprise two categories: montmorillonite with chemical formula $Si_{12}Mg_8O_{30}(OH)_4(OH_2)_4{\cdot}8H_2O$ and laponite (synthetic hectorite) with chemical formula $Na^{+0.7}[(Si_8Mg_{5.5}Li_{0.3})O_{20}(OH)_4]^{-0.7}$; and Sepiolite-polygorskite that is composed of sepiolite with chemical formula $Si_{12}Mg_8O_{30}(OH)_4(OH_2)_4{\cdot}8H_2O$, having an architecture like montmorillonite with small differences in its morphology [24].

In the last years, polymer/clay nanocomposites incorporating drugs have been studied to provide new strategies for various applications in the regenerative medicine field [25]. The most studied nanoclays used in the synthesis of collagen-based biomaterials envisaged for medical area are laponite, halloysite, and montmorillonite [25–27]. For example, Yu et al. [28] prepared a chitosan-collagen/organomontmorillonite composite loaded with *Callicarpa nudiflora* as a wound dressing membrane. Moreover, Wang et al. [29] obtained composite fibers doped with amoxicillin using poly (lactic-co-glycolic acid) copolymer and laponite. Another set of polymer/clay nanocomposites based on multilayered polylactic acid/halloysite/gentamicin membranes for bone regeneration, was obtain by Pierchala and collaborators [30]. In a previous study [31], a polyester and acrylate-based composite with hydroxyapatite and halloysite nanotubes was developed and characterized envisaging medical applications. Another hybrid collagen-based hydrogel with embedded montmorillonite (Dellite HPS, Dellite 67G, Cloisite 93A) nanoparticles was developed by Nistor et al. [32].

Montmorillonite (MMT) is a natural biomaterial that has grown relevant due to its high availability, good internal surface area, high cation exchange capability, good adsorption and swelling ratio, excellent biocompatibility. Additionally, montmorillonite is an FDA approved material [33–35]. Several research studies proved that the introduction of clays into polymers matrices not only influenced the mechanical properties of the new designed composites, but also the modulated swelling ratio, degradation rate, and drug release [19,36,37]. The literature data about the conformational change in type II collagen structure induced by Cloisites, which is essential for understanding the new properties of clay mineral–collagen nanocomposites, are deficient.

In this regard, the purpose of the present study was to obtain, characterize, and investigate novel composite biomaterials for semi-hard tissue based on type II collagen with several types of clays that will be further loaded with gentamicin bioactive agent. The structures of the different types of Cloisites are provided in the scheme below (Scheme 1). The commercial clays: Cloisite 20A, Cloisite 15A, Cloisite 93A, and Cloisite 30B are organically modified montmorillonites with quaternary ammonium salts of fatty acids, while Cloisite Na represents the commercial name of montmorillonite without any organomodification [38]. Through organomodification process or cation exchange reaction, the hydrophilic surface of montmorillonite is converted to hydrophobic state. Thus, hydrophobic functional moieties beneficially increase the interactions between clay and nonpolar molecules [39].

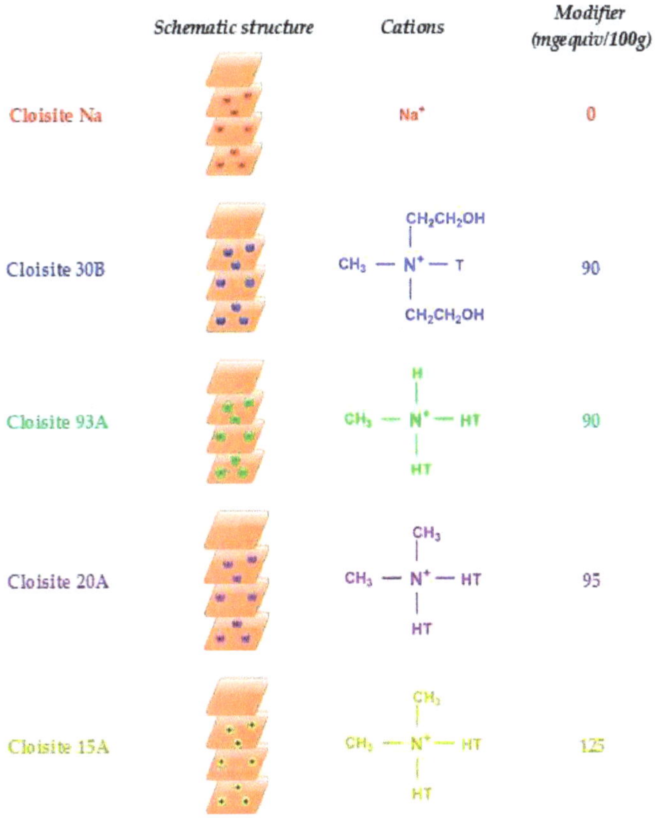

Scheme 1. Schematic structures of the different types of mineral clays.

Although several studies regarding the use of different natural or synthetic clays with collagen are available, none of them provides a systematic comparison between the uses of Cloisite clay type series (Cloisite Na, Cloisite 20A, Cloisite 15A, Cloisite 93A, and Cloisite 30B) in the synthesis and characterization of type II collagen-based biomaterials. Therefore, our study offers valuable information about the importance of clay type selection in the preparation of collagen-based biomaterials when a fixed concentration of clay is used. We expect that the inclusion of mineral clays to provide enhanced mechanical stability serving as reinforcing agents for the biopolymer matrix. Moreover, our study includes investigations about the influence of clay type on the release of gentamicin from gentamicin loaded collagen–clay composites and bactericidal and biocompatibility studies of the prepared nanocomposite materials. To the best of our knowledge, our study is the first systematic report investigating the inclusion of natural or functionalized clay in a type II collagen matrix for cartilaginous tissue regeneration, representing a first for the composite community.

2. Results and Discussion

2.1. FTIR Analyses

The structure of the composite biomaterials was determined by infrared spectrometry and are presented in Figure 1. The spectra of collagen/clay composite biomaterials indicated the characteristic infrared bands of specific components.

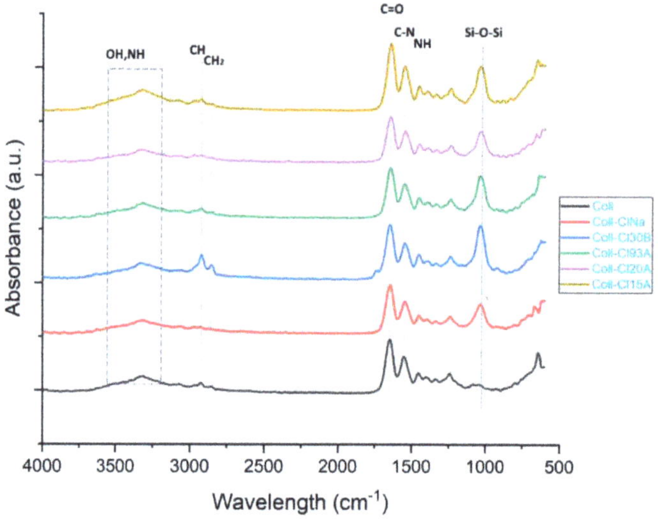

Figure 1. FTIR spectra of the obtained collagen/clay composite biomaterials.

The collagen macromolecule presents a specific triple helix conformation characterized, in infrared spectra, by the amide bands [21]. The peaks around 3319 cm^{-1} and 2928 cm^{-1}, are attributed to amide A and B bands, mostly associated with the NH stretching vibrations, OH groups, and CH asymmetric vibration [20,32]. The amide I band at 1648 cm^{-1} is assigned to the stretching vibrations of peptide C=O groups. The amide II is attributed with the peak at 1551 cm^{-1} arises to CN stretching vibrations. The Amide III band positioned at 1240 cm^{-1} is assigned to the NH bending vibrations from amide linkages [32].

FTIR spectra confirmed the inclusion of clay in the collagen polymeric matrix without any denaturation of triple helical conformation where the specific peaks of clay corresponding to Si-O-Si stretching vibration and CH_2 groups from the hydrocarbonate chains of the clay organic modifiers were found in the collagen/clay composite biomaterials at 1040–1048 cm^{-1} and, respectively, at 2800–2900 cm^{-1}.

2.2. X-ray Diffraction Analyses

The X-ray diffraction patterns of collagen/clay composite biomaterials are presented in Figure 2. Collagen diffraction patterns exhibit two major diffraction lines at two Bragg angles as follows: at ~7.5° a diffraction line generally assigned to triple helix molecular chains and at ~20° a diffraction line attributed to unordered components of collagen [40].

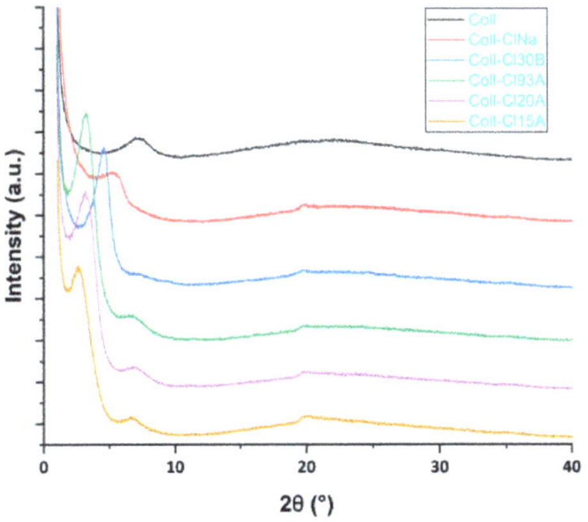

Figure 2. X-ray diffraction patterns of composite samples.

Usually, the mineral clay nanoparticles have a great miscibility with polymeric network and they can basically allow collagen insertion between clay layers [33]. According to XRD analyses, all the composite samples revealed a slight change in the 2-theta values pointing toward a homogenous distribution of clay layers inside the collagen matrix with the obtaining of mainly intercalated collagen–clay structures. Cloisite sodium sample exhibited a better compatibility with the collagen matrix as revealed by the broadening and shifting of Cloisite sodium specific peak.

2.3. SEM Analyses

SEM images (Figure 3) indicated a porous structure with interconnected pores for all the analyzed collagen-based samples.

The neat collagen sample presented a spongious structure with smaller pores than collagen/clay composite materials. The addition of mineral clay nanoparticles in polymeric matrix produces a disturbed porous structure, and somewhat larger pores with clay aggregates were visualized.

In order to quantify the possible changes in pore sizes, the average pore diameter (Dmed) was calculated using Scandium software after measuring 100 pores of each collagen-based sample. The presence of the clays in the architectural structure of collagen affected the polymeric network assembly according the calculated Dmed. The porosity of collagen/clay composite biomaterials varied depending on clay nanoparticles sort. Thus, Coll sample presented the minimum pore size with Dmed = 132 μm while the samples with mineral clays exhibited slightly higher values starting from Dmed = 147 μm for unmodified clay sample (Coll-ClNa) to Dmed ~160 to 170 μm for organomodified mineral clays containing samples [33]. These findings are in good agreement with other studies that observed greater pore sizes when clay particles are added to the biopolymer matrix [41–43].

2.4. Thermogravimetrical Analyses

In order to confirm that the addition of mineral clay nanoparticles in polymeric matrix improved the thermal stability of collagen biomaterials, TGA investigations were performed. Thermal analyses could provide useful information firstly regarding mineral clay dispersion inside collagen matrix and secondly, insights related to supplementary physical and/or chemical crosslinking within the networks [44,45]. The resulted TGA thermograms of the collagen/clay composite biomaterials are presented in Figure 4.

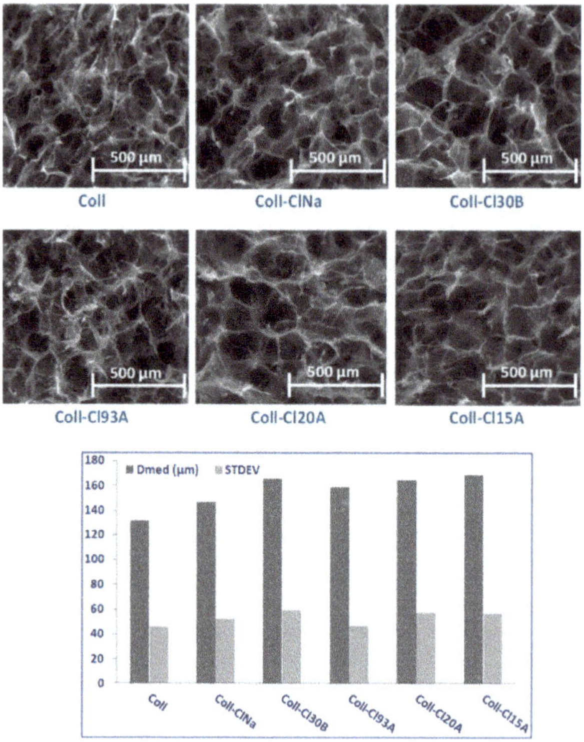

Figure 3. SEM images of collagen/clay composite biomaterials (250×) and calculated average pore diameter with standard deviation.

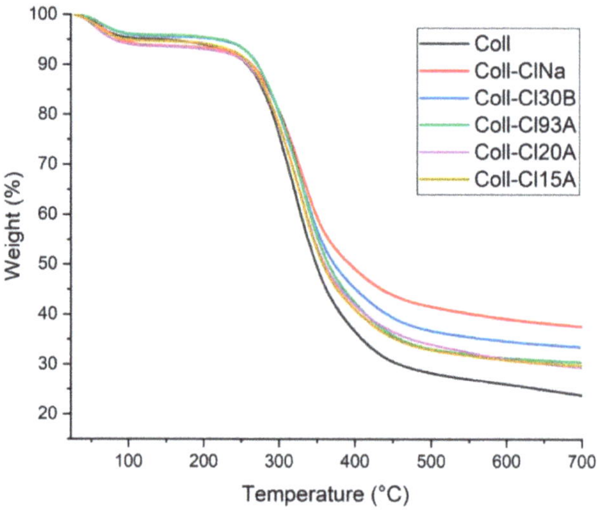

Figure 4. TGA curves of collagen/clay composite biomaterials.

The thermal stability of obtained composites has a significant role in defining the quality of the medical devices [28]. According to the obtained thermograms, for all the collagen/clay composite samples, the presence of the clays promoted an increase in their thermal stability. These results may indirectly point toward a denser structure possibly related to physical interactions established between nanoclays and polymer molecules [46]. TGA thermograms showed a multistep degradation for all samples. The first thermal transitional step appears in the range 45–150 °C and can be associated to the loss of water from the polymeric material [20,32]. The second thermal stage was recorded in the range 150–350 °C, which is associated with a gradual decomposition stage, correspondingly to the irreversible denaturation process [20].

In Table 1 are summarized the properties of the collagen/clay composite biomaterials.

Table 1. Thermogravimetric properties of the collagen/clay composite biomaterials.

Sample	$T_{10\%}$ (°C)	$T_{50\%}$ (°C)	Water Loss Step	Thermal Degradation Step	Residual Mass (%)
			$T_{max\%}$ (°C)	$T_{max\%}$ (°C)	
Coll	257.6	348.5	56.3	319.3	23.82
Coll-ClNa	263.7	393.2	64.8	327.2	37.59
Coll-C130B	271.6	372.7	61.0	326.1	33.51
Coll-C193A	271.2	364.2	64.3	329.0	30.44
Coll-C120A	259.0	359.7	56.3	326.6	29.41
Coll-C115A	262.7	357.6	58.7	326.5	29.76

Moreover, the increasing residual mass of composite biomaterials, according to the data presented in Table 1, confirms the embedding of mineral clays into the polymeric matrix [32]. The differences in the residual mass of composite materials are related with the organomodifier's presence, which gives greater residual mass for samples containing less hydrophobic clays. These findings are similar to those reported by Leon-Mancilla et al. [47] and the same enhanced thermal effect was demonstrated by other studies on polymer/clay nanocomposites. This phenomenon is generally related to the impediment of transport of gases in the nanocomposite sample caused by clay nanoplatelets that can act as a barrier retarding the decomposition process [48]. Moreover, these results could indirectly point interaction between clay nanoparticles and collagen matrix.

2.5. Swelling Studies

Generally, the biomaterials used for tissue regeneration must have specific characteristics for the development and maintenance of an optimal environment and water loss from the damaged tissue at an optimal ratio that is influenced by the water absorption capacity [28]. Swelling studies of all collagen samples indicated a very high ability to retain water, swelling degree ranging from 4500 to 5900% with respect to xerogel samples (Figure 5).

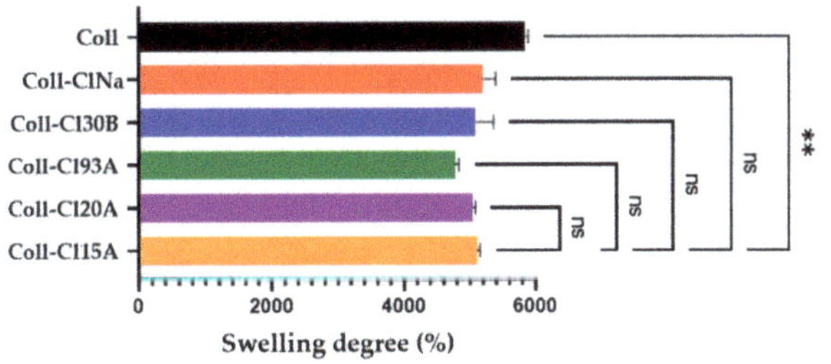

Figure 5. Equilibrium swelling degree of collagen-based samples (ns $p > 0.05$, ** $p \leq 0.01$).

The addition of mineral clay nanoparticles in the collagen polymeric matrix decreased the PBS equilibrium swelling degree of nanocomposite sample. This fact could be a consequence of the replacement of collagen with clay (in the synthesis stage) that did not absorb as much water as related collagen networks [49]. The swelling ability could be restricted also due the additional crosslinking caused by hydrogen bonding. Several researchers demonstrated clay–polymer interactions between the charged surface of clay nanosheets and certain functional groups from the polymer structure, yielding stronger networks [1].

Among nanocomposites samples, a very interesting is the fact that the Cl93A samples displayed the lowest swelling degree. Analyzing the structure of the several clays, Cloisite 93A structure presents a distinct sulfate counter anion of quaternary ammonium salt when compared with the other clay types, which present chloride as counter anion. Therefore, it is very likely that Cl93A could have generated a more crosslinked nanocomposite structure because of sulfate binding, which involves direct hydrogen bonding with positively charged amino groups from collagen polymeric networks, as other studied demonstrated [50].

Overall, the inclusion of clay into the collagen networks led to the limitation of hydrogel swelling most likely due collagen–clay interactions.

2.6. Biodegradation

For biomedical applications an ideal scaffold should present a suitable degradation rate to match the regenerating process of the damaged tissue [49]. The biodegradation of collagen structure can be achieved using collagenase solutions, which are composed of enzymes that are able to destroy the collagen triple helix conformation under the biological conditions of pH and temperature [51].

All the hydrogel samples presented a good stability for a long period of time, retaining more than 50% of the samples' mass after a long period of 50 days (Figure 6).

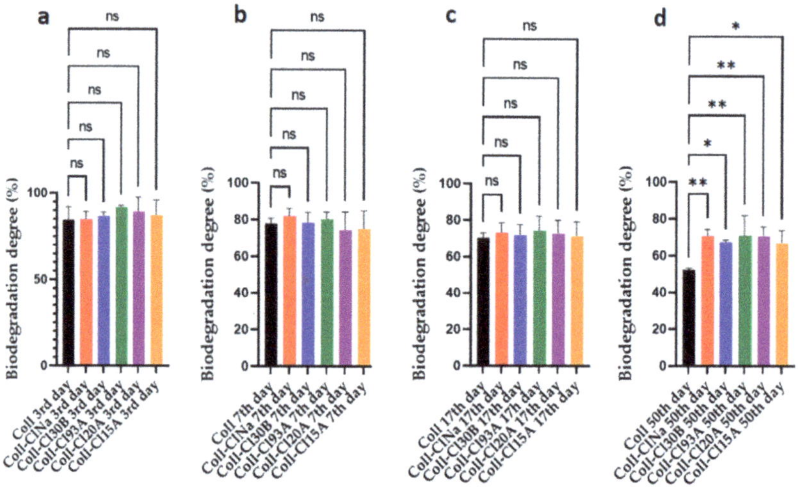

Figure 6. Biodegradation degree as function of time for the composite samples: (**a**). third day; (**b**). 7th day, (**c**). 17th day; (**d**). 50th day (ns $p > 0.05$, * $p \leq 0.05$, ** $p \leq 0.01$).

The addition of the mineral clays led to a decrease in the grade of enzymatic degradation by conserving more of the matrix ultrastructure comparing to the neat collagen sample. The interaction between mineral clays and collagen ultrastructure may consume some hydrophilic groups such as NH_2, which prevented macromolecular hydrolyzation, reinforcing the stability of the obtained biomaterials [49]. The most stable hydrogels were Coll-Cl93A and Coll-Cl20A nanocomposite samples. Biodegradation findings are also supported by swelling studies, which indicated a more crosslinked structure due additional H bonding brought on by nanoclays, especially Cl93A clay type.

The obtained nanocomposites could be suitable scaffolds for cartilaginous tissue regeneration as these retain their mass up to more than 65% after 50 days. Therefore, we expect that the biodegradable scaffolds will remain stable up to 3 months, the minimum period considered for cartilage regeneration [52].

2.7. Mechanical Tests

Collagen/clay composite samples gave rise to different mechanical behaviors when compared to the neat collagen sample. Earlier studies also demonstrated that layered silicates induce enhanced mechanical properties when included in different polymer matrices. However, these properties are strongly dependent on clay concentration and platelet distribution into the polymeric matrix [53]. In our case, the addition of mineral clay in the polymer matrix improved the mechanical properties of the dried samples (Figure 7). Increased mechanical stability and a stronger structure were evidenced, and the nanoclay platelets acted as an elastic solid under stress conditions.

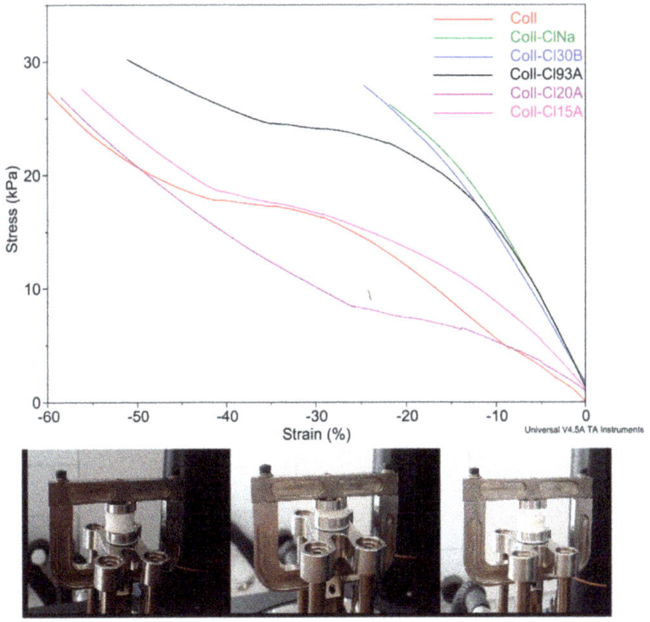

Figure 7. DMA mechanical properties of dried collagen/clay composite biomaterials.

Amongst the five clays used in the synthesis, ClNa produced the most resistant nanocomposite sample to compression. The Coll-Cl30B dried sample had a similar behavior as Coll-ClNa, while the composite obtained with the most hydrophobic clays had a lower resistance under the stress applied compared to the pure collagen sample. This behavior was probably due to the presence of different hydrophobic modifiers, which induced preferential distribution of clay platelets inside the collagen matrix, causing mostly intercalated clay structures as observed by X-ray diffractograms [54].

Moreover, the collagen dried sample had the highest distortion under stress, while the composites samples, especially those obtained with hydrophilic clays, deformed much less (almost three times) than the neat sample (Table 2). Very probably, the organic groups induced a slight elasticity of the composite samples, which recovered better and faster after mechanical stress (Table 2).

Table 2. Behavior of dried samples under stress applied. Revert to the initial form after stress condition.

Sample	Sample Distortion under Stress Condition (Force Applied = 5 N), (%)	Revert after 10 s, (%)	Revert after 30 min, (%)
Coll	62.79	56.45	88.02
Coll-ClNa	20.99	90.66	99.12
Coll-Cl30B	25.68	89.95	94.34
Coll-Cl93A	49.80	68.15	90.52
Coll-Cl20A	58.63	85.12	93.80
Coll-Cl15A	56.08	56.45	88.02

The compression tests performed on wet samples revealed that the presence of the inorganic filler also led to significant improvements in the mechanical strength of the nanocomposite samples (Figure 8). Especially, the presence of ClNa and Cl30B clays led to a significant increase in compressive strength of the composite wet samples against collagen neat sample. Thus, the same behavior from xerogel samples was also preserved to the hydrogel samples, the composite samples being more resistant to mechanical stress than the pure collagen, with emphasis on the samples obtained with the most hydrophilic clays.

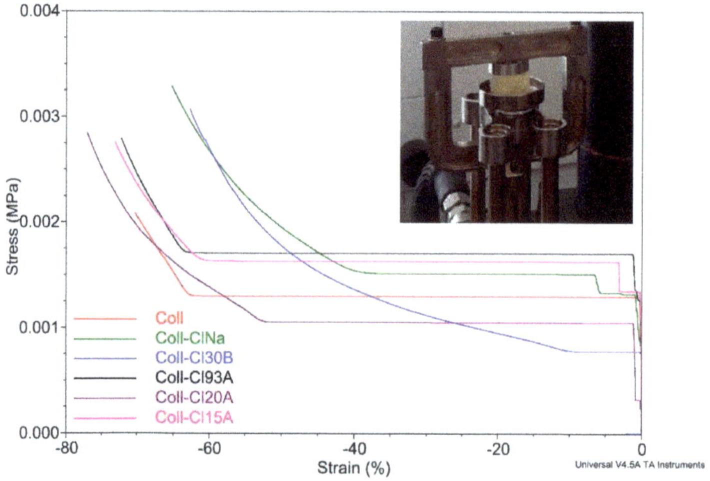

Figure 8. DMA stress–strain curves for the collagen/clay composite hydrogels swollen in PBS.

These results are in good agreement with earlier studies where layered silicates included in a polymer matrix tend to increase the intermolecular forces and dissipate the energy in the whole material under stress conditions [49,53]. Moreover, a higher dispersion of clay nanoplatelets and their interaction with the polymeric matrix were demonstrated to have direct consequences on the compressive strength of the final hydrogel-based nanocomposite materials [54].

Considering that the compression modules of human articular cartilage may vary from 0.1 to 2 MPa, depending on location, DMA results indicate that the synthesized hydrogel nanocomposites scaffolds could withstand the mechanical environment of the cartilaginous tissue [55].

2.8. Drug Release

Gentamicin is one of the most commonly utilized and tested antibiotics in drug delivery systems, and furthermore it has previously been accepted for clinical use [56]. Gentamicin is an antibiotic obtained from *Micromonospora purpurea*, which prevents infection, being efficient against a broad spectrum of Gram-positive and Gram-negative bacteria species [57]. Moreover, gentamicin was demonstrated to promote faster healing process when used along halloysite clay [58]. Considering these aspects, gentamicin was selected and used in our study as a model drug to evaluate clay influence over drug delivery process. The in vitro gentamicin kinetic profiles from collagen/clay composite biomaterials were represented as a drug cumulative released percentage as a function of time (Figure 9).

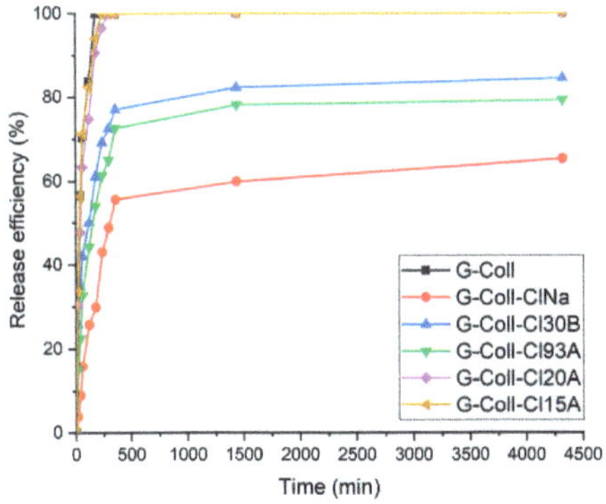

Sample	Release efficiency, %
G-Coll	100
G-Coll-ClNa	65 ± 0.26
G-Coll-Cl30B	85 ± 0.34
G-Coll-Cl93A	79 ± 0.40
G-Coll-Cl20A	100
G-Coll-Cl15A	100

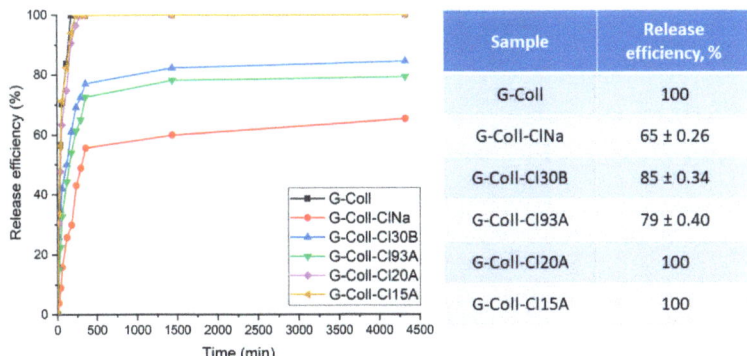

Figure 9. Gentamicin release profile as a function of time.

The release profiles had the same trend for all the samples loaded with gentamicin. Thus, the samples presented an initial burst release in the first hours, followed by a gradually and prolonged drug delivery over the next 72 h. It is worth mentioning that all nanocomposite samples presented a delayed gentamicin release when compared with the collagen-gentamicin sample. Thus, the most rapid release was recorded for the samples G0-Coll followed by G-Coll-Cl20A and G-Coll-Cl15A. Further, the samples obtained with the most hydrophilic clays, G-Coll-Cl30B, G-Coll-Cl93A, and G-Coll-ClNa presented the most retarded burst effect. The cumulative gentamicin released percentage after 72 h has varied between 60 and 80% depending on the type of clay. This extended drug release offers a local shielding antibacterial effect over a longer period of time, essential for tissue repair, and is correlated with the degradation results.

2.9. *Antimicrobial Activity*

The most significant feature of biomaterials is the anticipation of microorganisms' infection as bacteria [28]. The collagen/clay composite biomaterials loaded with gentamicin were tested for microbial activity against two bacterial strains, including *Escherichia coli* and *Staphylococcus aureus* according to SR EN ISO 20645/2005—Control of the antibacterial activity. The evaluation of the samples is based on the absence or presence of bacterial multiplication in the contact area between the inoculum and the sample and on the appearance of a possible inhibition zone around the samples (Figure 10) [59].

An insufficient effect was obtained for the sample without gentamicin and inclusion of mineral clays (Coll) which did not present antimicrobial activity against the bacterial strains. The inhibitions areas produced by all the formulations loaded with gentamicin showed diameters ranging between 6 and 10.5 mm when tested against *Staphylococcus aureus* and 3.5 and 11 mm against *Escherichia coli* after 24 h of incubation. Additionally, it can be observed that the largest zone of inhibition for *Staphylococcus aureus* was presented by the sample G-Coll-Cl20A (10.5 mm), and the largest zone of inhibition for *Escherichia coli* was exhibited by the sample G-Coll (11 mm), which does not have any addition of mineral clay nanoparticles in polymeric matrix. These results are in good agreement with gentamicin release studies where for G-Coll, G-Coll-Cl15A, and G-Coll-Cl20A samples, the most intense burst release and greater amount of gentamicin was recorded within 24 h, thus allowing an effective inhibition of the bacterial strains.

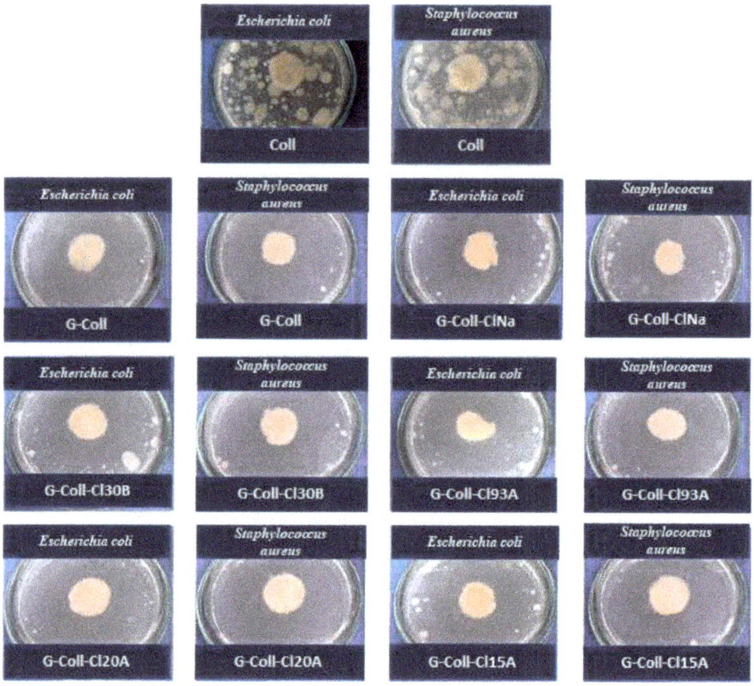

Figure 10. Antimicrobial activity against *Escherichia coli* and *Staphylococcus aureus*.

The results summarized in Table 3 revealed that all composite samples loaded with gentamicin presented microbiological activity and do not allow the development of aerobic germs for any of the bacteria tested.

Table 3. Evaluation of the antimicrobial activity of the composite samples loaded with gentamicin.

Sample	Inhibition Area (mm)	Bacterial Strain	Evaluation	SD (Standard Deviation) for Three Determinations
Coll	Absent	*Staphylococcus aureus*	Insufficient effect	0
	Absent	*Escherichia coli*	Insufficient effect	0
G-Coll	10	*Staphylococcus aureus*	Satisfactory effect	0.3
	11	*Escherichia coli*	Satisfactory effect	0.1
G-Coll-ClNa	7.5	*Staphylococcus aureus*	Satisfactory effect	0.1
	8.5	*Escherichia coli*	Satisfactory effect	0.1
G-Coll-Cl30B	6	*Staphylococcus aureus*	Satisfactory effect	0.1
	5	*Escherichia coli*	Satisfactory effect	0.1
G-Coll-Cl93A	9.5	*Staphylococcus aureus*	Satisfactory effect	0.1
	3.5	*Escherichia coli*	Satisfactory effect	0.1
G-Coll-Cl20A	10.5	*Staphylococcus aureus*	Satisfactory effect	0.1
	9	*Escherichia coli*	Satisfactory effect	0.2
G-Coll-Cl15A	10	*Staphylococcus aureus*	Satisfactory effect	0.1
	6	*Escherichia coli*	Satisfactory effect	0.1

2.10. Cellular Viability—MTT Tests

In order to test the biocompatibility of the new collagen composites we used the MTT assay, which is recognized as a proper method for measuring the cytotoxicity of new biomaterials [60]. The results depicted in the Figure 11 revealed a viability of 82.1 ± 0.61%; 86.8 ± 1.75; 69.3 ± 0.39; 55.4 ± 3.51; and 55.76 ± 0.36 for Coll-ClNa; Coll-Cl30B; Coll-Cl93A; Coll-Cl20A, and Coll-Cl15A, respectively. Thus, the results depicted in the Figure 11 revealed that the Coll-ClNa, Coll-CI30B, and Coll-CI93A composites presented an accepted viability (higher than 70%) in comparison with the control Coll composite. These composites are non-toxic so they could be recommended for biomedical application (ISO 10993-12:2009(E) standard (Biological evaluation of the medical devices. Part 5).

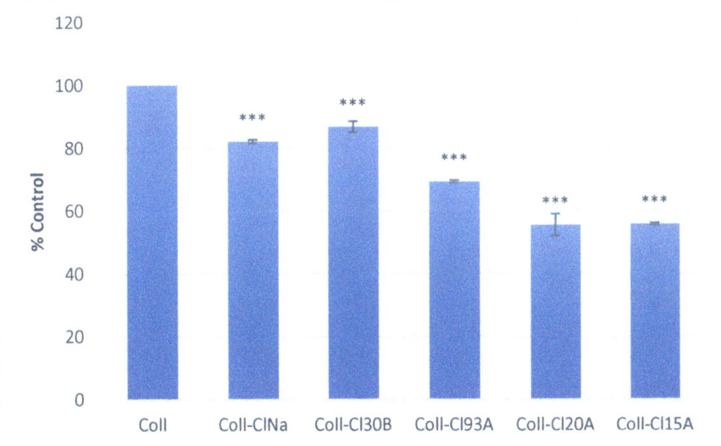

Figure 11. Biological evaluation of the obtained samples, *** $p \leq 0.001$.

In order to test the biocompatibility of the new collagen composites, we used the MTT assay, which is recognized as a proper method for measuring the cytotoxicity of new biomaterials [60].

The results depicted in the Figure 11 revealed that the Coll-ClNa, Coll-CI30B, and Coll-CI93A composites presented an accepted viability (higher than 70%) in comparison with the control Coll composite. These composites are non-toxic so they could be recommended for biomedical application (ISO 10993-12:2009(E) standard (Biological evaluation of the medical devices. Part 5). Our results could be related with organic modifier type, which, in a certain concentration, could influence the safety profile of the resulted collagen-based nanocomposite materials. Thus, the biological evaluation of the composites was found in good agreement with literature data, which suggested that a good biocompatibility occurs only in composites samples with a specific concentration of clay in the polymeric matrices [44]. The specific concentration refers to the recipe used in the synthesis and could range from 0.01 to 7% *w/v* [43].

3. Materials and Methods

3.1. Materials

Type II collagen gel was obtained from bovine cartilage by alkaline treatments. Each batch of cartilage was supplied from the same cattle farm and type II collagen gels with the same characteristics were extracted by following a patented protocol in the Collagen Department, Skin, and Footwear Research Institute [61]. Gentamicin was purchased from Fluka (Milwaukee, WI, USA). Type I collagenase extracted from *Clostridium histolyticum* was procured from Sigma-Aldrich, Darmstadt, Germany, and glutaraldehyde (GA) from

Merck, Darmstadt, Germany. The nanoclays were received from Southern Clay Products (Gonzales, TX, USA,).

3.2. Preparation of New Collagen/Clay Composite Biomaterials

Mineral clays were solubilized in ultrapure water and were kept under magnetically stirring for 15 h. Afterwards, the clay dispersion was ultrasonicated for 2 min. Type II collagen and the gentamicin solution were added and homogenized, at 24 °C, to obtain 100 g of gel for each sample in accordance with the composition given in Table 4.

Table 4. The composition of the new collagen/clay composite biomaterials.

Sample	Collagen (%)	ClNa (%)	Cl30B (%)	Cl93A (%)	Cl20A (%)	Cl15A (%)	Gentamicin (GE) (%)	GA (%)
Coll	1.5	-	-	-	-	-	-	0.16
Coll-ClNa	1.5	0.375	-	-	-	-	-	0.16
Coll-Cl30B	1.5	-	0.375	-	-	-	-	0.16
Coll-Cl93A	1.5	-	-	0.375			-	0.16
Coll-Cl20A	1.5	-	-	-	0.375		-	0.16
Coll-Cl15A	1.5	-	-	-	-	0.375	-	0.16
G-Coll	1.5	-	-	-	-	-	0.2	0.16
G-Coll-ClNa	1.5	0.375	-	-	-	-	0.2	0.16
G-Coll-Cl30B	1.5	-	0.375	-	-	-	0.2	0.16
G-Coll-Cl93A	1.5	-	-	0.375	-	-	0.2	0.16
G-Coll-Cl20A	1.5	-	-	-	0.375	-	0.2	0.16
G-Coll-Cl15A	1.5	-	-	-	-	0.375	0.2	0.16

All the percentages are reported to 100 g sample.

The composite hydrogels were freeze-dried using Delta 2–24 LSC (Martin Christ, Osterode, Germany) instrument and spongious forms were obtained and characterized. The obtained 3D composite biomaterials can be observed in Figure 12.

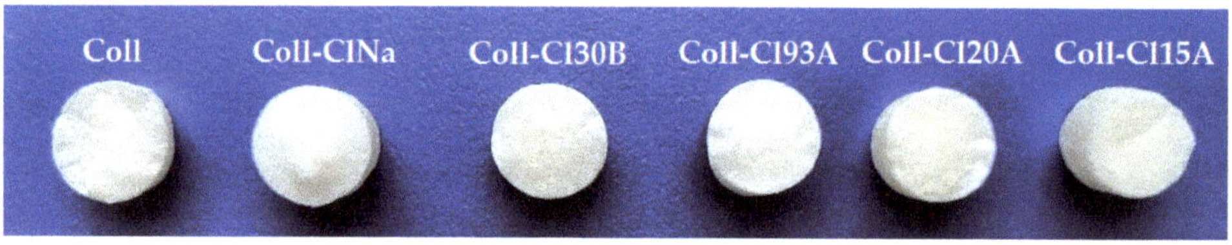

Figure 12. Obtained collagen/clay composite biomaterials (without gentamicin).

The freeze-dried composite scaffolds were evaluated by Fourier-transform infrared spectroscopy, X-ray diffraction, scanning electron microscopy, differential scanning calorimetry, thermo gravimetric analysis, swelling ratio, biodegradation ratio, mechanical tests, drug release, antimicrobial tests, and cellular viability.

3.3. Methods

3.3.1. Fourier-Transform Infrared Spectroscopy (FTIR)

FTIR analysis was accomplished on a Vertex 70 Bruker FTIR spectrometer (Billerica, MA, USA) using an attenuated total reflectance (ATR) addition. For all the obtained biomaterials, the FTIR spectra were recorded in the ATR-FTIR method (in triplicate) at a resolution of 4 cm^{-1} in the 600–4000 cm^{-1} wavenumber range.

3.3.2. X-ray Diffraction (XRD)

The obtained biomaterials were analyzed using an X-ray diffractometer (RigakuUltima IV, Tokyo, Japan) with CuKα radiation (λ = 1.5406 Å), operated at 40 kV and 30 mA. The assessment was performed in uninterrupted mode, at ~23 °C ± 1 and atmospheric pressure. The data were collected over the 2thetawith 1–50° and a scanning speed of 1°/min. The samples were evaluated in a dried powder form.

3.3.3. Scanning Electron Microscopy (SEM)

All the samples were studied using an environmental scanning electron microscopy (ESEM-FEI Quanta 200, Eindhoven, The Netherlands). Moreover, to obtain the secondary electrons images, a gaseous secondary electron detector (GSED) was utilized with the established parameters: 25–30 kV accelerating voltage, magnifications between 2000 and 5000× for the section of obtained biomaterials and the pressure on 2 torr (vacuum conditions).

3.3.4. Thermo Gravimetric Analysis (TGA)

The thermal properties of obtained collagen/clay composite biomaterials were evaluated in triplicate with a NETZSCH TG 209 F1 Libra instrument (Selb, Germany) (controlled atmosphere with a flow rate of nitrogen about 20 mL/min, scanning from 25 to 700 °C and a heating rate of 10 °C/min). Instead of analysis, all composite biomaterials were assessed, the mass ranging between 4 and 5 mg and then they were introduced into aluminum containers.

3.3.5. Swelling Ratio

The swelling ratio of the obtained composites was evaluated by incubation in ultrapure water and temperature of 37 °C. After a predefined time, the samples were taken out and surface adsorbed water was removed by filter paper. The swelling ratio was definite as the ratio of weight increase (w—w0) to the initial weight (w0). Each sample was tested in triplicate.

3.3.6. Biodegradation

The biodegradation behavior of each the obtained samples was assessed by placing the specimens (already swelled in PBS) in a collagenase solution. The hydrogels were maintained at 37 °C for up to 50 days. The wet samples were weighted periodically in order to determine the biodegradation degree. The measurements were performed in triplicate. The biodegradation degree of the hydrogels was calculated as the ratio of weight decrease (w—w0) reported to the initial weight (w0).

3.3.7. Mechanical Tests

Dynamic mechanical analysis of the samples was achieved using a DMA Q800 (TA Instruments, New Castle, DE, USA). Measurements were made at 37 °C, in compression mode, using round sponge samples with a diameter of 15 mm and a thickness of 10 mm. All the equilibrium swelled samples were compressed with a ramp force of 0.01 N/min, from 0.01 to 1.5 N. The dried samples were compressed with a Ramp force of 0.1 N/min from 0.01 to 5 N. The method used to evaluate both dried samples and hydrogel samples was the Compression modulus. All the tests were realized in triplicate.

3.3.8. Drug Release

In vitro drug release kinetic of gentamicin from the design scaffolds was investigated by immersion in containers with a volume of 15 mL ultrapure water. The recipients were additionally introduced in an orbital mixer (Benchmark Scientific, Sayreville, NJ, USA) at 300 rpm, and 37 °C. A 5 mL sample was collected at fixed time intervals and then examined by UV–VIS spectroscopy (SHIMADZU UV-3600 instrument). To preserve a constant volume, after each sampling, 5 mL of fresh ultrapure water were added to every flask. The release efficiency (*RE*) was determined using Equation (1) [62]:

$$RE(\%) = \frac{amount\ of\ released\ GE}{amount\ of\ loaded\ GE} \times 100 \quad (1)$$

3.3.9. Antimicrobial Activity

The control of the antimicrobial activity was tested against the *Staphylococcus aureus* (Gram positive) and *Escherichia. coli* (Gram negative) strains. All the steps of this evaluation were described in our previous work [63]. The samples, placed on the surface of the nutrient medium were analyzed after 24 h of incubation at 37 °C. Bioactivity was determined by determining the diameter of inhibition zones in (mm). Each measurement was repeated for three times and the mean of the diameter of the inhibition areas was calculated.

3.3.10. Cellular Viability—MTT Tests

In order to assess the biological effect of the collagen samples, the MG63 cell line (CLS) was used. The cells were cultured in Earle's minimum essential medium (MEM) containing L-glutamine (Biochrom, Merck Milipore, Burlington, MA, USA) and supplemented with 10% fetal bovine serum (FBS), 1% penicillin and streptomycin antibiotics, and 1% non-essential amino acids in standard conditions of temperature and humidity (37 ± 2 °C, 5 ± 1% CO_2 and more than 90% humidity).

The samples were sterilized by gamma irradiation. Afterwards, 2.5×10^5 cells in 500 μL were directly seeded onto each sample. The cells were allowed to attach for about 30 min and afterwards cell culture medium was added in order to cover the whole structure. The cells were incubated in standard conditions of temperature and humidity during 5 days.

The cellular viability was quantitatively measured using the MTT tetrazolium-salt assay (Serva, Heidelberg, Baden-Wuerttemberg, Germany). For this, at the corresponding time-point, the medium was removed and gently replaced with fresh culture medium containing 10% MTT solution (5 mg/mL in PBS). The cells were incubated for another 3 h in standard conditions, and afterwards the supernatant was replaced with DMSO in order to solubilize the grown formazan crystals. The absorbance corresponding to each sample was measured at 570 nm wavelength using a microplate reader.

In order to eliminate any possible interferences, two "Blanks" samples with and without the material and no cells, were used (according to ISO 10993-12 and ISO 10993-5). The absorbance of the blank containing only the solubilizing agent (DMSO) and the absorbance of the blank containing the material and DMSO were mostly the same, results showing that the material does not interfere with the absorbance measurement.

All experiments were performed in triplicate and the data was presented as mean ± SEM. The statistical analysis was performed using a two-tailed Student's test, where values of $^{*}p \leq 0.05$, $^{**}p \leq 0.01$, $^{***}p \leq 0.001$ were considered as statistically significant.

4. Conclusions

Novel Collagen/Clay nanocomposite biomaterials were prepared using five different types of clay. Morphological analyses demonstrated spongiest structures with increased pore dimensions as a result of nanoclay embedding. Mainly intercalated collagen–clay structures with a homogenous distribution of clay layers inside the collagen matrix were obtained as demonstrated by XRD analyses. FTIR spectra confirmed the inclusion of clay in the collagen polymeric matrix without any denaturation of triple helical conformation.

The addition of clay nanoparticles into the collagen matrix promoted improved mechanical properties and decreased biodegradation and swelling ratios when compared with the neat collagen sample. The in vitro gentamicin kinetic profiles revealed retarded burst release of gentamicin as function of clay type. All the samples presented good microbiological activity after the inclusion of mineral clay nanoparticles not allowing the development of aerobic germs for any of the bacteria tested. Cellular viability tests showed good biocompatibility of the novel Coll-ClNa, Coll-Cl30B, and Coll-Cl93A collagen/clay composites.

Thus, our paper presents a preliminary study that aimed to investigate several types of clay of fixed concentration. Following the valuable results obtained, ClNa, Cl30B, and Cl93A will be further used for the development of reinforced hydrogels by varying their concentrations where their influence will be investigated in terms of antimicrobial and drug release properties.

Based on the results presented in our study, the performances of the new collagen-based composites recommend them as promising biomaterials for future applications in the biomedical field.

Author Contributions: Conceptualization, M.M.M. and R.I.; formal analysis, R.I., M.M.M., R.L.A., I.C.G., M.G.A.K., D.I.S., R.C.P., E.A., C.M.N., S.P., R.C., and M.I.; investigation, R.L.A., I.C.G., M.G.A.K., D.I.S., R.C.P., E.A., C.M.N., and S.P.; writing—original draft preparation, M.M.M., R.L.A., M.G.A.K., D.I.S., and R.C.P.; writing—review and editing, R.I. and H.I.; visualization, M.M.M.; supervision, R.I. and H.I. All authors have read and agreed to the published version of the manuscript.

Funding: The article was funded by University Politehnica of Bucharest, PubArt program.

Institutional Review Board Statement: Not applicable.

Informed Consent Statement: Not applicable.

Data Availability Statement: Not applicable.

Acknowledgments: The study was financially supported by Nucleu Program 2019–2022, projects codes PN 19 17 03 02 and PN 19060203. This work was supported by a grant of the Ministry of Research, Innovation and Digitization, CNCS/CCCDI—UEFISCDI, project number PN-III-P2-2.1-PED-2019-4216, within PNCDI III.

Conflicts of Interest: The authors declare no conflict of interest.

References

1. Reyna-Valencia, A.; Chevallier, P.; Mantovani, D. Development of a collagen/clay nanocomposite biomaterial. *Mater. Sci. Forum* **2012**, *706*, 461–466. [CrossRef]
2. Cui, Z.K.; Kim, S.; Baljon, J.J.; Wu, B.M.; Aghaloo, T.; Lee, M. Microporous methacrylated glycol chitosan montmorillonite nanocomposite hydrogel for bone tissue engineering. *Nat. Commun.* **2019**, *10*, 3523. [CrossRef] [PubMed]
3. Shen, Y.; Zhan, Y.; Tang, J.; Xu, P.; Johnson, P.A.; Radosz, M.; Van Kirk, E.A.; Murdoch, W.J. Multifunctioning pH-responsive nanoparticle from hierarchical self-assembly of polymer brush for cancer drug delivery. *AIChE J.* **2008**, *54*, 2979–2989. [CrossRef]
4. Geanaliu-Nicolae, R.E.; Andronescu, E. Blended natural support materials-collagen based hydrogels used in biomedicine. *Materials* **2020**, *13*, 5641. [CrossRef] [PubMed]
5. An, B.; Lin, Y.-S.; Brodsky, B. Collagen interactions: Drug design and delivery. *Adv. Drug Deliv. Rev.* **2016**, *97*, 69–84. [CrossRef] [PubMed]
6. Chvapil, M.; Kronenthal, R.L.; Van Winkle, W. Medical and surgical applications of collagen. *Int. Rev. Connect. Tissue Res.* **1973**, *6*, 1–61.
7. Antoine, E.E.; Vlachos, P.P.; Rylander, M.N. Review of collagen I hydrogels for bioengineered tissue microenvironments: Characterization of mechanics, structure, and transport. *Tissue Eng. Part B Rev.* **2014**, *20*, 683–696. [CrossRef]
8. Ahmadi, F.; Oveisi, Z.; Mohammadi-Samani, S.; Amoozgar, Z. Chitosan based hydrogels: Characteristics and pharmaceutical applications. *Res. Pharm. Sci.* **2015**, *10*, 1–16.
9. Chvapil, M. Collagen sponge: Theory and practice of medical applications. *J. Biomed. Mater. Res.* **1977**, *11*, 721–741. [CrossRef]
10. Bahram, M.; Mohseni, N.; Moghtader, M. *An Introduction to Hydrogels and Some Recent Applications*; IntechOpen: London, UK, 2016.
11. Parenteau-Bareil, R.; Gauvin, R.; Berthod, F. Collagen-based biomaterials for tissue engineering applications. *Materials* **2010**, *3*, 1863–1887. [CrossRef]

12. Andonegi, M.; Heras, K.L.; Santos-Vizcaino, E.; Igartua, M.; Hernandez, R.M.; de la Caba, K.; Guerrero, P. Structure-properties relationship of chitosan/collagen films with potential for biomedical applications. *Carbohydr. Polym.* **2020**, *237*, 116159. [CrossRef] [PubMed]
13. Lin, K.; Zhang, D.; Macedo, M.H.; Cui, W.; Sarmento, B.; Shen, G. Advanced collagen-based biomaterials for regenerative biomedicine. *Adv. Funct. Mater.* **2019**, *29*, 1804943. [CrossRef]
14. Valencia, G.A.; Luciano, C.G.; Lourenço, R.V.; Quinta Barbosa Bittante, A.M.; do Amaral Sobral, P.J. Morphological and physical properties of nano-biocomposite films based on collagen loaded with laponite. *Food Packag. Shelf Life* **2019**, *19*, 24–30. [CrossRef]
15. Albu, M.G.; Titorencu, I.; Ghica, M.V. Collagen-based drug delivery systems for tissue engineering. *Biomater. Appl. Nanomed.* **2011**, *17*, 333–358.
16. Cao, H.; Xu, S.Y. Purification and characterization of type II collagen from chick sternal cartilage. *Food Chem.* **2008**, *108*, 439–445. [CrossRef] [PubMed]
17. Gelse, K.; Poschl, E.; Aigner, T. Collagens-structure, function, and biosynthesis. *Adv. Drug Deliv. Rev.* **2003**, *55*, 1531–1546. [CrossRef] [PubMed]
18. Silva, T.H.; Moreirasilva, J.; Marques, A.L.; Domingues, A.; Bayon, Y.; Reis, R.L. Marine origin collagens and its potential applications. *Mar. Drugs* **2014**, *12*, 5881–5901. [CrossRef] [PubMed]
19. Fulya, B.; Onur, A.; Merih, O.; Funda, T.; Ozge, B.; Ozkan, A. Effects of native type II collagen treatment on knee osteoarthritis: A randomized controlled trial. *Eurasian J. Med.* **2016**, *48*, 95–101.
20. Marin, M.M.; Albu Kaya, M.G.; Vlasceanu, G.M.; Ghitman, J.; Radu, I.C.; Iovu, H. The effect of crosslinking agents on the properties of type II collagen biomaterials. *Mater. Plast.* **2020**, *57*, 166–180. [CrossRef]
21. Su, D.; Wang, C.; Cai, S.; Mu, C.; Li, D.; Lin, W. Influence of palygorskite on the structure and thermal stability of collagen. *Appl. Clay Sci.* **2012**, *62*, 41–46. [CrossRef]
22. Carretero, M.I.; Gomes, C.S.F.; Tateo, F. Clays, drugs, and human health. In *Developments in Clay Science*; Bergaya, F., Lagaly, G., Eds.; Elsevier: Cambridge, MA, USA, 2013; Volume 5.
23. Zhou, Y.; LaChance, A.M.; Smith, A.T.; Cheng, H.F.; Liu, Q.F.; Sun, L.Y. Multifunctional materials: Strategic design of clay-based multifunctional materials: From natural minerals to nanostructured membranes. *Adv. Funct. Mater.* **2019**, *29*, 1807611. [CrossRef]
24. Mousa, M.; Evans, N.; Oreffo, R.O.; Dawson, J. Clay nanoparticles for regenerative medicine and biomaterial design: A review of clay bioactivity. *Biomaterials* **2018**, *159*, 204–2014. [CrossRef]
25. Gaharwar, A.K.; Cross, L.M.; Peak, C.W.; Gold, K.; Carrow, J.K.; Brokesh, A.; Singh, K.A. 2D nanoclay for biomedical applications: Regenerative medicine, therapeutic delivery, and additive manufacturing. *Adv. Mater.* **2019**, *31*, 1900332. [CrossRef]
26. Liu, M.X.; Fakhrullin, R.; Novikov, A.; Panchal, A.; Lvov, Y. Tubule nanoclay-organic heterostructures for biomedical applications. *Macromol. Biosci.* **2019**, *19*, 1800419. [CrossRef] [PubMed]
27. Chimene, D.; Kaunas, R.; Gaharwar, A.K. Hydrogel bioink reinforcement for additive manufacturing: A focused review of emerging strategies. *Adv. Mater.* **2019**, *32*, 1902026. [CrossRef]
28. Yu, X.; Guo, L.; Liu, M.; Cao, X.; Shang, S.; Liu, Z.; Huang, D.; Cao, Y.; Cui, F.; Tian, L. *Callicarpa nudiflora* loaded on chitosan-collagen/organomontmorillonite composite membrane for antibacterial activity of wound dressing. *Int. J. Biol. Macromol.* **2018**, *120*, 2279–2284. [CrossRef]
29. Wang, S.G.; Zheng, F.Y.; Huang, Y.P.; Fang, Y.T.; Shen, M.W.; Zhu, M.F.; Shi, X.Y. Encapsulation of amoxicillin within laponite-doped poly(lactic-co-glycolic acid) nanofibers: Preparation, characterization, and antibacterial activity. *ACS Appl. Mater. Interfaces* **2012**, *4*, 6393. [CrossRef]
30. Pierchala, M.K.; Makaremi, M.; Tan, H.L.; Pushpamalar, J.; Muniyandy, S.; Solouk, A.; Lee, S.M.; Pasbakhsh, P. Nanotubes in nanofibers: Antibacterial multilayered polylactic acid/halloysite/gentamicin membranes for bone regeneration application. *Appl. Clay Sci.* **2018**, *160*, 95–105. [CrossRef]
31. Torres, E.; Dominguez-Candela, I.; Castello-Palacios, S.; Valles-Lluch, A.; Fombuena, V. Development and characterization of polyester and acrylate-based composites with hydroxyapatite and halloysite nanotubes for medical applications. *Polymers* **2020**, *12*, 1703. [CrossRef] [PubMed]
32. Nistor, M.T.; Vasile, C.; Chiriac, A.P. Hybrid collagen-based hydrogels with embedded montmorillonite nanoparticles. *Mater. Sci. Eng. C* **2015**, *53*, 212–221. [CrossRef] [PubMed]
33. Jayrajsinh, S.; Shankar, G.; Agrawal, Y.K.; Bakre, L. Montmorillonite nanoclay as a multifaceted drug delivery carrier: A review. *J. Drug Deliv. Sci. Technol.* **2017**, *39*, 200–209. [CrossRef]
34. Meirelles, L.M.A.; Raffin, F.N. Clay and polymer-based composites applied to drug release: A scientific and technological prospection. *J. Pharm. Pharm. Sci.* **2017**, *20*, 115–134. [CrossRef]
35. Sharma, A.K.; Mortensen, A.; Schmidt, B.; Frandsen, H.; Hadrup, N.; Larsen, E.H.; Binderup, M.L. *In-vivo* study of genotoxic and inflammatory effects of the organo-modified Montmorillonite Cloisite® 30B. *Mutat. Res. Genet. Toxicol. Environ. Mutagenesis* **2014**, *770*, 66–71. [CrossRef]
36. Dawson, J.I.; Oreffo, R.O.C. Clay: New opportunities for tissue regeneration and biomaterial design. *Adv. Mater.* **2013**, *25*, 4069–4086. [CrossRef]
37. Takeno, H.; Nagai, S. Mechanical properties and structures of clay-polyelectrolyte blend hydrogels. *Gels* **2018**, *4*, 71. [CrossRef]
38. Liu, X.; Lu, X.; Su, Y.; Kun, E.; Zhang, F. Clay-polymer nanocomposites prepared by reactive melt extrusion for sustained drug release. *Pharmaceutics* **2020**, *12*, 51. [CrossRef]

39. Firdaus, M.Y.; Octaviani, H.; Herlini, H.; Fatimah, N.; Mulyaningsih, T.; Fairuuz, Z.; Bayu, A. Review: The comparison of clay modifier (cloisite types) in various epoxy-clay nanocomposite synthesis methods. *Mediterr. J. Chem.* **2021**, *11*, 54–74. [CrossRef]
40. Bak, S.Y.; Lee, S.W.; Choi, C.H.; Kim, H.W. Assessment of the influence of acetic acid residue on type I collagen during isolation and characterization. *Materials* **2018**, *11*, 2518. [CrossRef] [PubMed]
41. Leu Alexa, R.; Iovu, H.; Trica, B.; Zaharia, C.; Serafim, A.; Alexandrescu, E.; Radu, I.C.; Vlasceanu, G.; Preda, S.; Ninciuleanu, C.M.; et al. Assessment of naturally sourced mineral clays for the 3D printing of biopolymer-based nanocomposite inks. *Nanomaterials* **2021**, *11*, 703. [CrossRef] [PubMed]
42. García-Villén, F.; Ruiz-Alonso, S.; Lafuente-Merchan, M.; Gallego, I.; Sainz-Ramos, M.; Saenz-del-Burgo, L.; Pedraz, J.L. Clay minerals as bioink ingredients for 3D printing and 3D bioprinting: Application in tissue engineering and regenerative medicine. *Pharmaceutics* **2021**, *13*, 1806. [CrossRef]
43. Leu Alexa, R.; Ianchis, R.; Savu, D.; Temelie, M.; Trica, B.; Serafim, A.; Vlasceanu, G.M.; Alexandrescu, E.; Preda, S.; Iovu, I. 3D printing of alginate-natural clay hydrogel-based nanocomposites. *Gels* **2021**, *7*, 211. [CrossRef]
44. Ianchis, R.; Ninciuleanu, C.M.; Gifu, I.C.; Alexandrescu, E.; Nistor, C.L.; Nitu, S.; Petcu, C. Hydrogel-clay nanocomposites as carriers for controlled release. *Curr. Med. Chem.* **2020**, *27*, 919–954. [CrossRef]
45. Shen, J.; Li, N.; Ye, M. Preparation and characterization of dual-sensitive double network hydrogels with clay as a physical crosslinker. *Appl. Clay Sci.* **2015**, *103*, 40–45. [CrossRef]
46. Pereira, K.A.B.; Aguiar, K.L.N.P.; Oliveira, P.F.; Vicente, B.M.; Pedroni, L.G.; Mansur, C.R.E. Synthesis of hydrogel nanocomposites based on partially hydrolysed polyacrylamide, polyethyleneimine, and modified clay. *ACS Omega* **2020**, *5*, 4759–4769. [CrossRef] [PubMed]
47. León-Mancilla, B.H.; Araiza-Téllez, M.A.; Flores-Flores, J.O.; Piña-Barba, M.C. Physico-chemical characterization of collagen scaffolds for tissue engineering. *J. Appl. Res. Technol.* **2016**, *14*, 77–85. [CrossRef]
48. Coppola, B.; Cappetti, N.; Di Maio, L.; Scarfato, P.; Incarnato, L. 3D printing of PLA/clay nanocomposites: Influence of printing temperature on printed samples properties. *Materials* **2018**, *11*, 1947. [CrossRef]
49. Cao, X.; Wang, J.; Liu, M.; Chen, Y.; Cao, Y.; Yu, X. Chitosan-collagen/organomontmorillonite scaffold for bone tissue engineering. *Front. Mater. Sci.* **2015**, *9*, 405–412. [CrossRef]
50. Mertz, E.L.; Leikin, S. Interactions of inorganic phosphate and sulfate anions with collagen. *Biochemistry* **2004**, *43*, 14901–14912. [CrossRef] [PubMed]
51. Del Prado Audelo, M.L.; Gómez Lizárraga, K.K.; Gómez, D.M.G.; Martínez Hernández, H.; Rodríguez Fuentes, N.; Castell Rodríguez, A.E.; Montufar, E.B.; Piña Barba, M.C. Development of collagen-EDC scaffolds for skin tissue engineering: Physicochemical and biological characterization. *Int. J. Eng. Res. Sci.* **2016**, *2*, 73–83.
52. Le, H.; Xu, W.; Zhuang, X.; Chang, F.; Wang, Y.; Ding, J. Mesenchymal stem cells for cartilage regeneration. *J. Tissue Eng.* **2020**, *1*, 1–22. [CrossRef]
53. Ianchis, R.; Rosca, I.D.; Ghiurea, M.; Spataru, C.I.; Nicolae, C.A.; Gabor, R.; Raditoiu, V.; Preda, S.; Fierascu, R.C.; Donescu, D. Synthesis and properties of new epoxy-organolayered silicates nanocomposites. *Appl. Clay Sci.* **2015**, *103*, 28–33. [CrossRef]
54. Munteanu, T.; Ninciuleanu, C.M.; Gifu, I.C.; Trica, B.; Alexandrescu, E.; Gabor, A.R.; Preda, S.; Petcu, C.; Nistor, C.L.; Nitu, S.G.; et al. The effect of clay type on the physicochemical properties of new hydrogelclay nanocomposites. In *Current Topics in the Utilization of Clay in Industrial and Medical Applications*; Zoveidavianpoor, M., Ed.; IntechOpen: London, UK, 2018; pp. 147–165.
55. Zhang, L.; Hu, J.; Athanasiou, K.A. The role of tissue engineering in articular cartilage repair and regeneration. *Crit. Rev. Biomed. Eng.* **2009**, *37*, 1–57. [CrossRef]
56. Lukáč, P.; Hartinger, J.M.; Mlček, M.; Popková, M.; Suchý, T.; Šupová, M.; Závora, J.; Adámková, V.; Benáková, H.; Slanař, O.; et al. A novel gentamicin-releasing wound dressing prepared from freshwater fish *Cyprinus carpio* collagen cross-linked with carbodiimide. *J. Bioact. Compat. Polym.* **2019**, *34*, 246–262. [CrossRef]
57. Nemu, R.P.; Adhyapak, A.; Mannur, V.S.; Mastiholimath, V.S.; Powalkar, T. Development and validation of spectrophotometric method for determination of gentamicin and curcumin in bulk powder. *Int. J. Pharm. Sci. Rev. Res.* **2019**, *59*, 109–113.
58. Wali, A.; Gorain, M.; Inamdar, S.; Kundu, G.; Badiger, M. In vivo wound healing performance of halloysite clay and gentamicin-incorporated cellulose ether-PVA electrospun nanofiber mats. *ACS Appl. Biol. Mater.* **2019**, *2*, 4324–4334. [CrossRef]
59. Marin, M.M.; Albu-Kaya, M.G.; Stavarache, C.E.; Constantinescu, R.R.; Chelaru, C.; Ghitman, J.; Iovu, H. Extraction and studies on the properties of type II collagen as potential biomaterial in cartilage repair. *UPB Sci. Bull. Ser. B* **2021**, *83*, 229–238.
60. Ciapetti, G.; Cenni, E.; Pratelli, L.; Pizzoferrato, A. In vitro evaluation of cell/biomaterial interaction by MTT assay. *Biomaterials* **1993**, *14*, 359–364. [CrossRef]
61. Marin, M.M.; Albu Kaya, M.; Marin, S.; Danila, E.; Bumbeneci, G.; Aldea, C.; Coara, G.; Albu, L. *Process for Obtaining Collagen Extracts from Bovine Cartilage for Medical Applications*; CBI OSIM A 00840/26.10.2018; OSIM: Bucharest, Romania, 2018.
62. Radu, I.C.; Zaharia, C.; Hudita, A.; Tanasa, E.; Ginghina, O.; Marin, M.; Galateanu, B.; Costache, M. In vitro interaction of doxorubicin-loaded silk sericin nanocarriers with mcf-7 breast cancer cells leads to DNA damage. *Polymers* **2021**, *13*, 2047. [CrossRef] [PubMed]
63. Marin, M.M.; Albu Kaya, M.; Iovu, H.; Stavarache, C.E.; Chelaru, C.; Constantinescu, R.R.; Dinu-Pîrvu, C.E.; Ghica, M.V. Obtaining, evaluation, and optimization of doxycycline-loaded microparticles intended for the local treatment of infectious arthritis. *Coatings* **2020**, *10*, 990. [CrossRef]

International Journal of
Molecular Sciences

Article

Broad Spectrum Anti-Bacterial Activity and Non-Selective Toxicity of Gum Arabic Silver Nanoparticles

Adewale O. Fadaka [1], Samantha Meyer [2], Omnia Ahmed [3], Greta Geerts [3], Madimabe A. Madiehe [1], Mervin Meyer [1,*] and Nicole R. S. Sibuyi [2,*]

1 Department of Science and Innovation (DSI)/Mintek Nanotechnology Innovation Centre (NIC), Biolabels Research Node, Department of Biotechnology, University of the Western Cape (UWC), Bellville 7535, South Africa; afadaka@uwc.ac.za (A.O.F.); amadiehe@uwc.ac.za (M.A.M.)
2 Department of Biomedical Sciences, Faculty of Health and Wellness Sciences, Cape Peninsula University of Technology, Bellville 7535, South Africa; meyers@cput.ac.za
3 Department of Restorative Dentistry; University of the Western Cape, Bellville 7535, South Africa; 3689306@myuwc.ac.za (O.A.); ggeerts@uwc.ac.za (G.G.)
* Correspondence: memeyer@uwc.ac.za (M.M.); nsibuyi@uwc.ac.za (N.R.S.S.); Tel.: +27-21-9592032 (M.M.); +27-21-9592735 (N.R.S.S.)

Abstract: Silver nanoparticles (AgNPs) are the most commercialized nanomaterials and presumed to be biocompatible based on the biological effects of the bulk material. However, their physicochemical properties differ significantly to the bulk materials and are associated with unique biological properties. The study investigated the antimicrobial and cytotoxicity effects of AgNPs synthesized using gum arabic (GA), sodium borohydride ($NaBH_4$), and their combination as reducing agents. The AgNPs were characterized using ultraviolet-visible spectrophotometry (UV-Vis), dynamic light scattering (DLS), transmission electron microscopy (TEM), and Fourier-transform infrared spectroscopy (FT-IR). The anti-bacterial activity was assessed using agar well diffusion and microdilution assays, and the cytotoxicity effects on Caco-2, HT-29 and KMST-6 cells using MTT assay. The GA-synthesized AgNPs (GA-AgNPs) demonstrated higher bactericidal activity against all bacteria, and non-selective cytotoxicity towards normal and cancer cells. AgNPs reduced by $NaBH_4$ (C-AgNPs) and the combination of GA and $NaBH_4$ (GAC-AgNPs) had insignificant anti-bacterial activity and cytotoxicity at $\geq$50 µg/mL. The study showed that despite the notion that AgNPs are safe and biocompatible, their toxicity cannot be overruled and that their toxicity can be channeled by using biocompatible polymers, thereby providing a therapeutic window at concentrations that are least harmful to mammalian cells but toxic to bacteria.

Keywords: anti-bacteria; cytotoxicity; green synthesis; gum arabic; silver nanoparticles

Citation: Fadaka, A.O.; Meyer, S.; Ahmed, O.; Geerts, G.; Madiehe, M.A.; Meyer, M.; Sibuyi, N.R.S. Broad Spectrum Anti-Bacterial Activity and Non-Selective Toxicity of Gum Arabic Silver Nanoparticles. *Int. J. Mol. Sci.* **2022**, *23*, 1799. https://doi.org/10.3390/ijms23031799

Academic Editor: Helena Felgueiras

Received: 29 December 2021
Accepted: 28 January 2022
Published: 4 February 2022

1. Introduction

In the past, silver-based compounds were used as antimicrobial agents due to their microbicidal activities [1]. Their biomedical application was encouraged by the fact that silver ions (Ag^+) and their related compounds are less toxic towards mammalian cells while being highly toxic to microorganisms, such as bacteria and fungi [2,3]. Recent advances in the field of nanotechnology have influenced and increased the use of silver-based compounds at a nanometer size. Several physical and chemical methods have been reported for the synthesis of AgNPs [4,5], however, AgNPs produced by these methods lead to the production of noxious compounds that are toxic to cells and the environment. To overcome these toxic effects, green synthesis methods, using natural products as reducing and stabilizing agents, were developed [6]. Green synthesis methods produce nanoparticles (NPs) using eco-friendly and non-toxic biological agents, such as microorganisms (e.g., bacteria, yeasts, fungi, and algae) and plant extracts as reducing and stabilizing agents [1,7,8]. Plant-extract mediated green synthesis of NPs is often preferred over the microbial-mediated synthesis method due to the biohazards and laborious process associated with the latter [9,10]. The use of plant extracts in green synthesis is easier, more efficient, eco-friendly and incurs low cost in comparison with the chemical or microbial mediated synthesis methods. Plant materials are cost-effective as plants are renewable, readily available, and contain antioxidant-rich phytochemicals [4] that can play a major role in the reduction and stabilization of Ag^+ into bioactive AgNPs. The availability of plants makes the green method amenable to large-scale production of NPs. Over the last few years, there has been an upsurge in the application of plant-extract-reduced AgNPs on account of their immense antimicrobial efficacy, and they are perceived as future-generation therapeutic agents against drug-resistant microbes. Examples of plant-based AgNPs that have demonstrated good anti-bacterial properties and potential anticancer effects include those synthesized using *Chrysanthemum indicum L* [11], *Acacia leucophloea* [12] and *Ganoderma neojaponicum Imazeki* [13] extracts.

AgNPs have distinct and superior properties compared to their bulk materials, and this has afforded their integration into numerous consumer (e.g., cosmetic and household) and health products to prevent microbial infestation and growth. AgNPs are now present in commercial products used daily, such as toothpaste, sunburn lotions, food packaging, medical devices, and clothing [14,15]. In addition to the antimicrobial effects of AgNPs against infectious microbes [16], they are used in catalysis [17], disease treatment [18,19], and as additives in polymerizable dental material [20–22].

Polysaccharides have played a huge role in the application of nanomaterials, especially in biomedical applications. Polysaccharides derived from algae (*Pterocladia capillacae, Jania rubins, Ulva faciata,* and *Colpmenia sinusa*) [23] and plants (gum arabic, GA [24]) alike, were previously used as stabilizers and capping agents for nanomaterials, both chemical and green synthesized NPs, to enhance their biocompatibility and biosafety. The most widely explored polysaccharide-rich compounds are chitosan [25] and GA [24]. GA is a natural plant-based gum composed of a complex mixture of glycoproteins and polysaccharides, in addition to being a historical source of monosaccharides, arabinose and ribose. GA is considered a safe additive with no adverse effects [26] and has wide applications in the food (e.g., stabilizer, thickening agent and hydrocolloid emulsifier), textile (e.g., pottery, lithography, and cosmetics) and pharmaceutical industries [27]. In the field of nanotechnology, GA has been employed because of its biocompatibility and stabilization effects for nanomaterials [28,29], such as iron oxide NPs [30–32], gold nanoparticles (AuNPs) [33–35], carbon nanotubes [36], quantum dots [37], AgNPs [24], and chitosan NPs (CT-NPs). Cross-linking the carboxylic groups of GA with CT produced CTGA-NPs that had improved mechanical properties, and which consequently found application as a bone graft substitute for bone regeneration [38]. GA has also been used as a reducing agent for the synthesis of GA-AgNPs [6,39]. GA-AgNPs showed potential as promising candidates in the development of antioxidant, anti-inflammatory, antimicrobial [6] and anticorrosive agents [40]. This study demonstrated the anti-bacterial and cytotoxicity effects of AgNPs green-synthesized using GA.

2. Results and Discussion

GA is a non-toxic glycoprotein polymer commonly used as a stabilizer in the food and pharmaceutical industries. It has various pharmacological properties; apart from being used as an emulsifying agent, it has antioxidant, anti-diabetic, and anti-lipid peroxidation properties, among others [41,42]. The chemical composition of GA is complex and varies among species, where all have high levels of carbohydrates and very low protein content [43].

The GA species used in the current study (*Acacia senegal*) had negligible flavonols, flavanols, TPC, with no antioxidant, radical scavenging or reducing abilities at 4 mg/mL, as shown in Table 1. As such, GAE on its own was incapable of reducing a metal precursor into metallic NPs at temperatures $\leq$100 °C. Due to its high sugar content, solubility and binding capacity, GA has been used as a stabilizer for AuNPs [24,30]. It stabilizes NPs by binding to other biomolecules on their surface through its abundant carboxyl groups [30].

Table 1. Phytochemical analysis and antioxidant capacity of GAE.

Phytochemical Content	4 mg/mL GAE
Flavanols (mg/g)	0.0187
Flavonols (mg/g)	0.0019
TPC (mgGAE/g)	0.0003
DPPH (μmolTE/g)	0.0000
ORAC (μmolTE/g)	0.0000
FRAP (μmolAAE/g)	0.0000

2.1. Synthesis of GA-AgNPs

Synthesis of GA-AgNPs was first attempted at R_T and by boiling (~100 °C) solutions that contained 4 mg/mL GAE and various $AgNO_3$ concentrations (1–5 mM). No GA-AgNPs were formed at all the tested concentrations; there was no color change in the solution at R_T and a pinkish color was observed after boiling the solution (data not shown). The negligible phytochemical and lack of antioxidant contents reported for GAE in Table 1 provides a clear indication that the GAE at the concentration used in the current study was incapable of reducing $AgNO_3$ to form GA-AgNPs. Other studies attempted to synthesize GA-AgNPs by devising methods to potentiate the reducing abilities of GAE, by changing the GAE pH [44], and by using honey as a reducing agent, while using GA as a stabilizer for the AgNPs [40].

A novel, greener approach, using an autoclave method, was established for other gum species to produce sterile AgNPs without additional reducing agents or change of pH. This method was successful in the reduction of $AgNO_3$ by gum acacia [39], gum tragacant [45] and *piyar* gum [46]. The same method was adapted for the synthesis of GA-AgNPs in the current study and was optimized by first varying the concentrations of $AgNO_3$ (0.1–0.5 g/40 mL) then the GAE concentrations (2–6 mg/mL/40 mL). The optimized conditions (i.e., concentrations of GAE and $AgNO_3$) were further used in the combined approach, with $NaBH_4$ as an additional reducing agent, to synthesize GAC-AgNPs.

Using the green synthesis approach, the solution containing GAE and $AgNO_3$ was colorless before autoclaving and changed to brown after autoclaving (Figure 1A). The color intensity increased with increasing concentrations of $AgNO_3$ and GAE. In the combined approach, the samples turned yellow immediately after adding ice cold $AgNO_3$, then to a grayish green color for the C-AgNPs, and brown for the GAC-AgNPs (Figure 1B) after autoclaving. Based on the colors, the GAC-AgNPs were more stable than the C-AgNPs.

The color change was a first indication of formation of the AgNPs, which are reported to have yellow, orange or brown colors [46,47]. Thus, the brown color indicated that GAE at high temperature (120 °C) and pressure (15 psi) was able to reduce Ag^+ into Ag^0, and form GA-AgNPs and GAC-AgNPs. The GAE in the green synthesis approach acted as both a reducing and capping agent for the GA-AgNPs. It is very common in green synthesis, especially for plant-derived NPs, for the biomolecules found in the extracts to serve as reducing, capping and stabilizing agents [47,48]. Plants contain a lot of phytochemicals (e.g., alkaloids, flavonoids, terpenoids, etc.), enzymes/proteins, amino acids, polysaccharides, and vitamins, that can aid in the reduction of metal salts in a rapid and environmentally benign process. Green synthesis is quite advantageous, as it is cost-effective and can be easily scaled up to produce biocompatible AgNPs. Moreover, the medicinal efficacy of the extracts will be a valuable addition to the NPs and enhance their pharmacological activities [40,47,49].

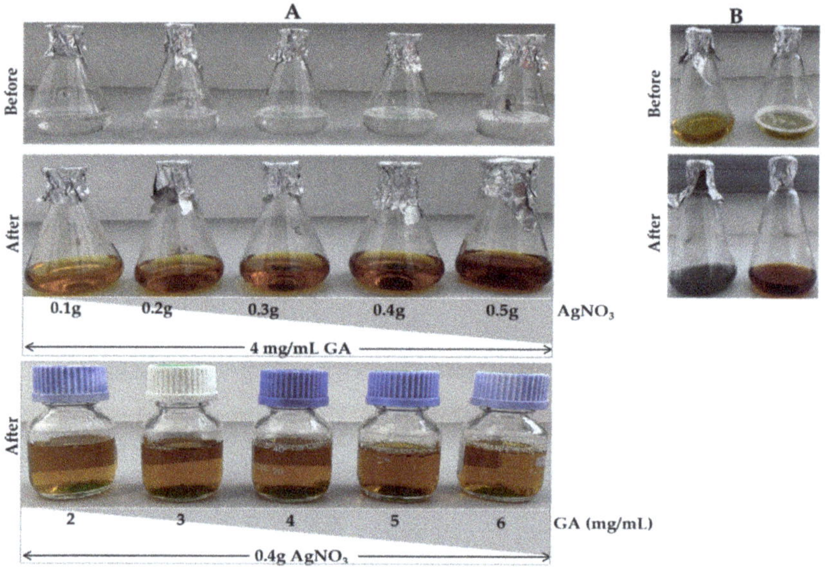

Figure 1. Synthesis of GA-AgNPs using green (**A**), chemical and combined (**B**) approaches.

2.2. Characterization of the AgNPs

2.2.1. Optical Properties of the AgNPs

UV-Vis spectrophotometry was used to confirm the formation of the AgNPs, which have a characteristic SPR around 400 nm [47,49]. Figure 2 shows the absorption spectra for the AgNPs produced via the green (GA-AgNPs), chemical (C-AgNPs) and combined (GAC-AgNPs) approaches. All the concentrations of GAE and $AgNO_3$ were able to synthesize AgNPs, which was confirmed by a characteristic SPR for AgNPs at ~400 nm. The peak intensity of the GA-AgNPs synthesized with 0.4 g $AgNO_3$ was higher than all the other concentrations (Figure 2A), which suggested that more AgNPs were formed at this concentration [48]. An amount of 0.4 g $AgNO_3$ was selected as an optimum concentration and used to optimize the concentration of GAE (2–6 mg/mL). The optimum GAE concentration was 4 mg/mL; both 4 and 5 mg/mL of GAE gave a similar spectral profile, indicating that GA-AgNPs of the same yield, size and shape were produced by the two concentrations (Figure 2B). Although 6 mg/mL showed higher biomass compared to all the GAE concentrations, there were some black precipitates after autoclaving the sample. The precipitates might have contained excess GAE and indicated that the extract concentration might be too high.

In the combined approach, $AgNO_3$ was reduced in the presence of GAE and a chemical reducing agent ($NaBH_4$) to produce GAC-AgNPs (Figure 2C). There are two assumptions as to how the GAC-AgNPs were produced, the first involves $NaBH_4$ acting as a reducing agent to form C-AgNPs (before autoclaving) which are then capped/stabilized by GAE to form GAC-AgNPs during the autoclave process. The second assumption is that GAE and $NaBH_4$ might have acted synergistically as reducing agents. The differences in the spectral profiles of the C-AgNPs$_A$ and GAC-AgNPs (Figure 2C) might have occurred as a result of the instability of C-AgNPs when exposed to high temperatures. The C-AgNPs synthesized at 70 °C were used in further studies (Figure 2D).

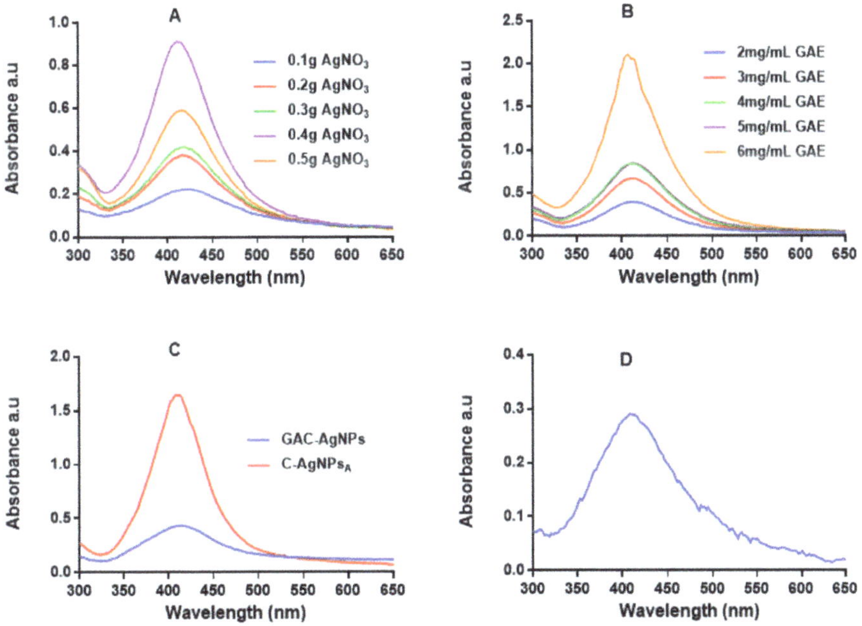

Figure 2. UV-Vis analysis of the AgNPs. The synthesis of GA-AgNPs was optimized using varying concentrations of $AgNO_3$ and 4 mg/mL GAE (**A**), varying GAE concentration and 0.4 g $AgNO_3$ (**B**), and by using $NaBH_4$ alone and in combination with 4 mg/mL GAE (**C**); all these solutions were autoclaved at 121 °C. C-AgNPs were synthesized at 70 °C (**D**).

2.2.2. Morphology and Size Distribution of the AgNPs

The morphology and core size of the AgNPs were analyzed by HRTEM. As shown in Figure 3A, the majority of the AgNPs were spherical in shape; their core size distribution varied from 1–30 nm.

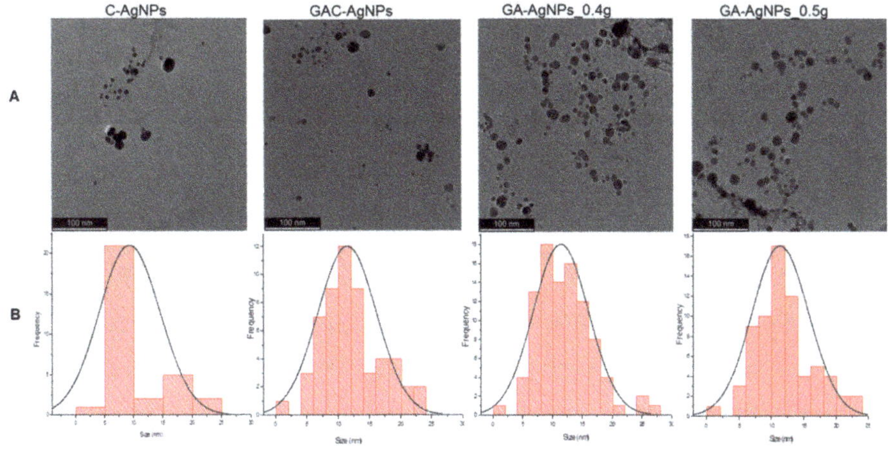

Figure 3. HRTEM micrographs of the AgNPs (**A**) and the AgNP core size distribution (**B**).

DLS analysis revealed a hydrodynamic diameter range from 87.22 nm for the C-AgNPs to 94.62 nm for the GA-AgNPs to 144.39 nm for the GAC-AgNPs (Table 2). These sizes vary from those obtained from the HRTEM as they account for both the core size and the molecules on the surface of the AgNPs [47]. The C-AgNPs had a smaller hydrodynamic size, followed by the GA-AgNPs, while the GAC-AgNPs were the largest in size. This indicates that the GAE played a crucial role in the synthesis of the GA-AgNPs as both reducing and capping agents.

Table 2. Physicochemical properties of the AgNPs.

AgNPs	λmax/SPR (nm)	Core Size (nm)	Hydrodynamic Size (nm)	ζ-Potential (mV)	Pdi
C-AgNPs	408	10 ± 1.69	87.22 ± 5.94	−30.50 ± 4.63	0.30 ± 0.03
GAC-AgNPs	414	12 ± 0.61	144.39 ± 4.99	+9.33 ± 17.23	0.55 ± 0.01
GA-AgNPs_0.4g	416	12 ± 0.47	76.21 ± 6.35	−29.60 ± 1.90	0.28 ± 0.03
GA-AgNPs_0.5g	414	12 ± 0.25	94.62 ± 10.06	−27.07 ± 3.71	0.23 ± 0.06

All the AgNPs had a negative zeta (ζ) potential, except for the GAC-AgNPs (9.33 mV). The polydispersity index (Pdi) indicated that GA-AgNPs, followed by C-AgNPs, were the most stable. Pdi serves as an indicator for the dispersity and stability of NPs, thus, NPs with a Pdi that is $\leq$0.05 are regarded as stable and monodispersed. Materials with a Pdi of $\geq$0.7 are classified as polydispersed, with broad size distribution and being less stable in suspension [47]. The GA-AgNPs_0.4g and GA-AgNPs_0.5g demonstrated similar physicochemical properties (Table 2), and the two were investigated further to determine if they have similar bioactivities as well.

2.2.3. FT-IR Analysis of GAE and AgNPs

FT-IR was used to identify the functional groups in GAE and those that were involved in the intermolecular interactions between the precursor ($AgNO_3$) and reducing agents ($NaBH_4$ and GAE). The intermolecular interactions between the samples occurs via hydrogen bonding or dipole–dipole interactions during synthesis and cause shifts in the frequency or absorption of the functional groups [50] that can be assigned to a particular biomolecule.

The dominant absorption bands at 3306–3321, 2139–2161, 1635–1636 and 695–667 cm^{-1} were identified in the FT-IR spectrum of all the AgNPs (Figure 4). These bands were associated with the alkyne C-H stretch (3320–3310), terminal alkyne monosubstituted (2140–2100), C≡C stretch (2260–2100), alkenyl C=C stretch (1680–1620), amide (1680–1630), secondary amine NH bend (1650–1550), alkyne C-H bend (680–610), organic nitrates (1640–1620), and aromatic C-H out-of-plane bend (900–670) [51].

The GAE FT-IR spectra had five major absorption peaks at 3514 cm^{-1} (3570–3200 cm^{-1} OH stretch), 2978 (CH_2 group in aliphatic chains), 2315, 1628 cm^{-1} (1650–1550 cm^{-1} secondary amine NH bend), and 1371 cm^{-1} (1380–1350 aliphatic nitro compounds) and 1065 cm^{-1}. The presence of different functional groups was a reflection of the phytochemical composition of the GAE; the OH bonds are attributed to alcohols or phenols and the N–H bond to amides which might be from the carbohydrates and proteins in GAE. The GAE FT-IR peaks showed similarity to those of other GA species, such as *Acacia senegal* and *Acacia seyal* [40,50,52]. Thus, the carbohydrates and proteins in GAE were responsible for the reduction, capping and stabilization of the GA-AgNPs and possibly the GAC-AgNPs.

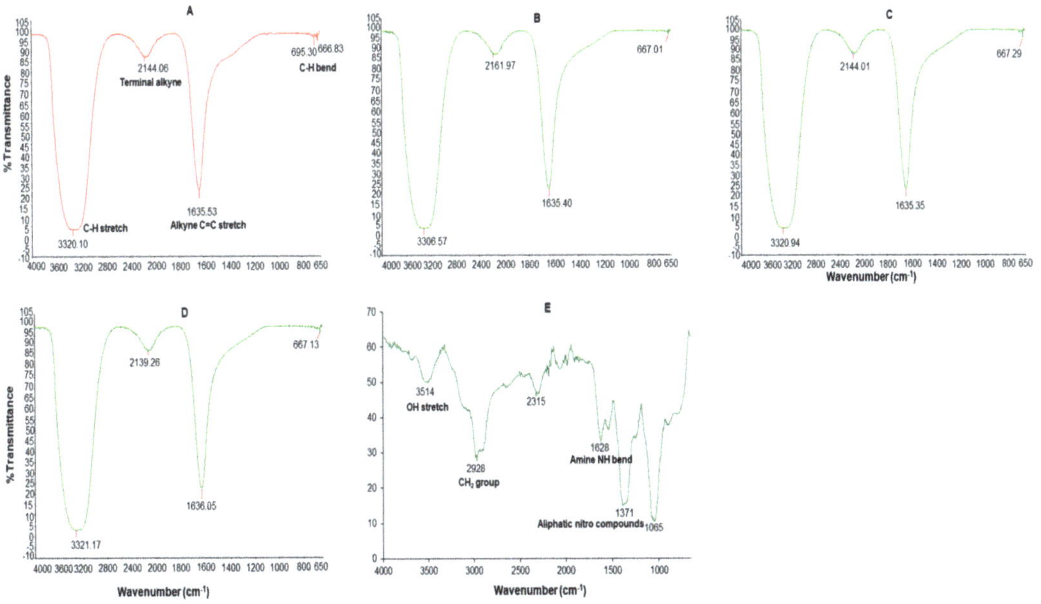

Figure 4. FT-IR spectra of C-AgNPs (**A**), GA-AgNPs_0.4g (**B**), GA-AgNPs_0.5g (**C**), GAC-AgNPs (**D**), and GAE (**E**).

2.3. Stability of GA-AgNPs

Stability of NPs in solutions other than water is crucial for bio-applications and requires NPs that can retain their physical characteristics when introduced into a biological environment. AgNPs are usually very stable in water; however, water is hypotonic and not a suitable vehicle for bioassays [53]. In addition to Pdi, the stability of AgNPs in suspension can also be predicted by their UV-Vis spectral profiles with a characteristic SPR at 400 nm [48]. AgNPs that are not stable will be recognized by aggregation or precipitation out of solution, and if the AgNPs precipitate they will not be useful as antimicrobial agents, as Ag^+ are known for this effect and have been used for the same purposes [54]. Stability of the AgNPs was assessed at hourly intervals for 6 hr after incubation at 37 °C, as shown in Figure 5A–C; the AgNPs were relatively stable in water, DPBS, and Mueller–Hinton broth (MHB). Cellular uptake of AgNPs is time and size dependent, where uptake and internalization of AgNPs by mammalian cells can occur within 0.5 h [55]. Following the growth kinetics of *Burkholderia pseudomallei*, the interaction and uptake of AgNPs by the bacterial species could be rapid, as the bacteria were killed within 5 min [56]. Biological assays, such as bacteria and cell culture, are performed at 37 °C and AgNPs can be used in culture media for bioassays without aggregation [57]. The components in the media can interact with the AgNPs and change their physicochemical properties and activity; hence, the AgNP-media interactions must be assessed to confirm NP stability before evaluating their activity [58]. Subjecting AgNPs to solutions with higher salt (NaCl) concentration, not only causes NP aggregation, but also a change in size and biological activity [59]. To improve on AgNP stability, biopolymers, such as GA and chitosan, were used as stabilizing agents; this led to plant-mediated synthesis of NPs with enhanced stability, biocompatibility and biological activity.

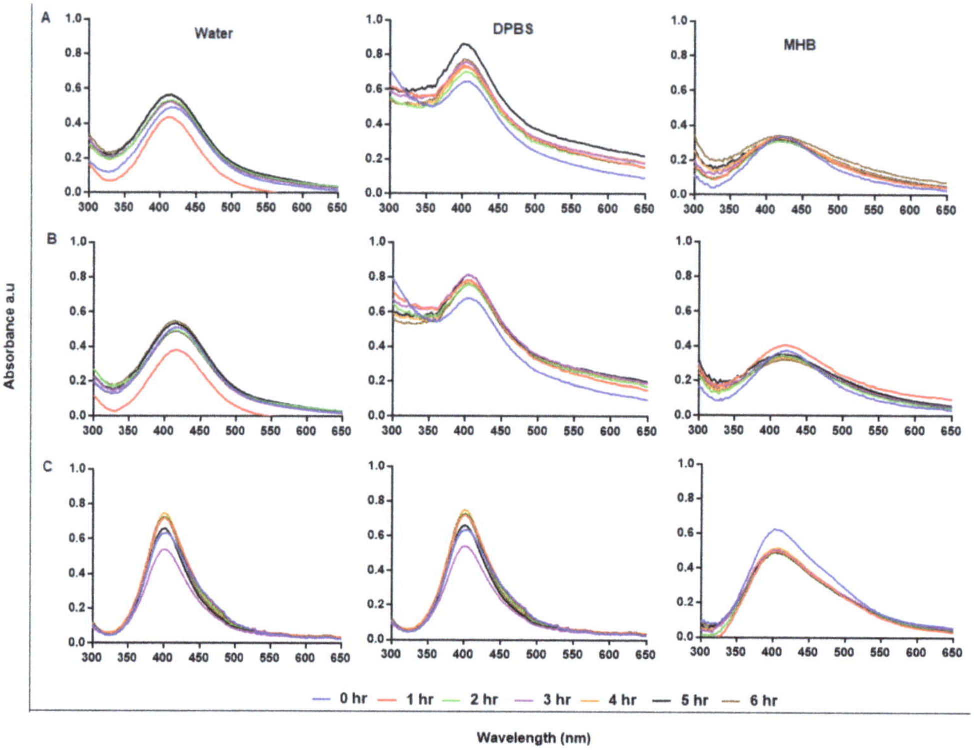

Figure 5. Assessment of AgNP stability in solution by UV-Vis. The GA-AgNPs_0.4g (**A**), GA-AgNPs_0.5g (**B**) and GAC-AgNPs (**C**) were diluted in water, DPBS and MHB and incubated at 37 °C for 1–6 h.

2.4. Anti-Bacterial Activity

Microbial resistance is among the leading factors responsible for death worldwide, due to the overwhelming abuse and misprescription of antibiotics [60,61]. Over the years, alternative antimicrobial agents effective against resistant strains have continually been sought [62,63]. Among others, AgNPs have displayed broad spectrum antimicrobial effects, even against multi-drug-resistant microbes. Of interest are the AgNPs produced through green synthesis, which are presumed to be biocompatible since they are reduced and coated by natural products [47–49,62,64].

The anti-bacterial effects of GAE and AgNPs were evaluated on Gram-positive (*S. aureus, MRSA, S. epidermidis, S. pyogenes*) and Gram-negative (*K. pneumoniae, E. coli*) bacteria. The susceptibility of the bacteria to the treatments was assessed through agar well diffusion and broth microdilution methods. Agar well diffusion demonstrated a lack of clearing zones (zone of inhibitions, ZOIs) in the bacteria that were exposed to MHB (negative control), GAE and GAC-AgNPs, indicating lack of anti-bacterial activity (Table 3) at the concentrations used in this test. Anti-bacterial activity of GAE was reported at concentrations ≥40 mg/mL for various GA species [65], while organic solvent GA extracts were effective from 0.25 to 2 mg/mL [66]. The GA-AgNPs and the C-AgNPs showed potency against the selected bacteria, both Gram-positive and Gram-negative strains; the highest anti-bacterial activity was observed with the GA-AgNPs when compared to the C-AgNPs. The two GA-AgNPs exhibited similar activity against the test bacteria. Similar effects were reported for GA-AgNPs synthesized using other GA species; the GA-AgNPs were potent against oral (*Streptococcus mutans*) [67] and fish (*Aeromonas hydrophila* and *P. aeruginosa*) [68] pathogens.

The activity of the GA-AgNPs in these pathogens was size, as well as concentration, dependent. C-AgNPs capped with citrate were reported to show size-dependent activity against *E. coli* and *S. aureus* [69].

Table 3. Anti-bacterial activity of the synthesized AgNPs.

Treatments	ZOI (mm)				
	S. aureus	*MRSA*	*S. epidermidis*	*K. pneumoniae*	*E. coli*
MHB	0	0	0	0	0
GAE	0	0	0	0	0
C-AgNPs	9.8	9.8	8.4	11	6.2
GAC-AgNPs	0	0	0	0	0
GA-AgNPs_0.4g	14.2	13.8	20	13.6	11.2
GA-AgNPs_0.5g	13	9.8	19	14.6	10.2

The MICs of the treatments were visually evaluated on the bacteria following microdilution assay. After 24 h treatment, GAE, C-AgNPs and GAC-AgNPs were unable to inhibit growth at all tested concentrations (6.25–100 µg/mL), as shown in Table 4. Bacterial growth inhibition was observed at 6.25–100 µg/mL for the two GA-AgNPs for all strains, with an MIC of 6.25 µg/mL, except for GA-AgNPs_0.4g effect in *E. coli* which had an MIC of 25 µg/mL. The MIC values were consistent with the GA-AgNPs reported by other studies; the NPs had an MIC of 10 µg/mL in *S. mutans* [67], 11–45 µg/mL in *P. aeruginosa* [44], 1.625 and 3.25 µg/mL for *A. hydrophila* and *P. aeruginosa*, respectively [68]. The results in the current study were further confirmed by the Alamar Blue assay, which quantifies the metabolic activity of cells. Only live bacteria can convert the blue resazurin dye into a pink and fluorescent resorufin. The color/fluorescent intensity is directly proportional to live bacteria [62,70].

Table 4. MIC of the AgNPs on test bacteria.

Treatments	MIC (µg/mL)					
	S. aureus	*MRSA*	*S. epidermidis*	*S. pyogenes*	*K. pneumoniae*	*E. coli*
GAE	>100	>100	>100	>100	>100	>100
C-AgNPs	>100	>100	>100	>100	>100	>100
GAC-AgNPs	>100	>100	>100	>100	>100	>100
GA-AgNPs_0.4g	6.25	6.25	6.25	6.25	6.25	25
GA-AgNPs_0.5g	6.25	6.25	6.25	6.25	6.25	6.25

Alamar Blue assay demonstrated reduction in bacterial growth with all treatments (Figure 6), including those that did not show ZOIs or MICs (i.e., GAE, C-AgNPs and GAC-AgNPs). The GAE showed stronger activity against Gram-positive bacteria, *S. pyogenes*, *MRSA* and *S. aureus* (Figure 6A). In contrast, *S. epidermidis* and the Gram-negative bacteria displayed some resistance towards these treatments. The GA-AgNPs were consistent in their activity, with significant effects being observed against all the strains above 6.25 µg/mL (Figure 6D,E).

The effects of GAE, C-AgNPs and GAC-AgNPs were not bactericidal, and their MBC values were undetermined. The GA-AgNPs had bactericidal effects on >60% of the selected strains, with MBCs ranging between 12.5 and 100 µg/mL (Table 5). The GA-AgNPs were active against the Gram-positive and Gram-negative bacteria and demonstrated similar trends in both antibiotic susceptible and resistant strains. This is a desirable property and implies that these NPs can be used as broad-spectrum anti-bacterial agents.

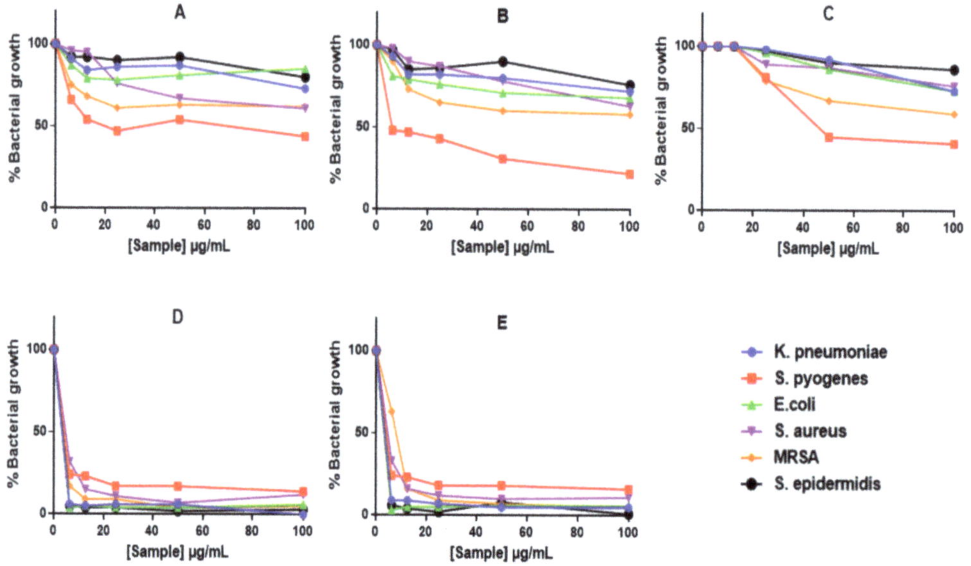

Figure 6. The anti-bacterial effects of GAE and AgNPs using Alamar Blue assay. Bacteria were treated with GAE (**A**), GAC-AgNPs (**B**), C-AgNPs (**C**), GA-AgNPs_0.4g (**D**), and GA-AgNPs_0.5g (**E**).

Table 5. MBC of the AgNPs on test bacteria.

Treatments	MBC (µg/mL)					
	S. aureus	*MRSA*	*S. epidermidis*	*S. pyogenes*	*K. pneumoniae*	*E. coli*
GAE	>100	>100	>100	>100	>100	>100
C-AgNPs	>100	>100	>100	>100	>100	>100
GAC-AgNPs	>100	>100	>100	>100	>100	>100
GA-AgNPs_0.4g	>100	12.5	100	>100	25	12.5
GA-AgNPs_0.5g	100	12.5	25	>100	12.5	12.5

2.5. *In Vitro Cytotoxicity of GA-AgNPs*

AgNPs have demonstrated unique properties compared to their bulk counterparts, and these have raised many concerns for biomedical application due to their ability to cross all cellular barriers and interact with important cellular organelles, such as the mitochondria and nucleus [7]. When inside cells, AgNPs can react with biomolecules, such as nucleic acids, proteins, enzymes, etc., resulting in dissolution and release of Ag^+. The Ag^+ are presumed to be responsible for the toxicity of the AgNPs [3].

The cytotoxicity of the AgNPs was investigated *in vitro* in two colon cancer (Caco-2 and HT-29) and non-cancerous (KMST-6) cells using 3-(4,5-dimethylthiazol-2-yl)-2,5-diphenyltetrazolium bromide (MTT) assay. The assay quantifies live cells by evaluating their mitochondrial metabolic activity, where live cells are able to reduce the MTT salt into the water-insoluble purple formazan. The color intensity of the dimethyl sulfoxide (DMSO)-dissolved formazan, which is measured by a spectrophotometer, is directly proportional to the amount of live cells [71]. As shown in Figure 7, GAE exhibited insignificant effects on the three cell lines. Of the four AgNPs, GAC-AgNPs were least toxic and showed selective effects to the non-cancer cells. Significant effects of GAC-AgNPs were observed on cancer cells at $\geq$50 µg/mL. The C-AgNPs were toxic to all cells at $\geq$50 µg/mL. GA-AgNPs were non-selective and were toxic against both cancer and non-cancer cells, with <15% viable cells at all concentrations.

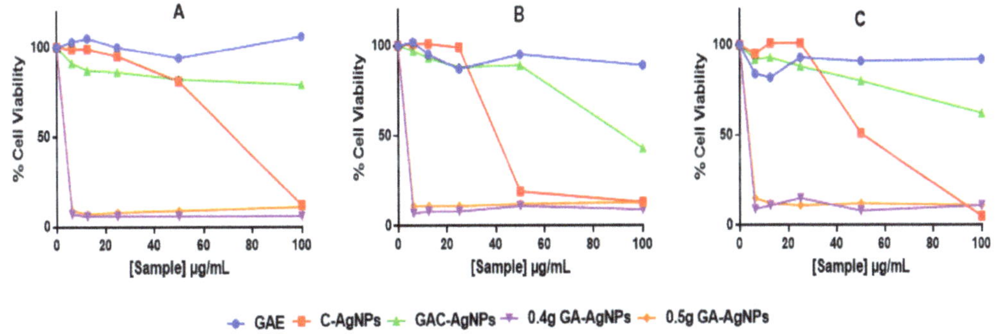

Figure 7. Cytotoxicity of the GAE, C-AgNPs, GAC-AgNPs and GA-AgNPs on KMST-6 (**A**), Caco-2 (**B**) and HT-29 (**C**) cells.

Therapeutic agents are deemed biocompatible when they have selective toxicity towards diseased cells or are at least cytotoxic at concentrations that are not toxic to normal cells. However, this was not the case with the GA-AgNPs, as these NPs were extremely toxic and nonspecific. The GA-AgNPs had an IC_{50} (Table 6) that was >5-fold lower than their MIC and MBC. Their toxicity was even higher to the non-cancer cells than the cancer cells, with the IC_{50} values of 0.67 µg/mL on the KMST-6 cells and 0.82–1.16 µg/mL on the colon cancer cells.

Table 6. The IC_{50} values of treatments against different cell lines.

Cell-Lines	IC_{50} (µg/mL)				
	GAE	C-AgNPs	GAC-AgNPs	GA-AgNPs_0.4g	GA-AgNPs_0.5g
KMST-6	>100	87.40	>100	0.67	0.90
Caco-2	>100	41.67	92.00	0.82	1.26
HT-29	>100	50.54	>100	1.16	1.55

The anti-bacterial effects of AgNPs have led to their use in several consumer and medical products. With an increased exposure rate to consumers who use, handle or manufacture these products, AgNPs can easily accumulate in human organs via inhalation, transdermal absorption, and ingestion [72]. Although it is known that over exposure to silver salts cases argyria [73], the chronic effects of AgNPs are still elusive and still under investigation. Based on their physicochemical properties, the biological effects of AgNPs can vary. Many studies have reported the biocompatibility, as well as toxicity, of AgNPs in *in vitro* and *in vivo* models [15,16,74]. The toxicity of AgNPs, which is often attributed to the leaching of Ag^{+} [75], has been demonstrated to be size and cell-specific [76]. Green synthesized *Annona muricata*-AgNPs were only toxic to acute monocytic leukemia (THP-1) and breast cancer (AMJ-13) cells, while sparing the normal breast epithelial (HBL) cells [74]. Poly(*N*-vinyl pyrrolidone)-coated AgNPs were not toxic to T cells at concentrations up to 50 ppm, but induced cell death of human mesenchymal stem cells (hMSCs) and monocytes at 30 and 50 ppm, respectively [3]. The anti-cancer properties of AgNPs were shown in several cancer cell lines; however, their toxicity towards both healthy and diseased cells is a huge concern for human health, as these NPs accumulate in biologically important organs, such as the liver, spleen, lung, kidney, and brain. Moreover, smaller size AgNPs are more toxic than larger sizes and surface coatings can be used to defer or control their activity [77].

3. Materials and Methods

3.1. Preparation of the GA Extracts

The GA extract (GAE) was prepared by dissolving a required amount of GA obtained from *Acacia senegal* (North Kordofan, Sudan) in hot water and filtering through 0.45 μm filters. The GAE was prepared fresh before use.

Phytochemical Analysis and Antioxidant Capacity

The amount of flavanols, flavonols, total polyphenolic content (TPC) and antioxidant capacity, was assessed using the ferric reducing antioxidant power (FRAP) assay kit (Sigma, St. Louis, MO, USA). An oxygen radical absorbance capacity (ORAC, Sigma) assay and 2,2-diphenyl-1-picrylhydrazyl (DPPH, Sigma) assay of 4 mg/mL GAE was quantified following standard biochemical methods as previously described [78].

3.2. Synthesis of AgNPs

The AgNPs were synthesized through: (a) chemical synthesis (C-AgNPs), (b) green synthesis (GA-AgNPs), and (c) a combined approach (GAC-AgNPs). All solutions were prepared in double-distilled water.

3.2.1. Chemical Synthesis

C-AgNPs were prepared following a previously described method with few modification [79]. Briefly, 10 mL of 2 mM $NaBH_4$ (Sigma) was added to 30 mL of double-distilled water and heated to 70 °C on a heating mantle while stirring. The solution was stirred vigorously at 250 rpm. Subsequently, 20 mL of 1 mM ice-cold silver nitrate ($AgNO_3$, Sigma) was added dropwise into $NaBH_4$ solution. The solution was removed from the heating mantle after a color change to yellow/brown and cooled to room temperature (R_T, ~25 °C).

3.2.2. Green Synthesis

GA-AgNP synthesis was adapted from a method by Venkatesham et al. [39]. A fixed concentration of GAE (4 mg/mL) was used to prepare GA-AgNPs by varying concentrations (0.1–0.5 g) of $AgNO_3$ in a final volume of 40 mL double-distilled water. The method was repeated, keeping the $AgNO_3$ (0.4 g) constant and varying the concentration of GAE (2–6 mg/mL). The samples were autoclaved at 121 °C and 15 psi for 20 min and removed after 60 min when the pressure had reduced to 0 psi.

3.2.3. Combined Approach

GAC-AgNPs were synthesized following the green synthesis method (Section 3.2.2) in a reaction mixture comprised of 20 mL of 1 mM silver $AgNO_3$, 4 mg/mL GAE and 10 mL of 2 mM $NaBH_4$ in a final volume of 40 mL. The synthesis was carried in the autoclave, as described in Section 3.2.2.

All the AgNPs (C-AgNPs, GA-AgNPs, and GAC-AgNPs) were washed twice and harvested by centrifugation at 9000 rpm for 30 min. The pellets were resuspended in double-distilled water and stored in amber bottles at R_T in the dark.

3.3. Characterization of the AgNPs

3.3.1. UV-Visible Spectrophotometer

The formation of AgNPs was monitored by measuring the UV-Vis spectrum of the reaction medium in the wavelength range from 300 to 650 nm using a POLARstar Omega plate reader (BMG LABTECH, Offenburg, Germany).

3.3.2. Dynamic Light Scattering (DLS)

The hydrodynamic size, surface charge, and Pdi of the AgNPs were analyzed by a Malvern NanoZS90 Zetasizer (Malvern Panalytical Ltd., Enigma Business Park, UK). The synthesized AgNPs were diluted 5-fold with double-distilled water; 1 mL aliquots were sampled in DLS cuvettes or DS1070 zeta cells (Malvern Panalytical Ltd.) and examined for size distribution and zeta potential, respectively. The particle diameters were assessed at a scattering angle of 90 °C at R_T. The data were represented as mean particle diameter of three measurements.

3.3.3. FT-IR

The infrared spectra of absorption or emission of the AgNPs and GAE in solution were identified using a Perkin Elmer Spectrum Two FT-IR spectrophotometer (Waltham, MA, USA) in the wavelength range 4000–500 cm^{-1}. The baseline corrections were performed for all spectra.

3.3.4. HRTEM

HRTEM analysis was performed by the addition of a drop of each AgNP solution on carbon-coated copper grids, then left to dry under ambient conditions. The shape and size of AgNPs were analyzed using TecnaiF20 HRTEM (FEI Company, Hillsboro, OR, USA) with an accelerating voltage of 300 kV at the Electron Microscope Unit (University of Cape Town, South Africa). In addition, the core size distribution of the AgNPs was calculated using ImageJ software (National Institutes of Health, Bethesda, MD, USA).

3.4. Assessment of the Stability of AgNPs

The stability of AgNPs over time was evaluated following a previous method [80], by measuring the UV–Vis profile hourly for 0–6 hr in water, Dulbecco's phosphate-buffered saline (DPBS; Lonza, Walkersville, MD, USA), and MHB (Sigma). The AgNPs were washed as before, and the pellets were resuspended in the test solutions and then incubated at 37 °C. Their UV–Vis profile (300–650 nm) was measured using a POLARstar Omega plate reader.

3.5. Anti-Bacterial Activity of the AgNPs

The anti-bacterial activity of the AgNPs was evaluated using Gram-negative and Gram-positive bacterial strains; i.e., *Klebsiella pneumoniae* (*K. pneumoniae*), *Escherichia coli* (*E. coli*), *Pseudomonas aeruginosa* (*P. aeruginosa*), *Staphylococcus aureus* (*S. aureus*), *Methicillin-resistant Staphylococcus aureus* (*MRSA*), *Staphylococcus epidermidis* (*S. epidermidis*), and *Streptococcus pyogenes* (*S. pyogenes*). All the bacterial strains were purchased from American Type Culture Collection (ATCC, Manassas, USA). The anti-bacterial activity was determined by agar well diffusion and microdilution assays according to the standards set by the Clinical and Laboratory Standard Institute with few modifications [81].

Bacterial colonies were cultured in MHB while shaking at 120 rpm overnight at 37 °C, then diluted at 1:100 in fresh MHB and cultured until reaching a 0.5 McFarland turbidity standard prior to experiments. The bacteria were used for anti-bacterial tests at 1.5×10^6 CFU/mL by diluting the 0.5 McFarland turbid suspensions to 1:150.

3.5.1. Agar Diffusion Assay

The bacterial cultures were streaked on Mueller–Hinton Agar (MHA; Sigma) plates at 1.5×10^6 CFU/mL using sterile cotton swabs. Wells of 6 mm diameter were made on the MHA plates, to which 20 µL of the AgNPs were added. The MHA plates were then incubated overnight at 37 °C. Ciprofloxacin (10 µg/mL; Sigma) was used as a positive control. The anti-bacterial activity of the AgNPs was determined by the presence of clear zones surrounding the wells. The diameter of the clear zones was measured using calipers after 24 hr.

3.5.2. Microdilution Assay

Microdilution assay was used to determine the minimum inhibitory concentration (MIC) [47,49] and minimum bactericidal concentration (MBC) [82] of the AgNPs following previously described protocols.

Minimum Inhibitory Concentration (MIC)

The MIC of the AgNPs required to inhibit the visual growth of the bacteria was determined according to the microdilution method [47,49]. The bacteria (1.5×10^6 CFU/mL) were exposed to different concentrations (0–100 μg/mL) of the AgNPs and incubated at 37 °C for 24 hr. The MIC values were visually observed, followed by measuring the optical density (OD) of the bacterial culture at 600 nm using a POLARstar plate reader. Bacterial growth was further evaluated by Alamar Blue colorimetric assay (Invitrogen, Eugene, Oregon, USA), where 10 μL of the dye was added to each well and incubated for 3 hr. The blue color was converted to a pink-purplish color by live bacteria that was quantifiable by measuring absorbance at 570 nm and a reference wavelength at 700 nm [83].

Minimum Bactericidal Concentration (MBC)

The MBC of the AgNPs was determined in the bacteria used for MIC, where a loopful of broth from the wells was spotted onto fresh MHA and incubated at 37 °C for 24 hr. The lowest concentration that exhibited no growth on the MHA was considered as the MBC.

3.6. Cytotoxicity Assay of the AgNPs

The effect of the AgNPs was evaluated by MTT assay, as previous described, on the human cell lines, KMST-6 normal skin fibroblasts, HT-29 and CaCo-2 colon carcinoma cells [80]. The cells were purchased from ATCC, and were cultured in Dulbecco's Modified Eagle's Medium (DMEM, Lonza) supplemented with 10% fetal bovine serum (Gibco, Waltham, Massachusetts, USA) and 1% penicillin-streptomycin cocktail (Lonza) and incubated at 37 °C. The cells were then seeded in 96 well plates at 1×10^5 cell/mL density, 100 μL in each well and incubated for 24 hr. The cells were treated with 0–500 μg/mL of the AgNPs and extracted in triplicates. The cell viability was assessed by adding 10 μL of 5 mg/mL of MTT (Sigma) solution to each well and incubated for 3 hr. Later, the MTT solution was discarded and 100 μL of DMSO was added to each well. The absorbance of the formazan product was measured at 570 nm with a reference at 700 nm using a POLARstar Omega plate reader. The concentration that inhibited 50% cell growth (IC_{50}) was further analyzed by Graphpad Prism 6.0.

3.7. Statistical Analysis

All the experiments were carried out in triplicate and the results were analysed using Graphpad Prism 6.0. The data are presented as means ± SD according to one-way ANOVA test followed by a post hoc, multiple comparisons (Tukey's) test. A p-value of <0.05 was considered statistically significant.

4. Conclusions

The growing interest in medical application of AgNPs has warranted greener methods for their synthesis to prevent toxicity and improve biocompatibility. Synthesis of AgNPs using plant extracts presents not only a greener method but a sustainable, reproducible and upscalable approach. However, for biomedical applications, the safety of plant-synthesized AgNPs must be authenticated. The current study demonstrated that GAE alone, and in the presence of a chemical reducing agent, produced AgNPs with distinct bioactivities. The GA-AgNPs demonstrated broad spectrum anti-bacterial effects on both Gram-positive and Gram-negative bacteria, and non-selective cytotoxicity on normal and colon cancer cells in the same concentration range. Interestingly, these effects were reduced in the GAC-AgNPs, suggesting that surface coating can be used to channel the effects of AgNPs. The selective and reduced cytotoxicity demonstrated by GAC-AgNPs towards colon cancer cells demonstrated that surface composition can be used to control the biodistribution, uptake and efficacy of AgNPs. AgNPs represent the next generation of antimicrobial agents, and have potential to help solve the antimicrobial resistance problem. Their biocompatibility can be enhanced by modifying the surface of AgNPs with targeting molecules or biocompatible molecules, such as PEG, for medical application.

Author Contributions: All authors made significant contributions to the submission of this manuscript. Conceptualization, A.O.F., S.M., G.G., M.A.M., M.M. and N.R.S.S.; supervision M.A.M., M.M. and N.R.S.S.; methodology, validation, writing—review and editing, S.M., O.A., G.G., M.A.M., M.M. and N.R.S.S.; funding acquisition, M.A.M. and M.M.; resources, S.M., M.A.M. and M.M.; project administration, formal analysis, investigation, A.O.F. and N.R.S.S.; writing—original draft preparation, A.O.F. All authors have read and agreed to the published version of the manuscript.

Funding: This research received no external funding.

Institutional Review Board Statement: Not applicable.

Informed Consent Statement: Not applicable.

Data Availability Statement: The data presented in the study can be requested from the authors.

Acknowledgments: The running costs and the APC for the study were covered by the DSI/Mintek NIC Biolabels Node at UWC. Adewale Fadaka has joined the Division of Pain Management (Department of Anesthesia, Cincinnati Children's Hospital Medical Centre, Ohio, USA), and Nicole Sibuyi is now at the Health Platform Diagnostic Unit (Advanced Materials Division, Mintek, Johannesburg, South Africa).

Conflicts of Interest: The authors declare no conflict of interest.

References

1. Iravani, S.; Korbekandi, H.; Mirmohammadi, S.V.; Zolfaghari, B. Synthesis of silver nanoparticles: Chemical, physical and biological methods. *Res. Pharm. Sci.* **2014**, *9*, 385–406. [PubMed]
2. Rauwel, P.; Küünal, S.; Ferdov, S.; Rauwel, E. A Review on the Green Synthesis of Silver Nanoparticles and Their Morphologies Studied via TEM. *Adv. Mater. Sci. Eng.* **2015**, *2015*, 682749. [CrossRef]
3. Greulich, C.; Braun, D.; Peetsch, A.; Diendorf, J.; Siebers, B.; Epple, M.; Köller, M. The toxic effect of silver ions and silver nanoparticles towards bacteria and human cells occurs in the same concentration range. *RSC Adv.* **2012**, *2*, 6981–6987. [CrossRef]
4. Chugh, D.; Viswamalya, V.S.; Das, B. Green synthesis of silver nanoparticles with algae and the importance of capping agents in the process. *J. Genet. Eng. Biotechnol.* **2021**, *19*, 126. [CrossRef]
5. Klaus-Joerger, T.; Joerger, R.; Olsson, E.; Granqvist, C.-G. Bacteria as workers in the living factory: Metal-accumulating bacteria and their potential for materials science. *TRENDS Biotechnol.* **2001**, *19*, 15–20. [CrossRef]
6. Helmy, A.; El-Shazly, M.; Seleem, A.; Abdelmohsen, U.; Salem, M.A.; Samir, A.; Rabeh, M.; Elshamy, A.; Singab, A.N.B. The synergistic effect of biosynthesized silver nanoparticles from a combined extract of parsley, corn silk, and gum arabic: In vivo antioxidant, anti-inflammatory and antimicrobial activities. *Mater. Res. Express* **2020**, *7*, 025002. [CrossRef]
7. Nqakala, Z.B.; Sibuyi, N.R.; Fadaka, A.O.; Meyer, M.; Onani, M.O.; Madiehe, A.M. Advances in Nanotechnology towards Development of Silver Nanoparticle-Based Wound-Healing Agents. *Int. J. Mol. Sci.* **2021**, *22*, 11272. [CrossRef]
8. Aboyewa, J.A.; Sibuyi, N.R.; Meyer, M.; Oguntibeju, O.O. Green synthesis of metallic nanoparticles using some selected medicinal plants from southern africa and their biological applications. *Plants* **2021**, *10*, 1929. [CrossRef]
9. Njagi, E.C.; Huang, H.; Stafford, L.; Genuino, H.; Galindo, H.M.; Collins, J.B.; Hoag, G.E.; Suib, S.L. Biosynthesis of iron and silver nanoparticles at room temperature using aqueous sorghum bran extracts. *Langmuir* **2011**, *27*, 264–271. [CrossRef]
10. Zargar, M.; Hamid, A.A.; Bakar, F.A.; Shamsudin, M.N.; Shameli, K.; Jahanshiri, F.; Farahani, F. Green synthesis and antibacterial effect of silver nanoparticles using *Vitex negundo* L. *Molecules* **2011**, *16*, 6667–6676. [CrossRef]
11. Arokiyaraj, S.; Arasu, M.V.; Vincent, S.; Prakash, N.U.; Choi, S.H.; Oh, Y.-K.; Choi, K.C.; Kim, K.H. Rapid green synthesis of silver nanoparticles from Chrysanthemum indicum L and its antibacterial and cytotoxic effects: An in vitro study. *Int. J. Nanomed.* **2014**, *9*, 379. [CrossRef] [PubMed]
12. Murugan, K.; Senthilkumar, B.; Senbagam, D.; Al-Sohaibani, S. Biosynthesis of silver nanoparticles using Acacia leucophloea extract and their antibacterial activity. *Int. J. Nanomed.* **2014**, *9*, 2431.
13. Gurunathan, S.; Raman, J.; Abd Malek, S.N.; John, P.A.; Vikineswary, S. Green synthesis of silver nanoparticles using Ganoderma neo-japonicum Imazeki: A potential cytotoxic agent against breast cancer cells. *Int. J. Nanomed.* **2013**, *8*, 4399.
14. Ipe, D.S.; Kumar, P.; Love, R.M.; Hamlet, S.M. Silver nanoparticles at biocompatible dosage synergistically increases bacterial susceptibility to antibiotics. *Front. Microbiol.* **2020**, *11*, 1074. [CrossRef]
15. Bilberg, K.; Hovgaard, M.B.; Besenbacher, F.; Baatrup, E. In vivo toxicity of silver nanoparticles and silver ions in zebrafish (*Danio rerio*). *J. Toxicol.* **2012**, *2012*, 293784. [CrossRef] [PubMed]
16. Qing, Y.; Cheng, L.; Li, R.; Liu, G.; Zhang, Y.; Tang, X.; Wang, J.; Liu, H.; Qin, Y. Potential antibacterial mechanism of silver nanoparticles and the optimization of orthopedic implants by advanced modification technologies. *Int. J. Nanomed.* **2018**, *13*, 3311–3327. [CrossRef]
17. Hu, C.; Lan, Y.; Qu, J.; Hu, X.; Wang, A. Ag/AgBr/TiO_2 visible light photocatalyst for destruction of azodyes and bacteria. *J. Phys. Chem. B* **2006**, *110*, 4066–4072. [CrossRef]

18. Durán, M.; Fávaro, W.J.; Islan, G.A.; Castro, G.R.; Durán, N. Silver nanoparticles for treatment of neglected diseases. In *Metal Nanoparticles in Pharma*; Springer: Cham, Switzerland, 2017; pp. 39–51.
19. Tăbăran, A.-F.; Matea, C.T.; Mocan, T.; Tăbăran, A.; Mihaiu, M.; Iancu, C.; Mocan, L. Silver nanoparticles for the therapy of tuberculosis. *Int. J. Nanomed.* **2020**, *15*, 2231–2258. [CrossRef]
20. Neves, P.B.A.d.; Agnelli, J.A.M.; Kurachi, C.; Souza, C.W.O.d. Addition of silver nanoparticles to composite resin: Effect on physical and bactericidal properties in vitro. *Braz. Dent. J.* **2014**, *25*, 141–145. [CrossRef]
21. Mahross, H.Z.; Baroudi, K. Effect of silver nanoparticles incorporation on viscoelastic properties of acrylic resin denture base material. *Eur. J. Dent.* **2015**, *9*, 207–212. [CrossRef]
22. Suzuki, T.Y.U.; Gallego, J.; Assunção, W.G.; Briso, A.L.F.; Dos Santos, P.H. Influence of silver nanoparticle solution on the mechanical properties of resin cements and intrarradicular dentin. *PLoS ONE* **2019**, *14*, e0217750. [CrossRef] [PubMed]
23. El-Rafie, H.; El-Rafie, M.; Zahran, M. Green synthesis of silver nanoparticles using polysaccharides extracted from marine macro algae. *Carbohydr. Polym.* **2013**, *96*, 403–410. [CrossRef] [PubMed]
24. Maziero, J.S.; Thipe, V.C.; Rogero, S.O.; Cavalcante, A.K.; Damasceno, K.C.; Ormenio, M.B.; Martini, G.A.; Batista, J.G.; Viveiros, W.; Katti, K.K. Species-Specific in vitro and in vivo Evaluation of Toxicity of Silver Nanoparticles Stabilized with Gum Arabic Protein. *Int. J. Nanomed.* **2020**, *15*, 7359. [CrossRef] [PubMed]
25. Rezazadeh, N.H.; Buazar, F.; Matroodi, S. Synergistic effects of combinatorial chitosan and polyphenol biomolecules on enhanced antibacterial activity of biofunctionalized silver nanoparticles. *Sci. Rep.* **2020**, *10*, 19615.
26. Johnson, W. Final report of the safety assessment of Acacia catechu gum, Acacia concinna fruit extract, Acacia dealbata leaf extract, Acacia dealbata leaf wax, Acacia decurrens extract, Acacia farnesiana extract, Acacia farnesiana flower wax, Acacia farnesiana gum, Acacia senegal extract, Acacia senegal gum, and Acacia senegal gum extract. *Int. J. Toxicol.* **2005**, *24*, 75–118.
27. Ali, B.H.; Ziada, A.; Blunden, G. Biological effects of gum arabic: A review of some recent research. *Food Chem. Toxicol.* **2009**, *47*, 1–8. [CrossRef]
28. Roque, A.C.A.; Bicho, A.; Batalha, I.L.; Cardoso, A.S.; Hussain, A. Biocompatible and bioactive gum Arabic coated iron oxide magnetic nanoparticles. *J. Biotechnol.* **2009**, *144*, 313–320. [CrossRef]
29. Williams, D.N.; Gold, K.A.; Holoman, T.R.P.; Ehrman, S.H.; Wilson, O.C. Surface Modification of Magnetic Nanoparticles Using Gum Arabic. *J. Nanoparticle Res.* **2006**, *8*, 749–753. [CrossRef]
30. Zhang, L.; Yu, F.; Cole, A.J.; Chertok, B.; David, A.E.; Wang, J.; Yang, V.C. Gum arabic-coated magnetic nanoparticles for potential application in simultaneous magnetic targeting and tumor imaging. *AAPS J.* **2009**, *11*, 693–699. [CrossRef]
31. Wilson, O.C., Jr.; Blair, E.; Kennedy, S.; Rivera, G.; Mehl, P. Surface modification of magnetic nanoparticles with oleylamine and gum Arabic. *Mater. Sci. Eng. C* **2008**, *28*, 438–442. [CrossRef]
32. Banerjee, S.S.; Chen, D.-H. Magnetic nanoparticles grafted with cyclodextrin for hydrophobic drug delivery. *Chem. Mater.* **2007**, *19*, 6345–6349. [CrossRef]
33. Kannan, R.; Rahing, V.; Cutler, C.; Pandrapragada, R.; Katti, K.K.; Kattumuri, V.; Robertson, J.D.; Casteel, S.J.; Jurisson, S.; Smith, C. Nanocompatible chemistry toward fabrication of target-specific gold nanoparticles. *J. Am. Chem. Soc.* **2006**, *128*, 11342–11343. [CrossRef] [PubMed]
34. Kattumuri, V.; Katti, K.; Bhaskaran, S.; Boote, E.J.; Casteel, S.W.; Fent, G.M.; Robertson, D.J.; Chandrasekhar, M.; Kannan, R.; Katti, K.V. Gum arabic as a phytochemical construct for the stabilization of gold nanoparticles: In vivo pharmacokinetics and X-ray-contrast-imaging studies. *Small* **2007**, *3*, 333–341. [CrossRef] [PubMed]
35. Aboyewa, J.A.; Sibuyi, N.R.; Meyer, M.; Oguntibeju, O.O. Gold Nanoparticles Synthesized Using Extracts of Cyclopia intermedia, Commonly Known as Honeybush, Amplify the Cytotoxic Effects of Doxorubicin. *Nanomaterials* **2021**, *11*, 132. [CrossRef]
36. Bandyopadhyaya, R.; Nativ-Roth, E.; Regev, O.; Yerushalmi-Rozen, R. Stabilization of individual carbon nanotubes in aqueous solutions. *Nano Lett.* **2002**, *2*, 25–28. [CrossRef]
37. Park, C.; Lim, K.H.; Kwon, D.; Yoon, T.H. Biocompatible quantum dot nanocolloids stabilized by gum Arabic. *Bull. -Korean Chem. Soc.* **2008**, *29*, 1277.
38. Ibekwe, C.A.; Oyatogun, G.M.; Esan, T.A.; Oluwasegun, K.M. Synthesis and characterization of chitosan/gum arabic nanoparticles for bone regeneration. *Am. J. Mater. Sci. Eng.* **2017**, *5*, 28–36.
39. Venkatesham, M.; Ayodhya, D.; Madhusudhan, A.; Veerabhadram, G. Synthesis of stable silver nanoparticles using gum acacia as reducing and stabilizing agent and study of its microbial properties: A novel green approach. *Int. J. Green Nanotechnol.* **2012**, *4*, 199–206. [CrossRef]
40. Solomon, M.M.; Gerengi, H.; Umoren, S.A.; Essien, N.B.; Essien, U.B.; Kaya, E. Gum Arabic-silver nanoparticles composite as a green anticorrosive formulation for steel corrosion in strong acid media. *Carbohydr. Polym.* **2018**, *181*, 43–55. [CrossRef]
41. Babiker, R.; Merghani, T.H.; Elmusharaf, K.; Badi, R.M.; Lang, F.; Saeed, A.M. Effects of gum Arabic ingestion on body mass index and body fat percentage in healthy adult females: Two-arm randomized, placebo controlled, double-blind trial. *Nutr. J.* **2012**, *11*, 1–7. [CrossRef]
42. Patel, S.; Goyal, A. Applications of natural polymer gum arabic: A review. *Int. J. Food Prop.* **2015**, *18*, 986–998. [CrossRef]
43. Musa, H.H.; Ahmed, A.A.; Musa, T.H. Chemistry, biological, and pharmacological properties of gum Arabic. In *Bioactive Molecules in Food*; Springer International Publishing AG: Cham, Switzerland, 2018; pp. 1–18.

44. Ansari, M.A.; Khan, H.M.; Khan, A.A.; Cameotra, S.S.; Saquib, Q.; Musarrat, J. Gum arabic capped-silver nanoparticles inhibit biofilm formation by multi-drug resistant strains of Pseudomonas aeruginosa. *J. Basic Microbiol.* **2014**, *54*, 688–699. [CrossRef] [PubMed]
45. Kora, A.J.; Arunachalam, J. Green fabrication of silver nanoparticles by gum tragacanth (*Astragalus gummifer*): A dual functional reductant and stabilizer. *J. Nanomater.* **2012**, *2012*, 69. [CrossRef]
46. Siddiqui, M.Z.; Chowdhury, A.R.; Singh, B.R.; Maurya, S.; Prasad, N. Synthesis, Characterization and Antimicrobial Evaluation of Piyar Gum-Induced Silver Nanoparticles. *Natl. Acad. Sci. Lett.* **2021**, *44*, 203–208. [CrossRef]
47. Majoumouo, M.S.; Sibuyi, N.R.S.; Tincho, M.B.; Mbekou, M.; Boyom, F.F.; Meyer, M. Enhanced anti-bacterial activity of biogenic silver nanoparticles synthesized from *Terminalia mantaly* Extracts. *Int. J. Nanomed.* **2019**, *14*, 9031. [CrossRef]
48. Simon, S.; Sibuyi, N.R.S.; Fadaka, A.O.; Meyer, M.; Madiehe, A.M.; du Preez, M.G. The antimicrobial activity of biogenic silver nanoparticles synthesized from extracts of Red and Green European pear cultivars. *Artif. Cells Nanomed. Biotechnol.* **2021**, *49*, 614–625. [CrossRef]
49. Dube, P.; Meyer, S.; Madiehe, A.; Meyer, M. Antibacterial activity of biogenic silver and gold nanoparticles synthesized from *Salvia africana-lutea* and *Sutherlandia frutescens*. *Nanotechnology* **2020**, *31*, 505607. [CrossRef]
50. Mamza, P.A.; Arthur, D.M.; Aliyu, M.J.; Desk, S. Purification, characterization and modification of gum arabic for possible use as additive for poly (vinyl chloride). *SDRP J. Comput. Chem. Mol. Model.* **2015**, *1*, 1–8.
51. Coates, J. Interpretation of infrared spectra, a practical approach. In *Encyclopedia of Analytical Chemistry*; John Wiley & Sons Ltd.: Chichester, UK, 2000.
52. Adam, H.; Siddig, M.A.; Siddig, A.A.; Eltahir, N.A. Electrical and optical properties of two types of Gum Arabic. *Sudan Med. Monit.* **2013**, *8*, 174.
53. Park, K.; Lee, Y. The stability of citrate-capped silver nanoparticles in isotonic glucose solution for intravenous injection. *J. Toxicol. Environ. Health Part A* **2013**, *76*, 1236–1245. [CrossRef]
54. Sim, W.; Barnard, R.T.; Blaskovich, M.; Ziora, Z.M. Antimicrobial silver in medicinal and consumer applications: A patent review of the past decade (2007–2017). *Antibiotics* **2018**, *7*, 93. [CrossRef] [PubMed]
55. Wu, M.; Guo, H.; Liu, L.; Liu, Y.; Xie, L. Size-dependent cellular uptake and localization profiles of silver nanoparticles. *Int. J. Nanomed.* **2019**, *14*, 4247. [CrossRef] [PubMed]
56. Siritongsuk, P.; Hongsing, N.; Thammawithan, S.; Daduang, S.; Klaynongsruang, S.; Tuanyok, A.; Patramanon, R. Two-phase bactericidal mechanism of silver nanoparticles against *Burkholderia pseudomallei*. *PLoS ONE* **2016**, *11*, e0168098. [CrossRef] [PubMed]
57. Tyavambiza, C.; Elbagory, A.M.; Madiehe, A.M.; Meyer, M.; Meyer, S. The Antimicrobial and Anti-Inflammatory Effects of Silver Nanoparticles Synthesised from Cotyledon orbiculata Aqueous Extract. *Nanomaterials* **2021**, *11*, 1343. [CrossRef] [PubMed]
58. Vazquez-Muñoz, R.; Bogdanchikova, N.; Huerta-Saquero, A. Beyond the nanomaterials approach: Influence of culture conditions on the stability and antimicrobial activity of silver nanoparticles. *ACS Omega* **2020**, *5*, 28441–28451. [CrossRef]
59. Liu, M.; Zhang, H.; Song, X.; Wei, C.; Xiong, Z.; Yu, F.; Li, C.; Ai, F.; Guo, G.; Wang, X. NaCl: For the safer in vivo use of antibacterial silver based nanoparticles. *Int. J. Nanomed.* **2018**, *13*, 1737. [CrossRef]
60. Fadaka, A.O.; Sibuyi, N.R.S.; Madiehe, A.M.; Meyer, M. Nanotechnology-based delivery systems for antimicrobial peptides. *Pharmaceutics* **2021**, *13*, 1795. [CrossRef]
61. Bakare, O.O.; Fadaka, A.O.; Klein, A.; Pretorius, A. Dietary effects of antimicrobial peptides in therapeutics. *All Life* **2020**, *13*, 78–91. [CrossRef]
62. Loo, Y.Y.; Rukayadi, Y.; Nor-Khaizura, M.-A.-R.; Kuan, C.H.; Chieng, B.W.; Nishibuchi, M.; Radu, S. In vitro antimicrobial activity of green synthesized silver nanoparticles against selected gram-negative foodborne pathogens. *Front. Microbiol.* **2018**, *9*, 1555. [CrossRef]
63. Singh, P.; Garg, A.; Pandit, S.; Mokkapati, V.; Mijakovic, I. Antimicrobial effects of biogenic nanoparticles. *Nanomaterials* **2018**, *8*, 1009. [CrossRef]
64. Ojo, O.A.; Oyinloye, B.E.; Ojo, A.B.; Afolabi, O.B.; Peters, O.A.; Olaiya, O.; Fadaka, A.; Jonathan, J.; Osunlana, O. Green synthesis of silver nanoparticles (AgNPs) using *Talinum triangulare* (Jacq.) Willd. leaf extract and monitoring their antimicrobial activity. *J. Bionanosci.* **2017**, *11*, 292–296. [CrossRef]
65. Baien, S.H.; Seele, J.; Henneck, T.; Freibrodt, C.; Szura, G.; Moubasher, H.; Nau, R.; Brogden, G.; Mörgelin, M.; Singh, M. Antimicrobial and immunomodulatory effect of gum arabic on human and bovine granulocytes against *Staphylococcus aureus* and *Escherichia coli*. *Front. Immunol.* **2020**, *10*, 3119. [CrossRef] [PubMed]
66. Al Alawi, S.M.; Hossain, M.A.; Abusham, A.A. Antimicrobial and cytotoxic comparative study of different extracts of Omani and Sudanese *Gum acacia*. *Beni-Suef Univ. J. Basic Appl. Sci.* **2018**, *7*, 22–26. [CrossRef]
67. Al-Ansari, M.M.; Al-Dahmash, N.D.; Ranjitsingh, A. Synthesis of silver nanoparticles using gum Arabic: Evaluation of its inhibitory action on Streptococcus mutans causing dental caries and endocarditis. *J. Infect. Public Health* **2021**, *14*, 324–330. [CrossRef] [PubMed]
68. El-Adawy, M.M.; Eissa, A.E.; Shaalan, M.; Ahmed, A.A.; Younis, N.A.; Ismail, M.M.; Abdelsalam, M. Green synthesis and physical properties of Gum Arabic-silver nanoparticles and its antibacterial efficacy against fish bacterial pathogens. *Aquac. Res.* **2021**, *52*, 1247–1254. [CrossRef]

69. Wu, Y.; Yang, Y.; Zhang, Z.; Wang, Z.; Zhao, Y.; Sun, L. A facile method to prepare size-tunable silver nanoparticles and its antibacterial mechanism. *Adv. Powder Technol.* **2018**, *29*, 407–415. [CrossRef]
70. Rampersad, S.N. Multiple applications of Alamar Blue as an indicator of metabolic function and cellular health in cell viability bioassays. *Sensors* **2012**, *12*, 12347–12360. [CrossRef] [PubMed]
71. Rai, Y.; Pathak, R.; Kumari, N.; Sah, D.K.; Pandey, S.; Kalra, N.; Soni, R.; Dwarakanath, B.; Bhatt, A.N. Mitochondrial biogenesis and metabolic hyperactivation limits the application of MTT assay in the estimation of radiation induced growth inhibition. *Sci. Rep.* **2018**, *8*, 1531. [CrossRef]
72. Liao, C.; Li, Y.; Tjong, S.C. Bactericidal and cytotoxic properties of silver nanoparticles. *Int. J. Mol. Sci.* **2019**, *20*, 449. [CrossRef]
73. Molina-Hernandez, A.I.; Diaz-Gonzalez, J.M.; Saeb-Lima, M.; Dominguez-Cherit, J. Argyria after silver nitrate intake: Case report and brief review of literature. *Indian J. Dermatol.* **2015**, *60*, 520. [CrossRef]
74. Jabir, M.S.; Saleh, Y.M.; Sulaiman, G.M.; Yaseen, N.Y.; Sahib, U.I.; Dewir, Y.H.; Alwahibi, M.S.; Soliman, D.A. Green Synthesis of Silver Nanoparticles Using Annona muricata Extract as an Inducer of Apoptosis in Cancer Cells and Inhibitor for NLRP3 Inflammasome via Enhanced Autophagy. *Nanomaterials* **2021**, *11*, 384. [CrossRef] [PubMed]
75. Chen, J.; Li, S.; Luo, J.; Wang, R.; Ding, W. Enhancement of the antibacterial activity of silver nanoparticles against phytopathogenic bacterium *Ralstonia solanacearum* by stabilization. *J. Nanomater.* **2016**, *2016*, 7135852. [CrossRef]
76. Van der Zande, M.; Undas, A.K.; Kramer, E.; Monopoli, M.P.; Peters, R.J.; Garry, D.; Antunes Fernandes, E.C.; Hendriksen, P.J.; Marvin, H.J.; Peijnenburg, A.A. Different responses of Caco-2 and MCF-7 cells to silver nanoparticles are based on highly similar mechanisms of action. *Nanotoxicology* **2016**, *10*, 1431–1441. [CrossRef] [PubMed]
77. Recordati, C.; De Maglie, M.; Bianchessi, S.; Argentiere, S.; Cella, C.; Mattiello, S.; Cubadda, F.; Aureli, F.; D'Amato, M.; Raggi, A. Tissue distribution and acute toxicity of silver after single intravenous administration in mice: Nano-specific and size-dependent effects. *Part. Fibre Toxicol.* **2015**, *13*, 1–17. [CrossRef]
78. Dube, P.; Meyer, S.; Marnewick, J.L. Antimicrobial and antioxidant activities of different solvent extracts from fermented and green honeybush (*Cyclopia intermedia*) plant material. *South Afr. J. Bot.* **2017**, *110*, 184–193. [CrossRef]
79. Mulfinger, L.; Solomon, S.D.; Bahadory, M.; Jeyarajasingam, A.V.; Rutkowsky, S.A.; Boritz, C. Synthesis and study of silver nanoparticles. *J. Chem. Educ.* **2007**, *84*, 322. [CrossRef]
80. Sibuyi, N.R.S.; Thipe, V.C.; Panjtan-Amiri, K.; Meyer, M.; Katti, K.V. Green synthesis of gold nanoparticles using Acai berry and Elderberry extracts and investigation of their effect on prostate and pancreatic cancer cells. *Nanobiomedicine* **2021**, *8*, 1849543521995310. [CrossRef]
81. Simo, A.; Drah, M.; Sibuyi, N.; Nkosi, M.; Meyer, M.; Maaza, M. Hydrothermal synthesis of cobalt-doped vanadium oxides: Antimicrobial activity study. *Ceram. Int.* **2018**, *44*, 7716–7722. [CrossRef]
82. Radhakrishnan, V.S.; Mudiam, M.K.R.; Kumar, M.; Dwivedi, S.P.; Singh, S.P.; Prasad, T. Silver nanoparticles induced alterations in multiple cellular targets, which are critical for drug susceptibilities and pathogenicity in fungal pathogen (*Candida albicans*). *Int. J. Nanomed.* **2018**, *13*, 2647. [CrossRef]
83. Tshweu, L.L.; Shemis, M.A.; Abdelghany, A.; Gouda, A.; Pilcher, L.A.; Sibuyi, N.R.; Meyer, M.; Dube, A.; Balogun, M.O. Synthesis, physicochemical characterization, toxicity and efficacy of a PEG conjugate and a hybrid PEG conjugate nanoparticle formulation of the antibiotic moxifloxacin. *RSC Adv.* **2020**, *10*, 19770–19780. [CrossRef]

International Journal of
Molecular Sciences

MDPI

Article

Synthesis of Novel Aminothiazole Derivatives as Promising Antiviral, Antioxidant and Antibacterial Candidates

Rūta Minickaitė [1], Birutė Grybaitė [1], Rita Vaickelionienė [1], Povilas Kavaliauskas [1,2,3,4,5], Vidmantas Petraitis [2,4,5], Rūta Petraitienė [2,4], Ingrida Tumosienė [1], Ilona Jonuškienė [1,*] and Vytautas Mickevičius [1]

1 Department of Organic Chemistry, Faculty of Chemical Technology, Kaunas University of Technology, Radvilėnų pl. 19, LT-50254 Kaunas, Lithuania; ruta.minickaite@ktu.edu (R.M.); birute.grybaite@ktu.lt (B.G.); rita.vaickelioniene@ktu.lt (R.V.); povilas.kavaliauskas@ktu.edu (P.K.); ingrida.tumosiene@ktu.lt (I.T.); vytautas.mickevicius@ktu.lt (V.M.)
2 Transplantation-Oncology Infectious Diseases Program, Division of Infectious Diseases, Department of Medicine, Weill Cornell Medicine of Cornell University, 527 East 68th Street, New York, NY 10065, USA; vip2007@med.cornell.edu (V.P.); rop2016@med.cornell.edu (R.P.)
3 Department of Microbiology and Immunology, University of Maryland Baltimore School of Medicine, 655 W. Baltimore Street, Baltimore, MD 21201, USA
4 Institute of Infectious Diseases and Pathogenic Microbiology, Birštono Str. 38A, LT-59116 Prienai, Lithuania
5 Biological Research Center, Veterinary Academy, Lithuanian University of Health Sciences, Tilžės St. 18, LT-47181 Kaunas, Lithuania
* Correspondence: ilona.jonuskiene@ktu.lt

Abstract: It is well-known that thiazole derivatives are usually found in lead structures, which demonstrate a wide range of pharmacological effects. The aim of this research was to explore the antiviral, antioxidant, and antibacterial activities of novel, substituted thiazole compounds and to find potential agents that could have biological activities in one single biomolecule. A series of novel aminothiazoles were synthesized, and their biological activity was characterized. The obtained results were compared with those of the standard antiviral, antioxidant, antibacterial and anticancer agents. The compound bearing 4-cianophenyl substituent in the thiazole ring demonstrated the highest cytotoxic properties by decreasing the A549 viability to 87.2%. The compound bearing 4-trifluoromethylphenyl substituent in the thiazole ring showed significant antiviral activity against the PR8 influenza A strain, which was comparable to the oseltamivir and amantadine. Novel compounds with 4-chlorophenyl, 4-trifluoromethylphenyl, phenyl, 4-fluorophenyl, and 4-cianophenyl substituents in the thiazole ring demonstrated antioxidant activity by DPPH, reducing power, FRAP methods, and antibacterial activity against *Escherichia coli* and *Bacillus subtilis* bacteria. These data demonstrate that substituted aminothiazole derivatives are promising scaffolds for further optimization and development of new compounds with potential influenza A-targeted antiviral activity. Study results could demonstrate that structure optimization of novel aminothiazole compounds may be useful in the prevention of reactive oxygen species and developing new specifically targeted antioxidant and antibacterial agents.

Keywords: thiazole; antiviral; oxidative stress; antioxidant; antibacterial; bioactivity

Citation: Minickaitė, R.; Grybaitė, B.; Vaickelionienė, R.; Kavaliauskas, P.; Petraitis, V.; Petraitienė, R.; Tumosienė, I.; Jonuškienė, I.; Mickevičius, V. Synthesis of Novel Aminothiazole Derivatives as Promising Antiviral, Antioxidant and Antibacterial Candidates. *Int. J. Mol. Sci.* **2022**, *23*, 7688. https://doi.org/10.3390/ijms23147688

Academic Editor: Helena Felgueiras

Received: 29 June 2022
Accepted: 8 July 2022
Published: 12 July 2022

1. Introduction

Progress in organic and medicinal chemistry allows for the design, synthesis and optimization of the structures of novel thiazole compounds. Thiazole compounds are widely used in the pharmaceutical industry for the design of therapeutics and novel biosensors for their antioxidant [1–3], antibacterial [4–6], anti-proliferative [7], antiparasitic [8], anti-inflammatory [9], analgesic [10], neuroprotective [11], antiviral (including SARS-CoV-2) [12], and anti-HIV activities [13]. Studies of thiazole-structure activities promote the improvement of their chemical/biochemical and therapeutic properties and anti-TB activity, mainly against resistant *Mycobacterium tuberculosis* (Mtb) strains [14].

Thiazole derivatives are important in designing and discovering pharmaceuticals, and they are incorporated into the structures of antimicrobial (acinitrazole and sulfathiazole) [15], antidepressant (pexole) [16], antineoplastic (bleomycin) [17], anti-HIV (ritonavir) [18], antiasthmatic (cinalukast) [19], antiulcer (nizatidine) [20], antibiotic (penicillin), thiamine (vitamin B1) [21], non-steroidal immunomodulatory (fanetizole) [22], anti-inflammatory (anetizole, meloxicam, fentiazac), analgesic, antineoplastic (tiazofurin, dasatinib), antifungal (ravuconazole), antiparasitic (nitazoxanide), anti-inflammatory (anetizole, meloxicam, fentiazac), and antiulcer (nizatidine) [23,24] drugs and agents. Thiazoles possess a polyoxygenated phenyl molecule that showed anti-fungal activity [25] and thiazolium also possesses bis-thiazolium salts that have been screened as potent antimalarial agents.

Novel thiazole compounds also participate in bioluminescent systems, which are focused on the substrate specificity of D-luciferin for luciferase. Previous studies have discovered that a thiazoline ring of the original structure should be conserved for emitting bioluminescence, whereas an aromatic ring and its substituents could be modified [26]. A thiazole ring containing firefly luciferin is responsible for the characteristic yellow-light emission from fireflies [27]. Bioluminescent systems have important roles in medicinal biology and clinical applications for the design of protein-based biosensors for detection of the SARS-CoV-2 virus [28].

Cancer is the leading disease and one of the significant healthcare challenges of the 21st century. It is important to mention that thiazole compounds could be used as highly versatile scaffolds for the development of anticancer agents [29,30]. A number of thiazole derivatives have been described to show potent anticancer activity by inhibiting tubulin polymerization [31,32]. Excessive reactive-oxygen species (ROS) production, oxidative stress, mitochondrial disfunction, and lipid peroxidation have also been implicated in cancer pathology. Oxidative stress is considered the starting point for tissues' chronic inflammation and cancer [33].

The demand of novel antioxidant agents has been increasing because of the long-term safety and a negative consumer perception about synthetic antioxidants such as butylhydroxyanisole, BHA, and butylhydroxytoluene, BHT, which showed toxic and carcinogenic side effects in animal models [34]. The discovery of compounds that can have both antimicrobial and antioxidant activities with no toxic effects on health is, therefore, highly awaited [35].

Camalexin (3-thiazol-2-yl-indole) is an indole alkaloid phytoalexin, which is induced by phytopathogens and accumulates in various *Brassicaceae* plant organs or tissues. Many studies have characterized that camalexin and its derivatives have been found to possess significant anticancer, antifungal, antiviral, and antibacterial activities [36]. Camalexin biosynthesis is dependent on cysteine, and glutathione reduced form (GSH) is the direct precursor of the thiazole ring [37].

Our research interest was focused on the design, synthesis, screening, and investigation of novel aminothiazole compounds for their influenza A-targeted antiviral, antioxidant, and antibacterial potential. To counter increasing drug resistance, thiazoles could be considered as a promising scaffold to generate novel bioactive derivatives.

Here, we discuss the important challenges for the understanding of aminothiazoles' activities and the current strategies for improving chemical, biological, and therapeutical characteristics, with the combination of three targets in one biomolecule structure.

2. Results

2.1. *Synthesis of Novel Aminothiazoles*

The starting compound **2** was synthesized from 4-aminoacetanilide (**1**) and acrylic acid. Initially, we used the method described in the literature [38]. Although the authors report a 77.4% yield, the reaction under the specified conditions yielded only 7% of the product. This led to the study of the above-mentioned reaction using different solvents.

Reactions were carried out in toluene, 1,4-dioxane, 2-propanol, and tetrahydrofuran (THF) at reflux for 24 h. The results are shown in Table 1.

Table 1. Reaction conditions for the synthesis of compound **2**.

Entry	Solvent	Temperature, °C	Reaction Time, h	Yield, %
A	Water	Reflux	5	7
B	Toluene		24	22
C	Dioxane			48
D	2-propanol			55
E	THF			70

The data demonstrate that a reaction in THF allowed the preparation of compound **2**, providing the highest yield of 70%. Triplets at 2.47 (CH_2CO) and 3.20 ($NHCH_2$), the singlet at 3.77 ($NHCH_2$), and a broad singlet at 11.81 (COOH) in ^1H NMR for the compound confirmed the formation of the β-alanine fragment in the structure.

The cyclization of β-alanine moiety to 2-thioxotetrahydropyrimidinedione **3** was performed by refluxing carboxylic acid **2** with potassium thiocyanate in acetic acid. Compound **3** was separated by dilution of the reaction mixture with water. The obtained product was applied for the preparation of thioureido acid **4** (Scheme 1). For this purpose, compound **3** was dissolved in hot, aqueous 5% sodium hydroxide, and the obtained solution of the carboxylic acid sodium salt was filtered off and transferred to an acidic form by acidifying the filtrate with acetic acid to pH 6.

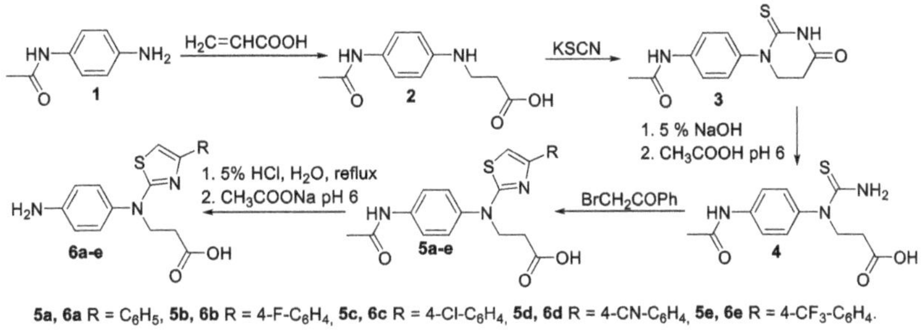

Scheme 1. Synthesis of compounds **2–6**.

The prepared thioureido acid **4** was applied for the synthesis of thiazoles **5a–e**. The products **5a–e** have been achieved by a reaction of thioureido acid **4** and the corresponding bromoacetophenone in water, with the presence of sodium carbonate in the reaction mixture. The ^1H NMR spectra of these compound singlets, in the range of 7.07–7.42 ppm (^{13}C, 102.09–106.41 ppm), and the additional peaks in the aromatic region, confirm the presence of a 4-arylthiazole moiety.

The next goal of this study was the transformation of the acetamide fragment to an amine group. Reactions occurred easily and rapidly and were completed after refluxing in aqueous 5% hydrochloric acid for 1 h. Products were isolated by neutralizing the reaction mixtures with sodium acetate to pH 6. By careful assignment of the peaks in the ^1H and ^{13}C NMR spectra, the structures **6** were elucidated. Comparison of the spectra of compounds **5** and **6** showed obvious differences, i.e., the spectra of the latter compounds do not contain singlets of the methyl group of the acetamide moiety, but broad singlets of amino group are visible at approximately 5.35 ppm. In addition, the additional proof of the new structure is the absence of the resonance of the carbonyl carbon of the CH_3CO fragment in the ^{13}C NMR spectra of compounds **6**, which are clearly visible in the analogous spectra of derivatives **5** at approximately 168.45 ppm.

To obtain thiazolone derivative **7**, a ring-closure reaction was carried out where thioureido acid **4** was reacted with monochloroacetic acid in an aqueous sodium carbonate solution, where acidification to pH 6 after completion of the reaction produced the target compound **7** (Scheme 2). The structure of 7 was approved based on the data of elemental analysis and NMR as well as IR spectroscopy.

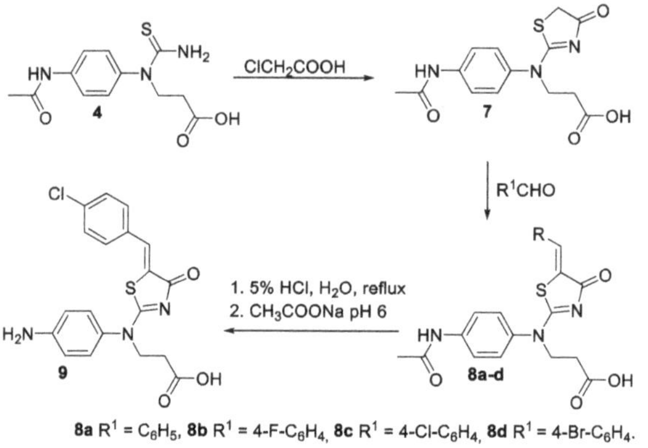

Scheme 2. Synthesis of thiazolone derivatives **7–9**.

The condensation of the obtained thiazolone **7** with various aromatic aldehydes was performed under analogous conditions, such as synthesis, instead of the monochloroacetic acid using the corresponding aromatic aldehydes. The reactions afforded 5-[(substituted phenyl)methylidene] thiazolones **8a–d**. The spectra of compounds **8** do not contain the proton singlet of the SCH_2, which arises at 3.91 (^1H) and 40.59 (^{13}C) ppm in the NMR spectra for compound 7. In the structure of compounds **8**, **a** = CHAr moiety is attached to the 5-position of the thiazole ring. The NMR spectra of formed molecules **8** show obvious differences in comparison with the NMR spectra of 7. The increase in spectral lines in the aromatic region of the ^1H (in the interval of 7.59–7.61 ppm for CH and in the range of 7.21–7.63 ppm for H_{Ar}) and ^{13}C (observed in the interval of 129–134 ppm) NMR spectra correspond to the number of hydrogen and carbon atoms of the new fragment. Then, 3-((4-aminophenyl)(4-(4-chlorobenzylidene)-5-oxo-4,5-dihydrothiazol-2-yl)amino)propanoic acid (**9**) was obtained by the deacetylation of compound **8c** in the aqueous 5% hydrochloric-acid solution. The formed amino group was confirmed by a broad singlet, which was visible at 5.61 ppm.

Next, 2-thioxotetrahydropyrimidinedione **3** was used to prepare derivative **10** with an amino group in its structure. For this reason, compound **3** was refluxed in an aqueous 5% HCl solution. Product **10** was isolated by neutralizing the reaction mixture with sodium acetate to pH 6.

The obtained product **10** was used for the preparation of thioureido acid **11** (Scheme 3). For this purpose, compound **10** was dissolved in a hot, aqueous 5% sodium hydroxide solution, then filtered off and acidified with acetic acid to pH 6, to transfer sodium salt to the acidic form. Comparison of the spectra of compounds **3** and **10** showed that the singlet of the methyl group of the acetamide moiety is absent, but a broad singlet of an amino group is visible at 5.20 ppm.

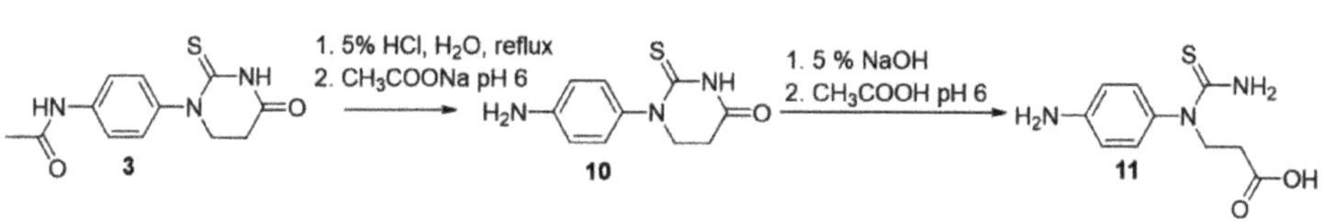

Scheme 3. Synthesis of compounds **10** and **11**.

2.2. *Study of Cytotoxic Activity of Compounds **3–11***

To explore the in vitro cytotoxicity of compounds **3–11**, we used A549 human pulmonary endothelial cells and a MTT viability assay. We exposed the cells to the fixed concentration of 100 µM of each compound for 48 h and subsequently measured the viability. Compounds **3–11** demonstrated overall favorable properties with low cytotoxicity. Among all tested compounds, **6d**, bearing 4-cianophenyl substituent in the thiazole ring, demonstrated the highest cytotoxic properties by decreasing the A549 viability to 87.2%. All compounds failed to reduce the A549 viability by 50%, suggesting good in vitro safety profiles (Figure 1).

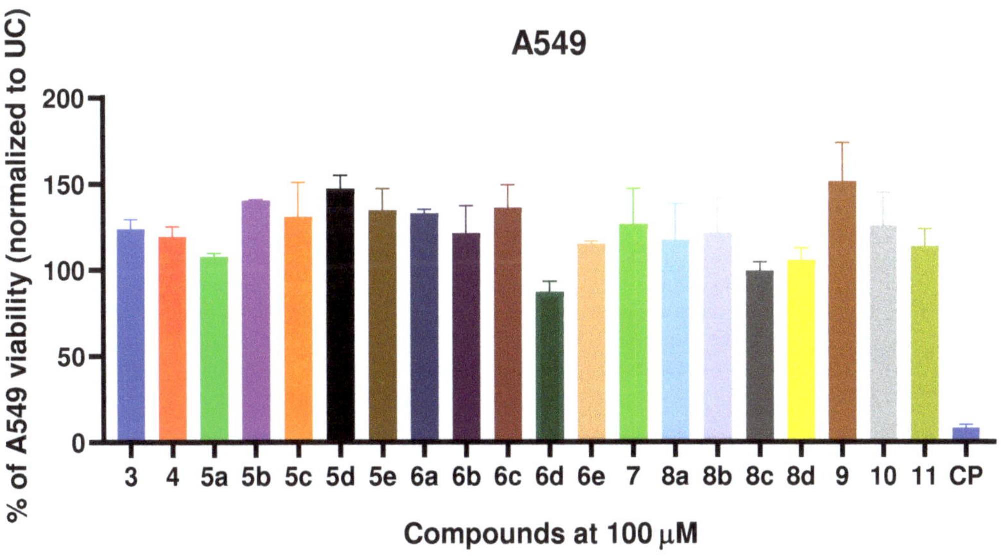

Figure 1. The in vitro cytotoxicity of compounds **3–11** on A549 human pulmonary cells. The A549 cells were treated with 100 µM of each compound or cisplatin (CP) that served as control for 48 h, and the post-treatment viability was measured by using MTT assay. The viability of untreated control (UC) was used for the post-treatment-viability normalization. Data are shown as mean ± SD from three experimental replicates.

2.3. *Study of Antiviral Activity of Compounds **3–11***

To explore the potential antiviral ability of synthesized compounds, we used an MDCK influenza in vitro infection model [39,40]. Prior to infection, we pretreated the MDCK cells with 100 µM of each compound, or oseltamivir and amantadine that served as antiviral controls. Compounds **3–11** showed structure-dependent antiviral activity against influenza A/Puerto Rico/8/34 H1N1 strain and were able to significantly ($p < 0.05$) restore MDCK viability in comparison to the untreated control (UC) (Figure 2). Compounds **8d**, **5e**, **5d**, and **6e** showed the highest antiviral activity ($p < 0.001$) in comparison to UC. The antiviral activity of compounds **8d**, **5e**, **5d**, and **6e** at 100 µM was similar or greater than oseltamivir and amantadine. Furthermore, compound **5e**, bearing 4-trifluoromethylphenyl substituent in the thiazole ring, showed significantly higher antiviral activity ($p < 0.0162$) than oseltamivir (Figure 2).

These data demonstrate that substituted aminothiazole derivatives are promising scaffolds for further optimization and the development of new compounds with potential influenza A targeted antiviral activity.

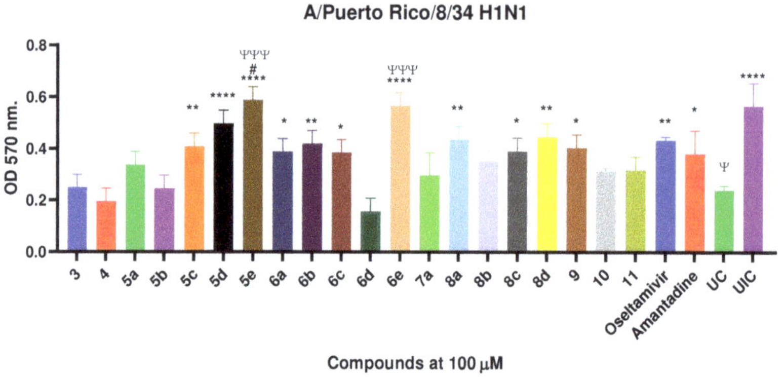

Figure 2. The in vitro antiviral activity of compounds **3–11** against the replication of influenza A/Puerto Rico/8/34 H1N1 strain in MDCK cells. MDCK cells were pretreated with compounds (100 μM) or antiviral control drugs (oseltamivir and amantadine) and infected with influenza A/Puerto Rico/8/34 H1N1 strain. After 24 h, the viability was measured using MTT assay. Uninfected control (UIC) cells were used as a comparison demonstrating the fully viable cells. * shows significant comparisons between test compounds and untreated control (UC), # shows significant comparisons between test compounds and oseltamivir, and Ψ shows significant comparisons between test compounds and amantadine. Statistical significance was tested with one-way ANOVA, and error bars show mean ± SD from three experiments. * $p < 0.05$, ** $p < 0.0021$, **** $p < 0.0001$, ΨΨΨ $p < 0.0001$.

2.4. Measurement of Antioxidant Activities

Ferric ion (Fe^{3+}) reduces the antioxidant power test (ferricyanide/Prussian blue assay). Bioactive compounds with antioxidant-reducing activity transfer an electron to ferricyanide's Perls Prussian blue complex, reducing $Fe[(CN)_6]_3$ to $Fe[(CN)_6]_2$ [41,42]. Increasing absorbance at 700 nm shows an increase in the reductive ability of the reaction complex [43].

The data obtained from the study (Figure 3) demonstrated that the compounds bearing 4-cianophenyl **6d**, 4-chlorophenyl **6c**, and 4-trifluoromethylphenyl **6e** substituents in the thiazole ring showed the highest ferric ion (Fe^{3+})-reducing power. The scaffolds of the compounds bearing 5-benzylidene **8a**, {5-[(4-bromophenyl)methylidene] **8d**, 5-[(4-chlorophenyl)methylidene] **8c**, 5-[(4-fluorophenyl)methylidene] **8b**, and 4-oxo-4,5-dihydro-1,3-thiazol-2-yl)amino] **7** in analyzed propanoic acid derivatives exhibited the lowest reducing antioxidant power.

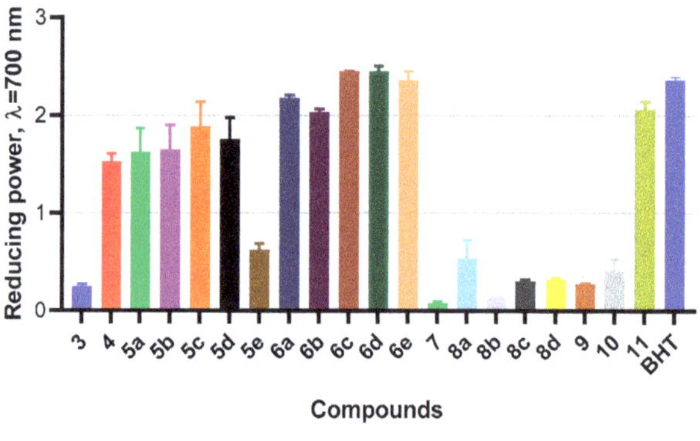

Figure 3. Evaluation of ferric ion (Fe^{3+}) reducing antioxidant power of **3–11** compounds and synthetic antioxidant BHT. Data are shown as mean ± SD from three experimental replicates.

Ferric-reducing antioxidant power (FRAP assay). The ferric ion reducing antioxidant power (FRAP)-reaction mechanism is focused on electron transfer (ET)-based bioassays. The FRAP technique is carried out at pH 3.6 and evaluates the reduction in ferric Fe^{3+} complex of 2,4,6-tripyridyl-*s*-triazine $Fe(TPTZ)^{3+}$ to the blue-colored ferrous (Fe^{2+}) complex $Fe(TPTZ)^{2+}$ by bioactive compounds.

Measuring the increasing absorption at 593 nm using a spectrophotometer monitors this reduction, and results are expressed as a Fe^{2+} μmol/L concentration. [44].

The results (Figure 4) of the study exhibited that compounds bearing 4-chlorophenyl **6c** (123.20 μmol/L), phenyl **6a** (114.18 μmol/L), 4-fluorophenyl **6b** (111.83 μmol/L), and 4-trifluoromethylphenyl **6e** (106.53 μmol/L) substituents in the thiazole ring showed the highest reduced FRAP power, in comparison with BHT (67.73 μmol/L). The compounds **8d**, **8c**, **8a**, **7**, and **8b** demonstrated the lowest FRAP power.

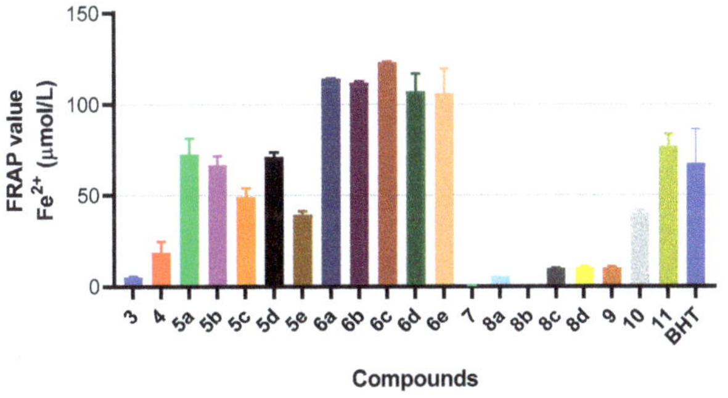

Figure 4. The ferric-reducing antioxidant power activity of **3–11** compounds and synthetic antioxidant BHT. Data are shown as mean ± SD from three experimental replicates.

DPPH radical-scavenging assay. The 1,1-Diphenyl-2-picrylhydrazyl (DPPH•) radical-scavenging assay has been one of the most commonly applied methods to determine antioxidant activity [45,46]. The DPPH test is based on either a hydrogen-atom transfer (HAT) or a single-electron transfer (SET) mechanism. Bioactive compounds are able to donate a hydrogen atom to reduce the stable DPPH• radical (a deep purple color) to the yellow-colored non-radical compound at 517 nm.

As seen from the results presented in Figure 5, the compounds bearing 4-fluorophenyl **6b** (83.63%) and 4-phenyl **6a** (52.04%) substituents in the thiazole ring, as well as 3-(1-(4-aminophenyl)thioureido)propanoic acid **11** (66.5%) and 3-[(4-acetamidophenyl)(carbamothioyl) amino]propanoic acid **4** (49.36%), possess a very high DPPH radical-scavenging ability in comparison with BHT (45.14%). The compounds **7, 8a,** and **8d** demonstrated low DPPH inhibition. The compounds **5a–5e** did not show antioxidant activity according to the DPPH method.

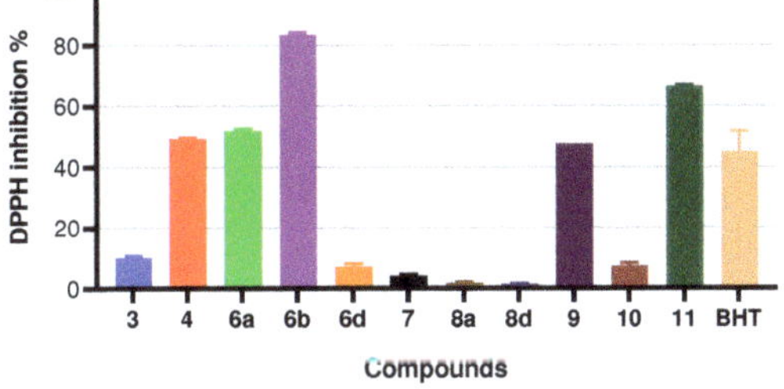

Figure 5. Antioxidant activity by DPPH assay of **3–11** compounds and synthetic antioxidant BHT. Data are shown as mean ± SD from three experimental replicates.

2.5. Evaluation of Antibacterial Activity

The novel derivatives were screened for their in vitro antibacterial activity against *Escherichia coli* (Gram-negative) and *Bacillus subtilis* (Gram-positive) bacteria strains. Antimicrobial tests were conducted using the agar well-diffusion method. Ciprofloxacin was used as the reference antibiotic for the in vitro antibacterial activity.

The results of the antibacterial study against *E. coli* (Figure 6) illustrated that the compounds bearing 4-cianophenyl **6d**, 4-fluorophenyl **6b**, 4-chlorophenyl **8c**, 4-trifluoromethylphenyl **5e**, and phenyl **6a** substituents in the thiazole ring showed the highest antibacterial activity against *E. coli*. The compounds **8b**, **8a**, **7**, **3**, **4**, **10**, and **11** showed the lowest antibacterial activity against *E. coli*.

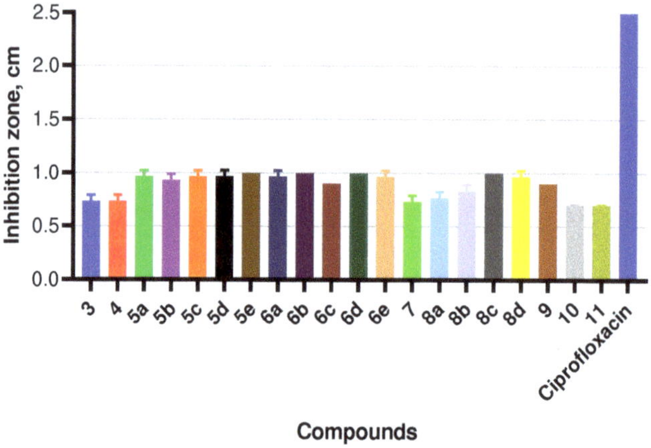

Figure 6. Antibacterial activity against *E. coli* of compounds **3–11** and control antibiotic Ciprofloxacin. Data are shown as mean ± SD from three experimental replicates.

The results of the antibacterial study against *B. subtilis* demonstrated (Figure 7) that the compounds bearing 4-cianophenyl **6d**, 4-fluorophenyl **6b**, 4-fluoro **5b**, 4-chlorophenyl **8c**, 4-trifluoromethylphenyl **5e**, and phenyl **6a** and **5a** substituents in the thiazole ring showed the highest antibacterial activity against this strain. The compounds **8a**, **8b**, **3**, **7**, **10**, **4**, and **11** showed the lowest antibacterial activity against *B. subtilis*.

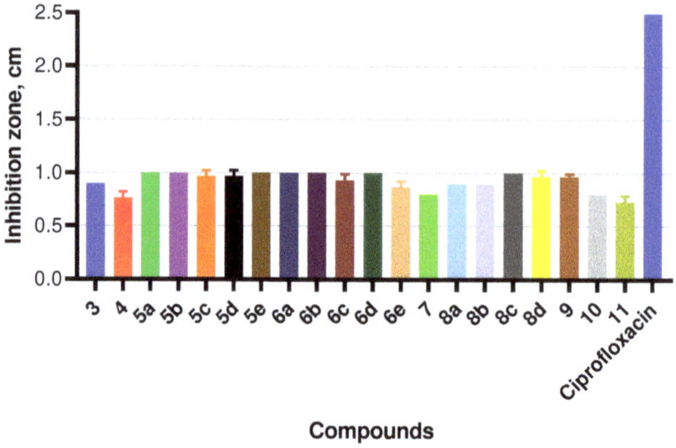

Figure 7. Antibacterial activity against *B. subtilis* of compounds **3–11** and control antibiotic Ciprofloxacin. Data are shown as mean ± SD from three experimental replicates.

3. Discussion

It is important to develop an understanding of these novel aminothiazole compounds by integrating their synthesis and biological activities (antiviral, antioxidant, antibacterial). The present study results demonstrated that the compound 3-{(4-aminophenyl)[4-(4-cianophenyl)-1,3-thiazol-2-yl]amino}propanoic acid (**6d**) showed the highest cytotoxic properties. Screening of the tested compounds for antiviral activity has revealed that the compounds 3-((4-aminophenyl){4-[4-(trifluoromethyl)phenyl]thiazol-2-yl}amino)propanoic acid (**6e**) and 3-{(4-acetamidophenyl)[4-(4-trifluoromethylphenyl)-1,3-thiazol-2-yl]amino} propanoic acid (**5e**) exhibited significant influenza A-targeted antiviral activity, in comparison with oseltamivir and amantadine. The principle of antioxidant activity is focused on the availability of electrons to neutralize any free radicals. Moreover, antioxidant activity is related to the nature of the hydroxylation pattern on the aromatic ring. Various antioxidant methods have been described to evaluate antioxidant properties of pharmaceuticals, antioxidants, and other bioactive samples [43]. The antioxidant bioassays should be based on the elucidation of the structure–antioxidant-activity relationship of the bioactive molecules. Screening of the reduction power of the bioactive compounds gives information not only about their reducing ability but also reveals their thermodynamic parameters. It was determined that thiazole compounds bearing 4-cyanophenyl **6d**, 4-chlorophenyl **6c**, and 4-trifluoromethylphenyl **6e** substituents in the thiazole ring showed the highest **6d** > **6c** > **6e** > **BHT** > **11** > **6a** > **6b** > **5c** antioxidant-reducing activity. The compounds **8a**, **8d**, **8c**, **8b**, and **7** demonstrated the lowest antioxidant-reducing power. It could be concluded that aminothiazole compounds bearing 4-chlorophenyl **6c**, 4-trifluoromethylphenyl **6e**, phenyl **6a**, 4-fluorophenyl **6b**, and 4-cianophenyl **6d** substituents in the thiazole ring exhibited the highest **6c** > **6a** > **6e** > **6b** > **6d** > **11** > **5a** > **5d** > **5b** > **BHT** reduced FRAP power. The model of scavenging the stable DPPH radical is a widely used method to evaluate the free-radical-scavenging ability of various samples. It is a stable nitrogen-centered free radical, the color of which changes from violet to yellow upon reduction by either the process of hydrogen or electron donation. It was determined that the thiazole compounds **6b** > **11** > **6a** > **4** > **BHT** showed the highest antioxidant activity by DPPH assay. The acquired results of the antibacterial activity showed that compounds bearing 4-cianophenyl **6d**, 4-fluorophenyl **6b**, 4-chlorophenyl **8c**, 4-trifluoromethylphenyl **5e, and** phenyl **6a** substituents in the thiazole ring have been indicated as the most active antibacterial agents against *E. coli*. The compounds **6d** = **6a** = **6b** = **8c** = **5a** = **5b** = **5e** > **5d** = **5c** = **8d** showed the highest antibacterial activity against *B. subtilis*. The antibacterial activity of the novel compounds could be related with the existence of electron-withdrawing groups in the thiazole ring.

4. Materials and Methods

4.1. Synthesis of Novel Compounds

Melting points were determined on a MEL-TEMP (Electrothermal, A Bibby Scientific Company, Burlington, NJ, USA) melting point apparatus and are uncorrected. FT-IR spectra (ν, cm^{-1}) were recorded on a Perkin–Elmer Spectrum BX FT–IR spectrometer (Perkin–Elmer Inc., Waltham, MA, USA) using KBr pellets. ^1H and ^{13}C-NMR spectra were recorded in DMSO-d_6 on a Bruker Avance III (400 MHz, 101 MHz and 700 MHz, 176 MHz) spectrometer. Chemical shifts (δ) are reported in parts per million (ppm) calibrated from TMS (0 ppm) as an internal standard for ^1H-NMR and DMSO-d_6 (39.43 ppm) for ^{13}C-NMR. The reaction course and purity of the synthesized compounds was monitored by TLC using aluminum plates coated with silica gel 60 F254 (MerckKGaA, Darmstadt, Germany). Reagents were obtained from Sigma-Aldrich (St. Louis, MO, USA).

N-[4-(acetylamino)phenyl]-*β*-alanine (**2**)

A mixture of 4-aminoacetanilide (**1**) (0.3 mol, 15 g), acrylic acid (0.45 mol, 30.88 mL), and THF (90 mL) was heated at reflux for 24 h. After completion of the reaction (TLC), it was cooled to room temperature, and the formed crystalline solid was filtered off and washed with THF.

Yield 47 g (70%). Melting point coincides with that given in the literature [38].
IR (KBr), ν, cm^{-1}: 2670 (OH), 3320 (NH), 1718, 1590 (2 C=O).
^{1}H NMR (400 MHz, DMSO-d_6) δ: 1.96 (s, 3H, CH_3), 2.47 (t, *J* = 6.9 Hz, 2H, CH_2CO), 3.20 (t, *J* = 8.7 Hz, 2H, NHC*H*$_2$), 3.77 (s, 1H, *N*HCH$_2$), 6.50 (d, *J* = 8.7 Hz, 2H, H_{Ar}), 7.27 (d, *J* = 8.7 Hz, 2H, H_{Ar}), 9.51 (s, 1H, NHCO), 11.81 (br s, 1H, COOH).
^{13}C NMR (101 MHz, DMSO-d_6) δ: 23.72 (CH_3), 33.83 (CH_2CO), 39.21 ($NHCH_2$), 112.04, 120.91, 128.81, 144.75, 167.28, 173.31 (C_{Ar}, CH_3CO, COOH).
Anal. Calcd. for $C_{11}H_{14}N_2O_3$, %: C 59.45; H 6.35; N 12.60. Found, %: C 59.56; H 6.31; N 12.71.
N-[4-(tetrahydro-4-oxo-2-thioxo-1(2*H*)-pyrimidinyl)phenyl]acetamide (**3**)
A mixture of *β*-alanine (**2**) (10 g, 45 mmol), potassium thiocyanate (13.10 g, 135 mmol), and acetic acid (25 mL) was heated at reflux for 24 h then cooled to room temperature and diluted with 100 mL of water. The formed precipitate was filtered off and washed with water. Yield 8.53 g (72%), m. p. 227−228 °C (from ethanol).
IR (KBr), ν, cm^{-1}: 3401−3115 (2 NH), 1683, 1598 (2 C=O).
^{1}H NMR (400 MHz, DMSO-d_6) δ: 2.05 (s, 3H, CH_3), 2.79 (t, *J* = 6.9 Hz, 2H, CH_2CO), 3.87 (t, *J* = 6.9 Hz, 2H, NCH_2), 7.25 (d, *J* = 8.6 Hz, 2H, H_{Ar}), 7.60 (d, *J* = 8.6 Hz, 2H, H_{Ar}), 10.05 (s, 1H, NH), 11.20 (s, 1H, NH).
^{13}C NMR (101 MHz, DMSO-d_6) δ: 23.99 (CH_3), 30.43 (CH_2CO), 48.88 (NCH_2), 119.36, 127.27, 138.35, 139.93, 166.97, 168.37, 179.40 (C_{Ar}, CH_3CO, $COCH_2$, C=S).
Anal. Calcd. for $C_{12}H_{13}N_3O_2S$, %: C 54.74; H 4.98; N 15.96. Found, %: C 54.84; H 5.03; N 15.84.
3-[(4-Acetamidophenyl)(carbamothioyl)amino]propanoic acid (**4**)
Compound **3** (7.90 g, 30 mmol) was dissolved in hot, aqueous 5% sodium hydroxide (22 mL), and the obtained solution was filtered off. After cooling to room temperature, the solution was acidified with acetic acid to pH 6. The formed solid was filtered off and washed with water.
Yield 7.93 g (94%), m.p. 137−138 °C (from ethanol).
IR (KBr), ν, cm^{-1}: 3404−3167 (NH, OH), 1657, 1596 (2 C=O).
^{1}H NMR (400 MHz, DMSO-d_6) δ: 2.06 (s, 3H, CH_3), 2.53 (t, *J* = 8.1 Hz, 2H, CH_2CO), 4.15 (t, *J* = 7.8 Hz, 2H, NCH_2), 6.40 (br. s, 2H, NH_2CS), 7.14 (d, *J* = 8.4 Hz, 2H, H_{Ar}), 7.66 (d, *J* = 8.4 Hz, 2H, H_{Ar}), 10.14 (s, 1H, NH), 12.22 (br. s, 1H, COOH).
^{13}C NMR (101 MHz, DMSO-d_6) δ: 24.02 (CH_3), 32.21 (CH_2CO), 50.38 (NCH_2), 120.04, 128.08, 136.21, 138.98, 168.45, 172.46, 181.68 (C_{Ar}, CH_3CO, COOH, C=S).
Anal. Calcd. for $C_{12}H_{15}N_3O_3S$, %: C 51.23; H 5.37; N 14.94. Found, %: C 51.38; H 5.47; N 14.77.
General procedure for the preparation of compounds **5a–e.**

To a solution of thioureido acid **4** (0.56 g, 2 mmol) and Na_2CO_3 (0.64 g, 6 mmol) in water (10 mL), the corresponding bromoacetophenone (2.4 mmol) was added, and the mixture was heated at reflux for 3 h. After completion of the reaction (TLC), the hot reaction mixture was filtered off, and the filtrate was acidified with acetic acid to pH 6. The formed precipitate was filtered off, washed with water, and purified by dissolving it in aqueous Na_2CO_3 solution (5 g, 40 mL of water), before filtering and acidifying the filtrate with acetic acid to pH 6.
3-[(4-Acetamidophenyl)(4-phenyl-1,3-thiazol-2-yl)amino]propanoic acid (**5a**)
Yield 0.53 g (69%), m. p. 132–133 °C.
IR (KBr), ν, cm^{-1}: 3305–3129 (NH, OH), 1694, 1632 (2 C=O).
^{1}H NMR (400 MHz, DMSO-d_6) δ: 2.07 (s, 3H, CH_3), 2.58 (t, *J* = 7.3 Hz, 2H, CH_2CO), 4.12 (t, *J* = 7.5 Hz, 2H, NCH_2), 7.10 (s, 1H, H_{Ar}), 7.28 (t, *J* = 7.3 Hz, 1H, H_{Ar}), 7.31–7.47 (m, 4H, H_{Ar}), 7.68 (d, *J* = 8.7 Hz, 2H, H_{Ar}); 7.86 (d, *J* = 7.8 Hz, 2H, H_{Ar}), 10.14 (s, 1H, NH).
^{13}C NMR (101 MHz, DMSO-d_6) δ: 24.01 (CH_3), 33.27 (CH_2CO), 49.10 (NCH_2), 102.49, 120.21, 125.66, 127.46, 127.63, 128.53, 134.73, 138.50, 139.28, 150.40, 168.43, 169.29, 173.16 (C_{Ar}, CH_3CO, COOH).

Anal. Calcd. For $C_{20}H_{19}N_3O_3S$, %: C 62.98; H 5.02; N 11.02. Found, %: C 63.05; H 5.19; N 11.10.

3-{(4-Acetamidophenyl)[4-(4-fluorophenyl)-1,3-thiazol-2-yl]amino}propanoic acid (**5b**)

Yield 0.52 g (65%), m. p. 125–126 °C.

IR (KBr), ν, cm-1: 3419–3112 (NH, OH), 1666, 1598 (2 C=O).

1H NMR (400 MHz, DMSO-d_6) δ: 2.06 (s, 3H, CH_3), 2.50–2.57 (signal of the CH_2CO (2H) overlaps with the DMSO-d_6), 4.09 (t, J = 7.4 Hz, 2H, NCH_2), 7.07 (s, 1H, H_{Ar}), 7.21 (t, J = 8.7 Hz, 2H, H_{Ar}), 7.36 (d, J = 8.5 Hz, 2H, H_{Ar}), 7.68 (d, J = 8.5 Hz, 2H, H_{Ar}), 7.89 (dd, J = 8.0, 5.9 Hz, 2H, H_{Ar}), 10.19 (s, 1H, NH).

13C NMR (101 MHz, DMSO-d_6) δ: 24.00 (CH_3), 33.94 (CH_2CO), 49.59 (NCH_2), 102.09, 115.24, 115.45, 120.21, 127.59, 127.67, 131.36, 138.47, 139.30, 149.35, 160.36, 162.78, 168.45, 169.40; 173.54 (C_{Ar}, CH_3CO, COOH).

Anal. Calcd. For $C_{20}H_{18}FN_3O_3S$, %: C 60.14; H 4.54; N 10.52. Found, %: C 60.26; H 4.47; N 10.43.

3-{(4-Acetamidophenyl)[4-(4-chlorophenyl)-1,3-thiazol-2-yl]amino}propanoic acid (**5c**)

Yield 0.52 g (63%), m. p. 194–195 °C.

IR (KBr), ν, cm^{-1}: 3294–3054 (NH, OH), 1672, 1600 (2 C=O).

^1H NMR (400 MHz, DMSO-d_6) δ: 2.07 (s, 3H, CH_3), 2.66 (t, J = 7.2 Hz, 2H, CH_2CO), 4.15 (t, J = 7.2 Hz, 2H, NCH_2), 7.19 (s, 1H, H_{Ar}), 7.37 (d, J = 8.7 Hz, 2H, H_{Ar}), 7.45 (d, J = 8.5 Hz, 2H, H_{Ar}), 7.69 (d, J = 8.7 Hz, 2H, H_{Ar}), 7.87 (d, J = 8.5 Hz, 2H, H_{Ar}), 10,13 (s, 1H, NH).

^{13}C NMR (101 MHz, DMSO-d_6) δ: 24.02 (CH_3), 32.35 (CH_2CO), 48.50 (NCH_2), 103.50, 120.28, 127.37, 127.75, 128.58, 128.88, 129.55, 131.93, 138.73, 139.00, 168.48, 169.55, 172.64 (C_{Ar}, CH_3CO, COOH).

Anal. Calcd. For $C_{20}H_{18}ClN_3O_3S$, %: C 57.76; H 4.36; N 10.10. Found, %: C 57.57; H 4.21; N 10.22.

3-{(4-Acetamidophenyl)[4-(4-cianophenyl)-1,3-thiazol-2-yl]amino}propanoic acid (**5d**)

Yield 0.66 g (81%). M. p. 181–182 °C.

IR (KBr), ν, cm^{-1}: 3332–2972 (NH, OH), 1688, 1605 (2 C=O).

^1H NMR (400 MHz, DMSO-d_6) δ: 2.07 (s, 3H, CH_3), 2.62 (t, J = 7.3 Hz, 2H, CH_2CO), 4.14 (t, J = 7.3 Hz, 2H, NCH_2), 7.37 (d, J = 8.7 Hz, 2H, H_{Ar}), 7.42 (s, 1H, H_{Ar}), 7.69 (d, J = 8.7 Hz, 2H, H_{Ar}), 7.85 (d, J = 8.3 Hz, 2H, H_{Ar}), 8.04 (d, J = 8.3 Hz, 2H, H_{Ar}), 10.13 (s, 1H, NH).

^{13}C NMR (101 MHz, DMSO-d_6) δ: 24.02 (CH_3), 32.82 (CH_2CO), 48.88 (NCH_2), 106.41, 109.51, 119.07, 120.28, 126.24, 127.74, 132.64, 138.74, 138.78, 138.97, 148.65, 168.48, 169.65, 172.87 (C_{Ar}, CH_3CO, COOH).

Anal. Calcd. For $C_{21}H_{18}N_4O_3S$, %: C 62.05; H 4.46; N 13.78. Found, %: C 61.97; H 4.53; N 13.57.

3-{(4-Acetamidophenyl)[4-(4-trifluoromethylphenyl)-1,3-thiazol-2-yl]amino}propanoic acid (**5e**)

Yield 0.84 g (94%), m. p. 205–206 °C.

IR (KBr), ν, cm^{-1}: 3407–3168 (NH, OH), 1741, 1707 (2 C=O).

^1H NMR (400 MHz, DMSO-d_6) δ: 2.07 (s, 3H, CH_3); 2.41 (t, J = 7.9 Hz, 2H, CH_2CO), 4,09 (t, J = 7.9 Hz, 2H, NCH_2), 7.32 (s, 1H, H_{Ar}), 7.36 (d, J = 8.6 Hz, 2H, H_{Ar}), 7.70 (d, J = 8.6 Hz, 2H, H_{Ar}), 7.73 (d, J = 8.3 Hz, 2H, H_{Ar}), 8.06 (d, J = 8.3 Hz, 2H, H_{Ar}), 10.35 (s, 1H, NH).

^{13}C NMR (101 MHz, DMSO-d_6) δ: 23.99 (CH_3), 35.09 (CH_2CO), 50.32 (NCH_2), 104.94, 120.24, 123.06, 125.53, 126.15, 127.59, 138.50, 138.55, 139.25, 148.88, 168.50, 169.66, 173.68, 174.42 (C_{Ar}, CH_3CO, COOH).

Anal. Calcd. For $C_{21}H_{18}N_3F_3O_3S$, %: C 56.12; H 4.04; N 9.35. Found, %: C 56.04; H 4.09; N 9.31.

General procedure for the preparation of derivatives **6a–e**

A solution of the corresponding compound **5a–e** (1.5 mmol) in aqueous 5% hydrochloric acid (20 mL) was refluxed for 1 h, cooled down, and evaporated under reduced pressure; then, the residue was dissolved in water, and the solution was neutralized with sodium acetate to pH 6. The formed precipitate was filtered off and recrystallized from 2-propanol.

3-[(4-Aminophenyl)(4-phenylthiazol-2-yl)amino]propanoic acid (**6a**)

Yield 0.45 g (88%), m. p. 194–195 °C.
IR (KBr), ν, cm^{-1}: 3294–3054 (NH, OH), 1672, 1600 (2 C=O).
^{1}H NMR (400 MHz, DMSO-d_6) δ: 2.63 (t, *J* = 6.5 Hz, 2H, CH_2CO), 4.08 (t, *J* = 7.0 Hz, 2H, NCH_2), 5.36 (br. s, 2H, NH_2), 6.63 (d, *J* = 8.2 Hz, 2H, H_{Ar}), 6.99–7.11 (m, 3H, H_{Ar}), 7.27–7.42 (m, 3H, H_{Ar}), 7.85 (d, *J* = 7.5 Hz, 2H, H_{Ar}), 12.22 (br. s, 1H, OH).
^{13}C NMR (101 MHz, DMSO-d_6) δ: 32.41 (CH_2CO), 48.41 (NCH_2), 102.38, 114.68, 125.61, 127.37, 128.50, 128.59, 132.60, 134.88, 148.64, 150.41, 170.64, 172.78 (C_{Ar}, COOH).
Anal. Calcd. for $C_{18}H_{17}N_3O_2S$, %: C 63.70; H 5.05; N 12.38. Found, %: C 57.57; H 4.21; N 10.22.
3-{(4-Aminophenyl)[4-(4-fluorophenyl)-1,3-thiazol-2-yl]amino}propanoic acid (**6b**)
Yield 0.46 g (86%), m. p. 194–195 °C.
IR (KBr), ν, cm^{-1}: 3294–3054 (NH, OH); 1672, 1600 (2 C=O).
^{1}H NMR (400 MHz, DMSO-d_6) δ: 2.62 (t, *J* = 7.3 Hz, 2H, CH_2CO), 4.06 (t, *J* = 7.3 Hz, 2H, NCH_2), 5.33 (br. s, 2H, NH_2), 6.62 (d, *J* = 8.5 Hz, 2H, H_{Ar}), 7.00–7.07 (m, 3H, H_{Ar}), 7.21 (t, *J* = 8.8 Hz, 2H, H_{Ar}), 7.88 (dd, *J* = 8.4, 5.8 Hz, 2H, H_{Ar}), 12.22 (br. s, 1H, OH).
^{13}C NMR (101 MHz, DMSO-d_6) δ: 32.40 (CH_2CO), 48.41 (NCH_2), 102.11, 114.67, 115.22, 15.43, 127.52, 127.60, 128.57, 131.50, 132.53, 148.66, 149.34, 160.31, 162.73, 170.73, 172.75 (C_{Ar}, COOH).
Anal. Calcd. for $C_{18}H_{16}FN_3O_2S$, %: C 60.49; H 4.51; N 11.76. Found, %: C 57.57; H 4.21; N 10.22.
3-{(4-Aminophenyl)[4-(4-chlorophenyl)-1,3-thiazol-2-yl]amino}propanoic acid (**6c**)
Yield 0.46 g (82%), m. p. 171–172 °C.
IR (KBr), ν, cm^{-1}: 3368–1974 (NH, OH), 1698 (C=O).
^{1}H NMR (400 MHz, DMSO-d_6) δ: 2.44–2.49 (signal overlaps with the DMSO-d_6, 2H, CH_2CO), 4.01 (t, *J* = 7.3 Hz, 2H, NCH_2), 5,34 (br s, 2H, NH_2), 6.62 (d, *J* = 8.3 Hz, 2H, H_{Ar}), 7.01 (d, *J* = 8.3 Hz, 2H, H_{Ar}), 7.08 (s, 1H, CH), 7.43 (d, *J* = 8.4 Hz, 2H, H_{Ar}), 7.86 (d, *J* = 8.4 Hz, 2H, H_{Ar}).
^{13}C NMR (101 MHz, DMSO-d_6) δ: 33.91 (CH_2CO), 49.37 (NCH_2), 102.82, 114.65, 127.28, 128.48; 128.54, 131.64, 132.71, 133.78, 148.53, 149.14, 170.75 (C_{Ar}, COOH).
Anal. Calcd. for $C_{18}H_{16}ClN_3O_2S$, %: C 57.83; H 4.31; N 11.24. Found, %: C 57.71; H 4.27; N 11.21.
3-{(4-Aminophenyl)[4-(4-cianophenyl)-1,3-thiazol-2-yl]amino}propanoic acid (**6d**)
Yield 0.44 g (81%), m. p. 171–172 °C.
IR (KBr), ν, cm^{-1}: 3368–1974 (NH, OH), 1698 (C=O).
^{1}H NMR (400 MHz, DMSO-d_6) δ: 2.62 (t, *J* = 6.6 Hz, 2H, CH_2CO), 4.08 (t, *J* = 6.6 Hz, 2H, NCH_2), 5,37 (br s, 2H, NH_2), 6.63 (d, *J* = 8.0 Hz, 2H, H_{Ar}), 7.04 (d, *J* = 8.0 Hz, 2H, H_{Ar}), 7.35 (s, 1H, CH), 7.84 (d, *J* = 7.8 Hz, 2H, H_{Ar}), 8.03 (d, *J* = 7.8 Hz, 2H, H_{Ar}), 12.26 (br. s, 1H, OH).
^{13}C NMR (101 MHz, DMSO-d_6) δ: 32.36 (CH_2CO), 48.44 (NCH_2), 106.24, 109.36, 114.69, 119.08, 126.17, 128.56, 132.32, 132.59, 138.93, 148.65, 148.76, 170.93, 172.73 (C_{Ar}, COOH).
Anal. Calcd. for $C_{19}H_{16}N_4O_2S$, %: C 62.62; H 4.43; N 15.37. Found, %: C 57.71; H 4.27; N 11.21.
3-((4-Aminophenyl){4-[4-(trifluoromethyl)phenyl]thiazol-2-yl}amino)propanoic acid (**6e**)
Yield 0.55 g (90%), m. p. 194–195 °C.
IR (KBr), ν, cm^{-1}: 3294–3054 (NH, OH); 1672, 1600 (2 C=O).
^{1}H NMR (400 MHz, DMSO-d_6) δ: 2.62 (t, *J* = 7.3 Hz, 2H, CH_2CO), 4.09 (t, *J* = 7.3 Hz, 2H, NCH_2), 5.36 (br. s, 2H, NH_2), 6.63 (d, *J* = 8.4 Hz, 2H, H_{Ar}), 7.04 (d, *J* = 8.4 Hz, 2H, H_{Ar}), 7.28 (s, 1H, CH), 7.74 (d, *J* = 8.2 Hz, 2H, H_{Ar}), 8.06 (d, *J* = 8.2 Hz, 2H, H_{Ar}), 12.27 (br. s, 1H, OH).
^{13}C NMR (101 MHz, DMSO-d_6) δ: 32.39 (CH_2CO), 48.40 (NCH_2), 105.18, 114.71, 123.06, 125.49, 125.53, 125.76, 126.10, 127.24, 127.55, 128.60, 132.37, 138.56, 148.77, 148.88, 170.98, 172.75 (C_{Ar}, COOH).
Anal. Calcd. for $C_{19}H_{16}F_3N_3O_2S$, %: C 56.01; H 3.96; N 10.31. Found, %: C 57.57; H 4.21; N 10.22.
3-[(4-Acetamidophenyl)(4-oxo-4,5-dihydro-1,3-thiazol-2-yl)amino]propanoic acid (**7**)

To a solution of thioureido acid **4** (8.44 g, 30 mmol) and sodium carbonate (9.02 g, 90 mmol) in water (35 mL), monochloroacetic acid (5.67 g, 60 mmol) was added, and the mixture was heated at reflux for 3 h. After completion of the reaction, the mixture was cooled down and acidified with acetic acid to pH 6. The formed precipitate was filtered off and washed with water.
Yield 6.75 g (70%), m. p. 133–134 °C (from ethanol).
IR (KBr), ν, cm^{-1}: 3542–3253 (NH, OH), 1716, 1694, 1667 (3 C=O).
^1H NMR (400 MHz, DMSO-d_6) δ: 2.07 (s, 3H, CH_3), 2.55 (t, *J* = 7.3 Hz, 2H, CH_2CO), 3.91 (s, 2H, SCH_2), 4.13 (t, *J* = 7.3 Hz, 2H, NCH_2), 7.37 (d, *J* = 8.6 Hz, 2H, H_{Ar}), 7.69 (d, *J* = 8.6 Hz, 2H, H_{Ar}), 10.18 (s, 1H, NH); 12.38 (br. s, 1H, COOH).
^{13}C NMR (101 MHz, DMSO-d_6) δ: 24.07 (CH_3), 31.94 (CH_2CO), 40.59 (SCH_2), 49.97 (NCH_2), 119.69, 128.60, 134.62, 140.24, 168.73, 171.99, 183.44, 187.06 (C_{Ar}, CH_3C=O, COOH, NC=O).
Anal. Calcd. for $C_{14}H_{15}N_3O_4S$, %: C 52.33; H 4.70; N 13.08. Found, %: C 52.54; H 4.68; N 13.16.
General procedure for the preparation of 3-{(4-acetamidophenyl)[5-(phenylmethyliden)-4-oxo-4,5-dihydro-1,3-thiazol-2-yl]amino}propanoic acids **8a–d.**

To a solution of compound **7** (1.6 g, 5 mmol) and sodium carbonate (2.12 g, 20 mmol) in water (10 mL), the corresponding benzaldehyde (4.7 mmol) was added, and the mixture was heated at reflux for 3 h. Then, the mixture was cooled down and acidified with acetic acid to pH 6. The formed was filtered off and washed with water. The purification was performed by dissolving in aqueous sodium carbonate solution (5 g, 60 mL of water) and filtering and acidifying the filtrate with acetic acid to pH 6.
3-[(4-Acetamidophenyl)(5-benzylidene-4-oxo-4,5-dihydro-1,3-thiazol-2-yl)amino]propanoic acid (**8a**)
Yield 1.76 g (86%), m. p. 227–228 °C.
IR (KBr), ν, cm^{-1}: 3419–3112 (NH, OH), 1673, 1599, 1685 (3 C=O).
^1H NMR (400 MHz, DMSO-d_6) δ: 2.09 (s, 3H, CH_3), 2.31 (t, *J* = 7.8 Hz, 2H, CH_2CO), 4.17 (t, *J* = 7.8 Hz, 2H, NCH_2), 7.21–7.54 (m, 7H, H_{Ar}), 7.60 (s, 1H, CH), 7.77 (d, *J* = 8.5 Hz, 2H, H_{Ar}), 10.60 (s, 1H, NH).
^{13}C NMR (101 MHz, DMSO-d_6) δ: 24.05 (CH_3), 35.10 (CH_2CO), 52.24 (NCH_2), 119.74, 128.68, 129.21, 129.39, 129.48, 129.67, 129.79, 133.79, 134.58, 140.54, 168.87, 173.35, 175.86, 179.69 (C_{Ar}, CH_3CO, COOH, NCO).
Anal. Calcd. for $C_{21}H_{19}N_3O_4S$, %: C 61.60; H 4.68; N 10.26. Found, %: C 61.35; H 4.55; N 10.33.
3-((4-Acetamidophenyl){5-[(4-fluorophenyl)methylidene]-4-oxo-4,5-dihydro-1,3-thiazol-2-yl}amino)propanoic acid (**8b**)
Yield 1.43 g (67%), m. p. 220–221 °C.
IR (KBr), ν, cm^{-1}: 3305–3115 (NH, OH), 1670, 1532, 1595 (3 C=O).
^1H NMR (700 MHz, DMSO-d_6) δ: 2.09 (s, 3H, CH_3), 2.40 (t, *J* = 7.6 Hz, 2H, CH_2CO), 4.18 (t, *J* = 7.6 Hz, 2H, NCH_2), 7.27 (t, *J* = 8.6 Hz, 3H, H_{Ar}), 7.38–7.55 (m, 4H, H_{Ar}), 7.61 (s, 1H, CH=), 7.75 (d, *J* = 8.4 Hz, 2H, H_{Ar}), 10.47 (s, 1H, NH).
^{13}C NMR (176 MHz, DMSO-d_6) δ: 24.06 (CH_3), 34.09 (CH_2CO), 51.53 (NCH_2), 116.23, 116.45, 119.77, 128.71, 128.88, 129.15, 129.18, 130.43, 131.72, 131.81, 134.49, 140.53, 161.22, 163.70, 168.86, 172.92, 175.96, 179.61 (C_{Ar}, CH, CH_3CO, COOH, NC=O).
Anal. Calcd. for $C_{21}H_{18}FN_3O_4S$, %: C 59.01; H 4.24; N 9.83. Found, %: C 51.35; H 4.11; N 11.89.
3-((4-Acetamidophenyl){5-[(4-chlorophenyl)methylidene]-4-oxo-4,5-dihydro-1,3-thiazol-2-yl}amino)propanoic acid (**8c**)
Yield 1.55 g (70%). m.p. 228–229 °C.
IR (KBr), ν, cm^{-1}: 3283–3123 (NH, OH), 1710, 1653, 1683 (3 C=O).
^1H NMR (400 MHz, DMSO-d_6) δ: 2.09 (s, 3H, CH_3), 2.55 (d, *J* = 7.4 Hz, 2H, CH_2CO), 4.21 (t, *J* = 7.4 Hz, 2H, NCH_2), 7.30–7.88 (m, 9H, H_{Ar} + CH), 10.32 (s, 1H, NH).

^{13}C NMR (101 MHz, DMSO-d_6) δ: 24.07 (CH_3), 32.64 (CH_2CO), 50.56 (NCH_2), 119.75, 128.72, 128.88, 129.29, 129.98, 131.08, 132.62, 134.26, 140.54, 168.80, 172.21, 176.12, 179.45 (C_{Ar}, CH_3CO, COOH, NCO).
Anal. Calcd. for $C_{21}H_{18}ClN_3O_4S$, %: C 56.82; H 4.09; N 9.47.
Found, %: C 51.35; H 4.11; N 11.89.
3-((4-Acetamidophenyl){5-[(4-bromophenyl)methylidene]-4-oxo-4,5-dihydro-1,3-thiazol-2-yl}amino)propanoic acid (**8d**)
Yield 1.61 g (66%), m. p. 243–244 °C.
IR (KBr), ν, cm^{-1}: 3279–3054 (NH, OH), 1708, 1653, 1683 (3 C=O).
^{1}H NMR (400 MHz, DMSO-d_6) δ: 2.09 (s, 3H, CH_3), 2.55 (d, J = 7.4 Hz, 2H, CH_2CO), 4.22 (t, J = 7.4 Hz, 2H, NCH_2), 7.38 (d, J = 8.4 Hz, 2H, H_{Ar}), 7.47 (d, J = 8.6 Hz, 2H, H_{Ar}), 7.59 (s, 1H, CH), 7.63 (d, J = 8.4 Hz, 2H, H_{Ar}), 7.74 (d, J = 8.6 Hz, 2H, H_{Ar}), 10.30 (s, 1H, NH).
^{13}C NMR (101 MHz, DMSO-d_6) δ: 24.10 (CH_3), 32.46 (CH_2CO), 50.45 (NCH_2), 119.82, 123.19, 128.76, 129.08, 130.08, 131.31, 132.27, 132.97, 134.29, 140.57, 168.89, 172.15, 176.22, 179.51 (C_{Ar}, CH_3CO, COOH, NCO).
Anal. Calcd. for $C_{21}H_{18}BrN_3O_4S$, %: C 51.65; H 3.72; N 8.60. Found, %: C 51.34; H 3.62; N 8.36.
3-((4-Aminophenyl)(4-(4-chlorobenzylidene)-5-oxo-4,5-dihydrothiazol-2-yl)amino) propanoic acid (**9**)
Compound **8c** (0.25 g, 0.56 mmol) was dissolved in 5% hydrochloric acid 6 mL, and the obtained mixture was refluxed for 1 h. Then, the mixture was cooled down and neutralized with sodium acetate to pH 6. The formed precipitate was filtered off.
Yield 0.23 g (92%). m. p. 192–193 °C (from 2-propanol).
IR (KBr), ν, cm^{-1}: 3401; 3050 (NH_2, OH), 1735, 1591 (2 CO).
^{1}H NMR (400 MHz, DMSO-d_6) δ: 2.54 (t, J = 7,5 Hz, 2H, CH_2CO), 4.15 (t, J = 7,6 Hz, 2H, NCH_2), 5.61 (br. s, 2H, NH_2), 6.64 (d, J = 8,2 Hz, 2H, H_{Ar}), 7.12 (d, J = 8,2 Hz, 2H, H_{Ar}), 7.48 (dd, J = 11,4, 5,0 Hz, 4H, H_{Ar}), 7.59 (s, 1H, CH).
^{13}C NMR (101 MHz, DMSO-d_6) δ: 32.23 (CH_2CO), 50.26 (NCH_2), 114.01, 127.47, 128.44, 128.78, 129.29, 130.45, 131.02, 132.74, 134.14, 150.09, 168.79, 176.62, 179.58 (C_{Ar}, COOH, NCO).
Anal. Calcd. for $C_{19}H_{16}ClN_3O_3S$, %: C 56.98; H 4.15; N 10.60.
Found, %: C 56.79; H 4.01; N 10.46.
1-(4-Aminophenyl)-2-thioxotetrahydropyrimidin-4(1*H*)-one (**10**)
Compound **3** (0.39 g, 1.5 mmol) was dissolved in 5% hydrochloric acid 15 mL, and the obtained mixture was boiled for 1 h. Then, the mixture was cooled down and neutralized with sodium acetate to pH 6. The formed precipitate was filtered off and washed with water.
Yield 0.23 g (70%). m. p. 219–220 °C (from 2-propanol).
IR (KBr), ν, cm^{-1}: 3399; 3325 (NH_2, NH); 1712 (CO).
^{1}H NMR (400 MHz, DMSO-d_6) δ: 2.75 (t, J = 6,9 Hz, 2H, CH_2CO), 3.80 (t, J = 6,9, Hz, 2H, NCH_2), 5.20 (br. s, 2H, NH_2), 6.54 (d, J = 8,4 Hz, 2H, H_{Ar}), 6.93 (d, J = 8,3 Hz, 2H, H_{Ar}), 11,06 (br. s, 1H, NH).
^{13}C NMR (101 MHz, DMSO-d_6) δ: 32.46 (CH_2CO), 50.45 (NCH_2), 119.82, 123.19, 128.76, 129.08, 130.08, 131.31, 132.27, 132.97, 134.29, 140.57, 168.89, 172.15, 176.22, 179.51 (C_{Ar}, CO, CS).
Anal. Calcd. for $C_{10}H_{11}ClN_3OS$, %: C 54,28; H 5,01; N 18,99.
Found, %: C 54.23; H 4.99; N 18.89.
3-(1-(4-Aminophenyl)thioureido)propanoic acid (**11**)
Compound **9** (0.5 g, 2,26 mmol) was dissolved in hot, aqueous 5% sodium hydroxide (10 mL), and the obtained solution was filtered off. After cooling to room temperature, the solution was acidified with 5% HCl to pH 6. The formed solid was filtered off and washed with water.
Yield 0.47 g (87%). m. p. 171–172 °C (from 2-propanol).
IR (KBr), ν, cm^{-1}: 3407; 3340; 3276 (2× NH_2, OH); 1742 (CO).

^{1}H NMR (400 MHz, DMSO-d_6) δ: 2.48–2.50 (signal of the CH_2CO (2H) overlaps with the DMSO-d_6), 4.12 (t, *J* = 6.9, Hz, 2H, NCH_2), 5.32 (br. s, 2H, NH_2CS), 6.59 (d, *J* = 8.5 Hz, 2H, H_{Ar}), 6.84 (d, *J* = 8.5 Hz, 2H, H_{Ar}), 7.45 (br. s., 2H, NH_2), 12.30 (br. s, 1H, OH).
^{13}C NMR (101 MHz, DMSO-d_6) δ: 32.26 (CH_2CO), 50.55 (NCH_2), 114.63, 128.02, 148.63, 172.59, 181.71 (C_{Ar}, CO, CS).
Anal. Calcd. for $C_{10}H_{13}N_3O_2S$, %: C 50.29; H 5.48; N 17.56.
Found, %: C 50.21; H 5.45; N 17.56.

4.2. Cell lines and Culture Conditions

MDCK cells were kindly provided by Dr. Mirella Salvatore (Department of Medicine, Division of Infectious Diseases, Weill Cornell Medicine of Cornell University) and were maintained in Dulbecco's MEM (Life Technologies, Burlington, ON, Canada) (DMEM) supplemented with 10% fetal blood serum (FBS), 100 U/mL penicillin, and 100 μg/mL streptomycin. A549 cells were obtained from American Type Culture Collection (ATCC, Manassas, VA, USA) and were cultured in Dulbecco's Modified Eagle Medium/Nutrient Mixture F-12 media supplemented with 10% FBS, 100 U/mL penicillin, and 100 μg/mL streptomycin.

4.3. Cytotoxicity Assay

The cytotoxicity of compounds **3–11** on A549 human lung cells were evaluated by using a commercial MTT assay (CyQUANT MTT Cell Viability Assay, Thermo Fisher Scientific, Eugene, Oregon, USA). A549 was plated to flat-bottomed 96-well plates (1 × 10^4 cells/well) and incubated overnight to facilitate the attachment. The compounds at fixed 100 μM concentration were added, and plates were further incubated for 48 h at 37 °C, 5% CO_2. After incubation, the commercial MTT reagent was added, and the % of viability was determined, in accordance with the description of the manufacturer, using untreated cells as a control. All experiments were performed in triplicate.

4.4. Viral Infection Assay

To determine the potential antiviral activity of compounds **3–11** on the virus replication in MDCK cells, we used virus-induced cell death as an experimental output. Briefly, MDCK cells were plated to flat-bottomed 96-well plates (1 × 10^4 cells/well) and incubated overnight to facilitate the attachment. After incubation, the media was removed, cells were gently washed twice with DPBS, and the compounds (100 μM) were dissolved in DMEM supplemented with 5% bovine serum albumin (BSA), 2 μg/mL TPCK-treated trypsin (Thermo Fisher Scientific, Rockford, Illinois, USA), 100 U/mL penicillin, and 100 μg/mL streptomycin. The oseltamivir and amantadine (100 μM) were used as a comparator. Cells were incubated with compounds for 1 h at 37 °C, 5% CO_2, and were then infected with influenza A/Puerto Rico/8/34 H1N1 strain at MOI 1:5. The infected cells were then further incubated for 24 h to facilitate the infection, and the remaining post-infection viability was measured by using MTT assay.

4.5. Measurement of Antioxidant Activities

4.5.1. Ferric ion (Fe^{3+}) Reducing Antioxidant Power (Fe^3 – Fe^{2+} Transformation Assay)

Newly synthesized compounds **3–11** of concentration 20 mM in 0.5 mL of DMSO were mixed with phosphate buffer (1.25 mL, 0.2 M, pH 6.6) and potassium ferricyanide [$K_3Fe(CN)_6$] (1.25 mL, 1%). The mixture was incubated at 50 °C for 20 min. Aliquots (1.25 mL) of trichloroacetic acid (10%) were added to the mixture, which was then centrifuged for 10 min at 9000 rpm. The upper layer of solution (1.25 mL) was mixed with distilled water (1.25 mL) and $FeCl_3$ (0.25 mL, 0.1%), and the absorbance was measured at 700 nm in a spectrophotometer [47,48]. Butylhydroxytoluene (BHT) was used as a positive control.

4.5.2. Ferric Reducing Antioxidant Power Assay (FRAP)

Reducing properties were investigated using the FRAP method, which is based on the reduction of a ferric-tripyridyl triazine complex to its ferrous-colored form in the presence of antioxidants [49]. The FRAP reagent contained 2.5 mL of 10 mM TPTZ (2,4,6-tripyridyl-*s*-triazine) solution in 40 mM HCl as well as 2.5 mL of $FeCl_3$ (20 mM) and 25 mL of acetate buffer (0.3 M, pH = 3.6). Then, 100 μL of analyzed compounds (20 mM) were mixed with 3 mL of the FRAP reagent. The absorbance of the reaction mixture was measured spectrophotometrically at 593 nm. For comprising the calibration curve, five concentrations of $FeSO_4 \cdot 7H_2O$ (5, 10, 15, 20, 25 μM) were used, and the absorbance was measured as a sample solution. Each experiment was repeated three times.

4.5.3. 1,1-Diphenyl-2-picrylhydrazyl (DPPH) Radical Scavenging Assay

The free-radical-scavenging activity of **3–11** compounds was measured by the DPPH method [48,50]. Firstly, a solution (20 mM) of **3–11** compounds was prepared in DMSO. Then, a 1 mM solution of DPPH in ethanol was prepared, and 1 mL of this solution was added to the solutions of the analyzed compounds. The mixture was vigorously stirred and allowed to stand at room temperature. After 20 min, the absorbance of the reaction mixture was measured at 517 nm with a UV-1280 spectrophotometer (Shimadzu, Kyoto, Japan). Each experiment was repeated three time.

4.6. Evaluation of Antibacterial Activity

Antibacterial activity of the compounds was screened by using the disk-diffusion method [51]. In this study, inhibition of bacterial growth was investigated against Gram-positive bacteria *Bacillus subtilis* and Gram-negative bacteria *Escherichia coli*. The solution (20 mM) of the compounds was prepared in DMSO. Bacterial cultures were cultivated in Petri dishes at 37 °C for 24 h on the Luria-Bertani (LB) agar medium. Then, 50 μL inoculum containing bacterial cells were spread across the LB agar medium. Sterile filter-paper disks were soaked in 25 μL of each compound solution, and then the disks were put on the LB agar medium. Ciprofloxacin (20 mM) was used as positive control, and DMSO was used as the negative control. Petri dishes were incubated aerobically at 37 °C and examined for zones of inhibition after 24 h. The inhibition zones (cm) were measured.

5. Conclusions

The obtained results revealed that selected aminothiazole compounds bearing 4-cyanophenyl, 4-chlorophenyl, and 4-trifluoromethylphenyl substituents in the thiazole ring could act, with a built-in capacity, on three targets, with the combination of a single structure with antiviral, antioxidant, and antibacterial activities. Among the synthesized compounds, 3-{(4-aminophenyl)[4-(4-cianophenyl)-1,3-thiazol-2-yl]amino}propanoic acid (**6d**) showed the highest cytotoxic properties. The selected compounds 3-((4-aminophenyl){4-[4-(trifluoromethyl)phenyl]thiazol-2-yl}amino)propanoic acid (**6e**) and 3-{(4-acetamidophenyl) amino}propanoic acid (**5e**) exhibited significant influenza A-targeted antiviral activity. Future work can be focused on application of thiazoles scaffolded in bioluminescent systems to develop novel substrates for luciferase.

Author Contributions: Conceptualization, R.M., V.M. and P.K.; methodology, R.M., B.G., I.J., I.T., R.V. and V.M.; formal analysis, V.M., B.G., P.K. and I.J.; investigation, R.M., I.J., B.G., P.K., V.P. and R.P.; resources, R.M., I.J. and V.M.; data curation, B.G., I.J., P.K., I.T. and V.M.; writing—original draft preparation, B.G.; I.J., P.K., V.P., R.P. and V.M.; writing—review and editing, I.J., B.G., P.K., V.P., R.P. and V.M.; supervision, V.M. and P.K. All authors have read and agreed to the published version of the manuscript.

Funding: This research was funded by the Doctoral Fund of Kaunas University of Technology No. A-410, approved 26th of June, 2019, and the European Regional Development Fund (Project No. 01.2.2-LMT-K-718-02-0023) under a grant agreement with the Research Council of Lithuania (LMTLT).

Institutional Review Board Statement: Not applicable.

Informed Consent Statement: Not applicable.

Data Availability Statement: Not applicable.

Acknowledgments: The authors thank the Research Council of Lithuania (LMTLT). This research was funded by the European Regional Development Fund (project no. 01.2.2-LMT-K-718-02-0023) under a grant agreement with the LMTLT.

Conflicts of Interest: The authors declare no conflict of interest.

References

1. Galstyan, A.S.; Martiryan, A.I.; Grigoryan, K.R.; Ghazaryan, A.G.; Samvelyan, M.A.; Ghochikyan, T.V.; Nenajdenko, V.G. Synthesis of Carvone-Derived 1,2,3-Triazoles Study of Their Antioxidant Properties and Interaction with Bovine Serum Albumin. *Molecules* **2018**, *23*, 2991. [CrossRef] [PubMed]
2. Yakan, H. Preparation, structure elucidation, and antioxidant activity of new bis(thiosemicarbazone) derivatives. *Turk. J. Chem.* **2020**, *44*, 1085–1099. [CrossRef] [PubMed]
3. Secci, D.; Carradori, S.; Petzer, A.; Guglielmi, P.; D'Ascenzio, M.; Chimenti, P.; Bagetta, D.; Alcaro, S.; Zengin, G.; Petzer, J.P.; et al. 4-(3-Nitrophenyl)thiazol-2-ylhydrazone derivatives as antioxidants and selective hMAO-B inhibitors: Synthesis, biological activity and computational analysis. *J. Enzym. Inhib. Med. Chem.* **2019**, *34*, 597–612. [CrossRef]
4. Rogolino, D.; Gatti, A.; Carcelli, M.; Pelosi, G.; Bisceglie, F.; Restivo, F.M.; Degola, F.; Buschini, A.; Montalbano, S.; Feretti, D.; et al. Thiosemicarbazone scaffold for the design of antifungal and antiaflatoxigenic agents: Evaluation of ligands and related copper complexes. *Sci. Rep.* **2017**, *7*, 11214. [CrossRef] [PubMed]
5. Cascioferro, S.M.; Parrino, B.; Carbone, D.; Schillaci, D.; Giovannetti, E.; Cirrincione, G.; Diana, P. Thiazoles, Their Benzofused Systems, and Thiazolidinone Derivatives: Versatile and Promising Tools to Combat Antibiotic Resistance. *J. Med. Chem.* **2020**, *63*, 7923–7956. [CrossRef] [PubMed]
6. Mohammad, H.; Reddy, P.V.N.; Monteleone, D.; Mayhoub, A.S.; Cushman, M.; Hammac, G.K.; Seleem, M.N. Antibacterial Characterization of Novel Synthetic Thiazole Compounds against Methicillin-Resistant Staphylococcus pseudintermedius. *PLoS ONE* **2015**, *10*, e0130385. [CrossRef] [PubMed]
7. Ferroni, C.; Pepe, A.; Kim, Y.S.; Lee, S.; Guerrini, A.; Parenti, M.D.; Tesei, A.; Zamagni, A.; Cortesi, M.; Zaffaroni, N.; et al. 1,4-Substituted Triazoles as Nonsteroidal Anti-Androgens for Prostate Cancer Treatment. *J. Med. Chem.* **2017**, *60*, 3082–3093. [CrossRef] [PubMed]
8. dos Santos, B.M.; Gonzaga, D.T.G.; da Silva, F.C.; Ferreira, V.F.; Garcia, C.R.S. *Plasmodium falciparum* Knockout for the GPCR-Like PfSR25 Receptor Displays Greater Susceptibility to 1,2,3-Triazole Compounds That Block Malaria Parasite Development. *Biomolecules* **2020**, *10*, 1197. [CrossRef]
9. Geronikaki, A.; Hadjipavlou-Litina, D.; Zablotskaya, A.; Segal, I. Organosilicon-containing thiazole derivatives as potential lipoxygenase inhibitors and anti inflammatory agents. *Bioinorgan. Chem. Appl.* **2007**, *2007*, 092145. [CrossRef]
10. Almasirad, A.; Mousavi, Z.; Tajik, M.; Assarzadeh, M.J.; Shafiee, A. Synthesis, analgesic and anti-inflammatory activities of new methyl-imidazolyl-1,3,4-oxadiazoles and 1,2,4-triazoles. *DARU J. Pharm. Sci.* **2014**, *22*, 22. [CrossRef]
11. Huuskonen, M.T.; Tuo, Q.-Z.; Loppi, S.; Dhungana, H.; Korhonen, P.; McInnes, L.E.; Donnelly, P.S.; Grubman, A.; Wojciechowski, S.; Lejavova, K.; et al. The Copper bis(thiosemicarbazone) Complex CuII(atsm) Is Protective Against Cerebral Ischemia Through Modulation of the Inflammatory Milieu. *Neurotherapeutics* **2017**, *14*, 519–532. [CrossRef] [PubMed]
12. Sebastian, L.; Desai, A.; Shampur, M.N.; Perumal, Y.; Sriram, D.; Vasanthapuram, R. N-methylisatin-beta-thiosemicarbazone derivative (SCH 16) is an inhibitor of Japanese encephalitis virus infection in vitro and in vivo. *Virol. J.* **2008**, *5*, 64. [CrossRef] [PubMed]
13. McFadden, K.; Fletcher, P.S.; Rossi, F.; Kantharaju Umashankara, M.; Pirrone, V.; Rajagopal, S.; Gopi, H.N.; Krebs, F.C.; Martín-García, J.; Shattock, R.J.; et al. Antiviral Breadth and Combination Potential of Peptide Triazole HIV-1 Entry Inhibitors. *Antimicrob. Agents Chemother.* **2011**, *56*, 1073–1080. [CrossRef] [PubMed]
14. Papadopoulou, M.V.; Trunz, B.B.; Bloomer, W.D.; McKenzie, C.; Wilkinson, S.R.; Prasittichai, C.; Brun, R.; Kaiser, M.; Torreele, E. Novel 3-Nitro-1*H*-1,2,4-triazole-Based Aliphatic and Aromatic Amines as Anti-Chagasic Agents. *J. Med. Chem.* **2011**, *54*, 8214–8223. [CrossRef]
15. Borisenko, V.; Koll, A.; Kolmakov, E.; Rjasnyi, A. Hydrogen bonds of 2-aminothiazoles in intermolecular complexes (1:1 and 1:2) with proton acceptors in solutions. *J. Mol. Struct.* **2006**, *783*, 101–115. [CrossRef]
16. Maj, J.; Rogóż, Z.; Skuza, G.; Kołodziejczyk, K. Antidepressant effects of pramipexole, a novel dopamine receptor agonist. *J. Neural Transm.* **1997**, *104*, 525–533. [CrossRef]
17. Milne, G.W.A. *Ashgate Handbook of Autineoplastic Agents*, 1st ed.; Routledge: London, UK, 2000; p. 190.
18. De Souza, M.V.N.; De Almeida, M.V. Drugs: Anti-HIV: Past, present and future directions. *Quimica Nova* **2003**, *26*, 366–372. [CrossRef]
19. Chhabria, M.T.; Patel, S.; Modi, P.; Brahmkshatriya, P.S. Thiazole: A Review on Chemistry, Synthesis and Therapeutic Importance of its Derivatives. *Curr. Top. Med. Chem.* **2016**, *16*, 2841–2862. [CrossRef]

20. Knadler, M.P.; Bergstrom, R.F.; Callaghan, J.T.; Rubin, A. Nizatidine, an H2-blocker. Its metabolism and disposition in man. *Drug Metab. Dispos. Biol. Fate Chem.* **1986**, *14*, 175–182.
21. Dawood, K.M.; Raslan, M.A.; Abbas, A.A.; Mohamed, B.E.; Abdellattif, M.H.; Nafie, M.S.; Hassan, M.K. Novel Bis-Thiazole Derivatives: Synthesis and Potential Cytotoxic Activity Through Apoptosis with Molecular Docking Approaches. *Front. Chem.* **2021**, *9*, 694870. [CrossRef]
22. Lednicer, D.; Mitscher, L.A.; Georg, G.I. *The Organic Chemistry of Drug Synthesis*; Wiley: Hoboken, NJ, USA, 1990; p. 304.
23. Hassan, A.A.; Mohamed, N.K.; Aly, A.A.; Tawfeek, H.N.; Bräse, S.; Nieger, M. Synthesis and structure confirmation of 2,4-disubstituted thiazole and 2,3,4-trisubstituted thiazole as thiazolium bromide salts. *Mon. Für Chem. Chem. Mon.* **2020**, *151*, 1143–1152. [CrossRef]
24. Ayati, A.; Emami, S.; Asadipour, A.; Shafiee, A.; Foroumadi, A. Recent applications of 1,3-thiazole core structure in the identification of new lead compounds and drug discovery. *Eur. J. Med. Chem.* **2015**, *97*, 699–718. [CrossRef] [PubMed]
25. Beuchet, P.; Varache-Lembège, M.; Neveu, A.; Léger, J.-M.; Vercauteren, J.; Larrouture, S.; Deffieux, G.; Nuhrich, A. New 2-sulfonamidothiazoles substituted at C-4: Synthesis of polyoxygenated aryl derivatives and in vitro evaluation of antifungal activity. *Eur. J. Med. Chem.* **1999**, *34*, 773–779. [CrossRef]
26. Takakura, H. Molecular Design of D-Luciferin-Based Bioluminescence and 1,2-Dioxetane-Based Chemiluminescence Substrates for Altered Output Wavelength and Detecting Various Molecules. *Molecules* **2021**, *26*, 1618. [CrossRef] [PubMed]
27. Chowdhury, A.; Patel, S.; Sharma, A.; Das, A.; Meshram, P.; Shard, A. A perspective on environmentally benign protocols of thiazole synthesis. *Chem. Heterocycl. Compd.* **2020**, *56*, 455–463. [CrossRef]
28. Quijano-Rubio, A.; Yeh, H.-W.; Park, J.; Lee, H.; Langan, R.A.; Boyken, S.E.; Lajoie, M.J.; Cao, L.; Chow, C.M.; Miranda, M.C.; et al. De novo design of modular and tunable protein biosensors. *Nature* **2021**, *591*, 482–487. [CrossRef] [PubMed]
29. Sharma, P.C.; Bansal, K.K.; Sharma, A.; Sharma, D.; Deep, A. Thiazole-containing compounds as therapeutic targets for cancer therapy. *Eur. J. Med. Chem.* **2020**, *188*, 112016. [CrossRef]
30. Jain, S.; Pattnaik, S.; Pathak, K.; Kumar, S.; Pathak, D.; Jain, S.; Vaidya, A. Anticancer Potential of Thiazole Derivatives: A Retrospective Review. *Mini-Rev. Med. Chem.* **2018**, *18*, 640–655. [CrossRef]
31. Ohsumi, K.; Hatanaka, T.; Fujita, K.; Nakagawa, R.; Fukuda, Y.; Nihei, Y.; Suga, Y.; Morinaga, Y.; Akiyama, Y.; Tsuji, T. Syntheses and antitumor activity of cis-restricted combretastatins: 5-Membered heterocyclic analogues. *Bioorganic Med. Chem. Lett.* **1998**, *8*, 3153–3158. [CrossRef]
32. Sun, M.; Xu, Q.; Xu, J.; Wu, Y.; Wang, Y.; Zuo, D.; Guan, Q.; Bao, K.; Wang, J.; Wu, Y.; et al. Synthesis and bioevaluation of N,4-diaryl-1,3-thiazole-2-amines as tubulin inhibitors with potent antiproliferative activity. *PLoS ONE* **2017**, *12*, e0174006. [CrossRef]
33. Valko, M.; Leibfritz, D.; Moncol, J.; Cronin, M.T.D.; Mazur, M.; Telser, J. Free radicals and antioxidants in normal physiological functions and human disease. *Int. J. Biochem. Cell Biol.* **2007**, *39*, 44–84. [CrossRef]
34. Suh, H.-J.; Chung, M.-S.; Cho, Y.-H.; Kim, J.-W.; Kim, D.-H.; Han, K.-W.; Kim, C.-J. Estimated daily intakes of butylated hydroxyanisole (BHA), butylated hydroxytoluene (BHT) and*tert*-butyl hydroquinone (TBHQ) antioxidants in Korea. *Food Addit. Contam.* **2005**, *22*, 1176–1188. [CrossRef] [PubMed]
35. Martelli, G.; Giacomini, D. Antibacterial and antioxidant activities for natural and synthetic dual-active compounds. *Eur. J. Med. Chem.* **2018**, *158*, 91–105. [CrossRef]
36. Yamashita, N.; Taga, C.; Ozawa, M.; Kanno, Y.; Sanada, N.; Kizu, R. Camalexin, an indole phytoalexin, inhibits cell proliferation, migration, and mammosphere formation in breast cancer cells via the aryl hydrocarbon receptor. *J. Nat. Med.* **2022**, *76*, 110–118. [CrossRef]
37. Gupta, D.K.; Palma, J.M.; Corpas, F.J. *Antioxidants and Antioxidant Enzymes in Higher Plants*; Springer International Publishing AG: Manhattan, NY, USA, 2018; p. 269.
38. Rutkauskas, K.; Jakienė, E.; Beresnevičius, Z.J. Products of reaction of p-phenylenediamine with unsaturated carboxylic acids and their biological activity. *Cheminė Technol.* **2003**, *2*, 68–73.
39. Xue, J.; Chambers, B.S.; Hensley, S.E.; López, C.B. Propagation and Characterization of Influenza Virus Stocks That Lack High Levels of Defective Viral Genomes and Hemagglutinin Mutations. *Front. Microbiol.* **2016**, *7*, 326. [CrossRef] [PubMed]
40. Karakus, U.; Crameri, M.; Lanz, C.; Yángüez, E. Propagation and Titration of Influenza Viruses. *Methods Mol. Biol.* **2018**, *1836*, 59–88. [CrossRef]
41. Koksal, E.; Gulcin, I. Antioxidant Activity of Cauliflower (*Brassica oleracea* L.). *Turk. J. Agric. For.* **2008**, *32*, 65–78.
42. Bursal, E.; Gülçin, I. Polyphenol contents and in vitro antioxidant activities of lyophilised aqueous extract of kiwifruit (Actinidia deliciosa). *Food Res. Int.* **2011**, *44*, 1482–1489. [CrossRef]
43. Gulcin, İ. Antioxidants and antioxidant methods: An updated overview. *Arch. Toxicol.* **2020**, *94*, 651–715. [CrossRef]
44. Benzie, I.F.F.; Strain, J.J. Ferric reducing/antioxidant power assay: Direct measure of total antioxidant activity of biological fluids and modified version for simultaneous measurement of total antioxidant power and ascorbic acid concentration. *Methods Enzymol.* **1996**, *239*, 15–27. [CrossRef]
45. Gulcin, I.; Buyukokuroglu, M.E.; Oktay, M.; Kufrevioglu, O.I. On the in vitro antioxidative properties of melatonin. *J. Pineal Res.* **2002**, *33*, 167–171. [CrossRef] [PubMed]
46. Gülçin, I.; Oktay, M.; Küfrevioğlu, O.I.; Aslan, A. Determination of antioxidant activity of lichen *Cetraria islandica* (L) Ach. *J. Ethnopharmacol.* **2002**, *79*, 325–329. [CrossRef]

47. Jaishree, V.; Ramdas, N.; Sachin, J.; Ramesh, B. In vitro antioxidant properties of new thiazole derivatives. *J. Saudi Chem. Soc.* **2012**, *16*, 371–376. [CrossRef]
48. Sztanke, M.; Sztanke, K. Biologically important hydrazide-containing fused azaisocytosines as antioxidant agents. *Redox Rep.* **2017**, *22*, 572–581. [CrossRef]
49. Huang, D.; Ou, B.; Prior, R.L. The Chemistry behind Antioxidant Capacity Assays. *J. Agric. Food Chem.* **2005**, *53*, 1841–1856. [CrossRef]
50. Salar, U.; Khan, K.M.; Chigurupati, S.; Taha, M.; Wadood, A.; Vijayabalan, S.; Ghufran, M.; Perveen, S. New Hybrid Hydrazinyl Thiazole Substituted Chromones: As Potential α-Amylase Inhibitors and Radical (DPPH & ABTS) Scavengers. *Sci. Rep.* **2017**, *7*, 16980. [CrossRef]
51. Zaki, Y.H.; Al-Gendey, M.S.; Abdelhamid, A.O. A facile synthesis, and antimicrobial and anticancer activities of some pyridines, thioamides, thiazole, urea, quinazoline, β-naphthyl carbamate, and pyrano[2,3-d]thiazole derivatives. *Chem. Central J.* **2018**, *12*, 70. [CrossRef]

International Journal of
Molecular Sciences

Article

Antibacterial and Sporicidal Activity Evaluation of Theaflavin-3,3′-digallate

Ayuni Yussof, Brian Cammalleri, Oluwanifemi Fayemiwo, Sabrina Lopez and Tinchun Chu *

Department of Biological Sciences, Seton Hall University, South Orange, NJ 07079, USA;
mohamesi@shu.edu (A.Y.); cammalbr@shu.edu (B.C.); fayemiol@shu.edu (O.F.); lopezsac@shu.edu (S.L.)
* Correspondence: tinchun.chu@shu.edu

Abstract: Theaflavin-3,3′-digallate (TFDG), a polyphenol derived from the leaves of *Camellia sinensis*, is known to have many health benefits. In this study, the antibacterial effect of TFDG against nine bacteria and the sporicidal activities on spore-forming *Bacillus* spp. have been investigated. Microplate assay, colony-forming unit, BacTiter-Glo™, and Live/Dead Assays showed that 250 μg/mL TFDG was able to inhibit bacterial growth up to 99.97%, while 625 μg/mL TFDG was able to inhibit up to 99.92% of the spores from germinating after a one-hour treatment. Binding analysis revealed the favorable binding affinity of two germination-associated proteins, GPR and Lgt (GerF), to TFDG, ranging from −7.6 to −10.3 kcal/mol. Semi-quantitative RT-PCR showed that TFDG treatment lowered the expression of *gpr*, ranging from 0.20 to 0.39 compared to the control in both *Bacillus* spp. The results suggest that TFDG not only inhibits the growth of vegetative cells but also prevents the germination of bacterial spores. This report indicates that TFDG is a promising broad-spectrum antibacterial and anti-spore agent against Gram-positive, Gram-negative, acid-fast bacteria, and endospores. The potential anti-germination mechanism has also been elucidated.

Keywords: antibacterial; sporicidal; anti-germination; binding analysis; natural product; black tea polyphenol; theaflavin

Citation: Yussof, A.; Cammalleri, B.; Fayemiwo, O.; Lopez, S.; Chu, T. Antibacterial and Sporicidal Activity Evaluation of Theaflavin-3,3′-digallate. *Int. J. Mol. Sci.* **2022**, *23*, 2153. https://doi.org/10.3390/ijms23042153

Academic Editor: Helena Felgueiras

Received: 28 December 2021
Accepted: 10 February 2022
Published: 15 February 2022

1. Introduction

Many medical and scientific journal articles have documented the rising number of antibiotic-resistant bacteria and the multidrug resistance crisis linked to the overuse or abuse of antibiotics [1]. Vancomycin, for example, was first introduced to clinical practice in 1972, and unfortunately, vancomycin-resistant *S. aureus* (VRSA) was reported in 1979 [2]. In the United States, approximately 2.8 million people are infected with antibiotic-resistant bacteria yearly, and at least 35,000 die from the infection [3]. The problem of antibiotic resistance imposes a significant financial burden as evidenced by the number of methicillin-resistant *Staphylococcus aureus* (MRSA)-related issues that cost the US healthcare system around $3–4 billion annually [4].

The aromatic allure, taste, and health benefits of tea make it one of the most popular beverages worldwide [5]. Both black and green tea are derived from the leaves of *Camellia sinensis* but differ in the level of oxidation due to fermentation [5,6]. Black tea contains a lower level of catechins than green tea but makes up for it with a higher amount of theaflavin [6]. The major theaflavins present in black tea include theaflavin (TF), theaflavin-3-gallate (TF3G), theaflavin-3′-gallate (TF3′G), and theaflavin-3,3′-digallate (TFDG) [6].

Theaflavins (TFs) are the major polyphenols in black tea, showing great potential as an antimicrobial agent. A previous study demonstrated that 1 g of theaflavin mixture extract could contain up to 32.80% of TFDG [7]. As for cellular toxicity, theaflavin has little to no effect on human lung fibroblast tissue, CEM cells, A549, and Vero cells [8]. Compared to epigallocatechin gallate (EGCG), major catechin extracted from green tea, TF is more stable under non-favorable conditions, making it a better candidate for antimicrobial agents [8]. TFDG was chosen based on a study indicating that TFDG was the most effective in inhibiting *Streptococcus mutans* (*S. mutans*) growth compared to TF, TF3G, and TF3′G [9]. Most previous studies focused on the antioxidant properties of theaflavin. It has been documented that drinking six cups of black tea could significantly increase the antioxidant capacity within the cell [6]. The number of polyphenols in tea varies highly depending on the origin and the brewing technique. Previous studies reported that the level of TFDG ranges from 0.07 to 1.13 g per 100 g of dry leaves among Darjeeling, Assam, Sri Lankan, African, and Chinese tea samples [10]. The level of TFs is approximately 7 mg when brewing a standard US tea bag (2.25 g) in 100 mL of water for less than 2 min and can increase to 14 mg when brewed for more than 4 min [11]. A study using LDL conjugation compared the antioxidant properties of theaflavin to green tea polyphenols, including epicatechin (EC), epicatechin gallate (ECG), epigallocatechin (EGC), and EGCG. The result showed that TFDG > ECG > EGCG ≥ TF3′G ≥ TF3G > TF ≥ EC > EGC in terms of antioxidant properties [12]. Based on the promising results, interest has expanded into the antiviral and antibacterial effects of TFs [8,13–17]. One study indicated 125 μg/mL TFs was the minimum inhibitory concentration (MIC) against *Porphyromonas gingivitis* (*P. gingivalis*) and 250 μg/mL TFDG in *Clostridium perfringens* (*C. perfringens*) while in Hepatitis C virus (HCV), 25 μg/mL TF3 was acting directly on the virus to prevent viral entry into the cell [13,18,19]. Several research groups also investigated the beneficial effect of TFs on the bacterial population and signaling pathways in the oral cavity and gut [20,21]. Some antibacterial mechanisms of TFs have been suggested, including reducing biosynthetic and metabolic activities in *C. perfringens* and anti-hemolytic activity in *Staphylococcus aureus* (*S. aureus*) [13,17].

This study explores the antimicrobial effect against nine pathogenic and clinically significant bacteria. Gram-negative *Klebsiella aerogenes* (*K. aerogenes*) is typically associated with nosocomial outbreaks due to the emergence of multidrug-resistant strains [22]. *Escherichia coli* (*E. coli*), a mutualism in the gastrointestinal (GI) tract of humans, is a model organism for Gram-negative bacteria [23–29]. *Pseudomonas aeruginosa* (*P. aeruginosa*), another nosocomial pathogen found among cystic fibrosis patients with a high mortality rate [30,31], has high resistance to most antimicrobial agents [30]. Multidrug-resistant *Proteus mirabilis* (*P. mirabilis*) is resistant to almost all antibiotic classes, and its prevalence among UTI infections has significantly increased [32].

The "*Bacillus cereus* group" includes several species of closely related pathogenic species like *Bacillus anthracis* (*B. anthracis*) and *Bacillus cereus* (*B. cereus*) [33]. *B. anthracis* and *B. cereus* are the causative agents of anthrax and the emetic syndrome, respectively [33]. *Bacillus subtilis* (*B. subtilis*) is considered a model organism for cellular development, including spore formation, germination, and biofilm production [34,35]. *Bacillus* spores may remain dormant for years but can germinate in favorable conditions such as specific nutrient reintroduction [36–41]. *Staphylococcus aureus* (*S. aureus*) causes a variety of life-threatening diseases, including endocarditis, toxic shock syndrome (TSS), and osteomyelitis [41]. Group A *Streptococcus pyogenes* (*S. pyogenes*) is a beta-hemolytic strain that can cause a wide range of infections, from superficial epithelial infection to the more severe streptococcal TSS (STSS) [42,43].

Acid-fast *Mycobacterium tuberculosis* (*M. tuberculosis*) is the pathogenic bacterium that causes tuberculosis (TB) [44]. Over the past three decades, TB has re-emerged as a global health concern, and in 2019, it is estimated that 10 million people were infected with TB worldwide, and 1.4 million people died [45]. Since detecting multidrug-resistant *M. tuberculosis* (MDR TB), research agencies, non-profit agencies, and academia have spared no effort to develop new treatments [46,47].

This study focuses on the antibacterial and sporicidal activity of TFDG as it contains the highest antioxidant [12] and antiviral [8,19] effects among all theaflavins. Each species used poses a public health threat. Most previous reports centered on the antibacterial activities of green tea polyphenols or a mixture of theaflavins against one or a few species. On the other hand, our results demonstrate that TFDG could potentially serve as a broad-spectrum antimicrobial agent that can inhibit the growth of nine bacteria across Gram-positive, Gram-negative, and acid-fast groups and an antispore agent. The anti-germination mechanism of TFDG against two *Bacillus* spp. is also proposed. Both 2D and 3D structures of TFDG are displayed in Figure 1. The 3D structure is used for molecular docking analysis.

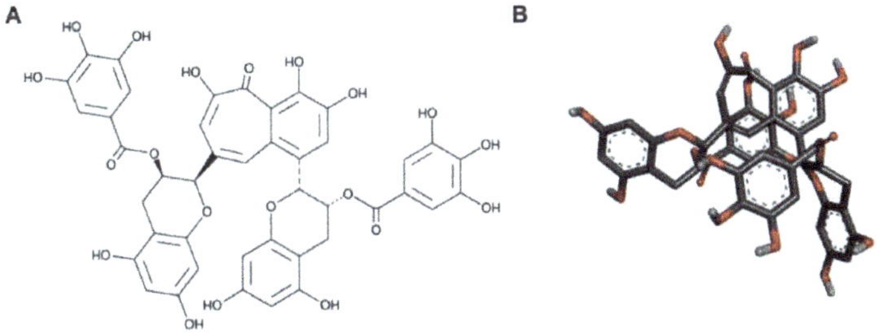

Figure 1. The (**A**) 2D and (**B**) 3D chemical structures of TFDG.

2. Results

2.1. Determination of MIC and Half-Maximal Inhibitory Concentration (IC_{50})

No bacterial growth was observed when treated with 250 μg/mL or higher TFDG, so the MIC was determined as 250 μg/mL. The IC_{50} for all bacteria is around 62.5 μg/mL. As for erythromycin, the IC_{50} ranged from 7 to 26 μg/mL, and the MIC should be greater than 45 μg/mL for the bacteria tested in this study (Supplementary Figures S1–S3).

2.2. Colony Forming Unit (CFU) Assay

Based on the microplate assay result, the effect of TFDG on the bacteria was further analyzed using CFU assay (Table 1). At the sixth hour, 62.5 μg/mL was able to inhibit the bacteria from 43.20% to 55.37% and ranged from 93.12% to 99.98% for 250 μg/mL TFDG. This correlates to the log reduction ranging from 0.25 to 0.35 for 62.5 μg/mL TFDG and from 1.17 to 3.69 for 250 μg/mL TFDG. Among nine bacteria tested, 250 μg/mL TFDG worked the best on *P. aeruginosa* (99.98 ± 0.01%). All the data were statistically significant ($p < 0.05$).

Table 1. Colony-forming unit (CFU/mL) with the log reduction and percent inhibition of different bacteria with TFDG.

		Bacteria	TFDG (μg/mL)	CFU/mL (Mean ± SD)	Log Reduction (Mean ± SD)	% Inhibition (Mean ± SD)
Gram-negative		*K. aerogenes*	0	$(9.86 \pm 0.09) \times 10^8$	0	0
			62.5	$(4.40 \pm 0.12) \times 10^8$	0.35 ± 0.02	55.37 ± 1.59%
			250	$(6.07 \pm 0.48) \times 10^7$	1.17 ± 0.03	93.12 ± 0.46%
		E. coli	0	$(1.09 \pm 0.06) \times 10^9$	0	0
			62.5	$(6.20 \pm 0.42) \times 10^8$	0.25 ± 0.01	43.20 ± 0.83%
			250	$(2.36 \pm 0.66) \times 10^7$	1.69 ± 0.12	97.87 ± 0.52%
		P. aeruginosa	0	$(7.01 \pm 0.07) \times 10^8$	0	0
			62.5	$(3.68 \pm 0.11) \times 10^8$	0.28 ± 0.01	47.50 ± 1.15%
			250	$(1.57 \pm 0.60) \times 10^5$	3.69 ± 0.21	99.98 ± 0.01%
		P. mirabilis	0	$(6.27 \pm 0.08) \times 10^9$	0	0
			62.5	$(3.17 \pm 0.05) \times 10^9$	0.30 ± 0.00	49.39 ± 0.23%
			250	$(1.57 \pm 0.39) \times 10^7$	2.62 ± 0.13	99.75 ± 0.07%
Gram-positive	Spore former	*B. cereus*	0	$(6.54 \pm 0.13) \times 10^8$	0	0
			62.5	$(3.32 \pm 0.08) \times 10^8$	0.29 ± 0.01	49. 16 ± 1.65%
			250	$(6.00 \pm 1.63) \times 10^5$	3.05 ± 0.13	99.91 ± 0.03%
		B. subtilis	0	$(6.89 \pm 0.09) \times 10^8$	0	0
			62.5	$(3.35 \pm 0.08) \times 10^8$	0.31 ± 0.01	51.40 ± 0.72%
			250	$(3.33 \pm 0.82) \times 10^5$	3.34 ± 0.13	99.95 ± 0.01%
	Non-spore former	*S. aureus*	0	$(4.69 \pm 0.12) \times 10^9$	0	0
			62.5	$(2.10 \pm 0.18) \times 10^9$	0.35 ± 0.04	55.20 ± 4.62%
			250	$(3.03 \pm 1.23) \times 10^6$	3.24 ± 0.24	99.93 ± 0.03%
		S. pyogenes	0	$(4.33 \pm 0.02) \times 10^9$	0	0
			62.5	$(2.24 \pm 0.05) \times 10^9$	0.29 ± 0.01	48.28 ± 0.85%
			250	$(3.47 \pm 0.09) \times 10^6$	3.10 ± 0.01	99.92 ± 0.05%
Acid-fast		*M. smegmatis*	0	$(4.11 \pm 0.07) \times 10^9$	0	0
			62.5	$(2.02 \pm 0.05) \times 10^9$	0.31 ± 0.02	50.88 ± 1.92%
			250	$(1.33 \pm 0.34) \times 10^6$	3.50 ± 0.11	99.97 ± 0.01%

2.3. BacTiter-Glo™ Microbial Cell Viability Assay

62.5 μg/mL TFDG was able to inhibit up to 59.82 ± 6.19% of cell viability based on the ATP level compared to the control, while 250 μg/mL TFDG was able to inhibit up to 99.33 ± 0.16% of bacteria (Table 2).

Table 2. Relative fluorescence unit (RFU) with the log reduction and percent inhibition of different bacteria treated with TFDG based on BacTiter-Glo^{TM} assay.

		Bacteria	TFDG (μg/mL)	RFU (Mean ± SD)	Log Reduction (Mean ± SD)	% Inhibition (Mean ± SD)
Gram-negative		*K. aerogenes*	0	$(1.90 \pm 0.46) \times 10^{6}$	0	0
			62.5	$(9.17 \pm 2.01) \times 10^{5}$	0.31 ± 0.01	$51.52 \pm 1.63\%$
			250	$(1.51 \pm 0.73) \times 10^{4}$	2.14 ± 0.12	$99.25 \pm 0.22\%$
		E. coli	0	$(1.67 \pm 0.09) \times 10^{6}$	0	0
			62.5	$(7.89 \pm 1.08) \times 10^{5}$	0.33 ± 0.04	$53.00 \pm 4.48\%$
			250	$(1.15 \pm 0.19) \times 10^{4}$	2.17 ± 0.09	$99.31 \pm 0.14\%$
		P. aeruginosa	0	$(1.67 \pm 0.36) \times 10^{6}$	0	0
			62.5	$(8.07 \pm 1.91) \times 10^{5}$	0.32 ± 0.02	$51.97 \pm 2.74\%$
			250	$(6.16 \pm 2.84) \times 10^{4}$	1.48 ± 0.30	$95.87 \pm 2.39\%$
		P. mirabilis	0	$(1.52 \pm 0.05) \times 10^{6}$	0	0
			62.5	$(7.05 \pm 0.36) \times 10^{5}$	0.34 ± 0.02	$53.77 \pm 1.69\%$
			250	$(3.52 \pm 2.45) \times 10^{4}$	1.78 ± 0.37	$97.71 \pm 1.58\%$
Gram-positive	Spore former	*B. cereus*	0	$(2.03 \pm 1.00) \times 10^{6}$	0	0
			62.5	$(7.58 \pm 2.80) \times 10^{5}$	0.40 ± 0.07	$59. 82 \pm 6.19\%$
			250	$(1.28 \pm 0.48) \times 10^{5}$	1.18 ± 0.08	$93.24 \pm 1.26\%$
		B. subtilis	0	$(2.30 \pm 0.32) \times 10^{6}$	0	0
			62.5	$(1.09 \pm 0.21) \times 10^{5}$	0.33 ± 0.03	$52.81 \pm 3.47\%$
			250	$(4.82 \pm 1.41) \times 10^{4}$	1.69 ± 0.07	$97.94 \pm 0.35\%$
	Non-spore former	*S. aureus*	0	$(7.74 \pm 2.02) \times 10^{6}$	0	0
			62.5	$(3.66 \pm 1.08) \times 10^{6}$	0.33 ± 0.03	$53.12 \pm 3.11\%$
			250	$(8.55 \pm 3.73) \times 10^{4}$	1.98 ± 0.29	$98.71 \pm 0.76\%$
		S. pyogenes	0	$(4.43 \pm 0.99) \times 10^{6}$	0	0
			62.5	$(2.15 \pm 0.42) \times 10^{6}$	0.31 ± 0.05	$50.81 \pm 5.81\%$
			250	$(1.01 \pm 0.80) \times 10^{5}$	1.83 ± 0.50	$97.72 \pm 1.41\%$
	Acid-fast	*M. smegmatis*	0	$(1.83 \pm 0.25) \times 10^{6}$	0	0
			62.5	$(9.09 \pm 0.59) \times 10^{5}$	0.30 ± 0.04	$49.82 \pm 4.42\%$
			250	$(1.24 \pm 0.42) \times 10^{4}$	2.19 ± 0.12	$99.33 \pm 0.16\%$

2.4. Live/Dead Bacterial Viability Assay

Figures 2–4 show the bacterial viability when treated with various concentrations of TFDG after 6 h. Overall, the control bacteria were primarily green and maintained normal morphology. Cells treated with 62.5 μg/mL TFDG showed a mixture of live, impaired, and dead cells. Most cells appeared to be smaller and more clumped together when compared to the control except for the *M. smegmatis*, which had less aggregation. Cells treated with 250 μg/mL TFDG were mainly non-viable. The cell numbers were significantly less than the control. The cell morphology appeared smaller and/or segmented with TFDG treatment.

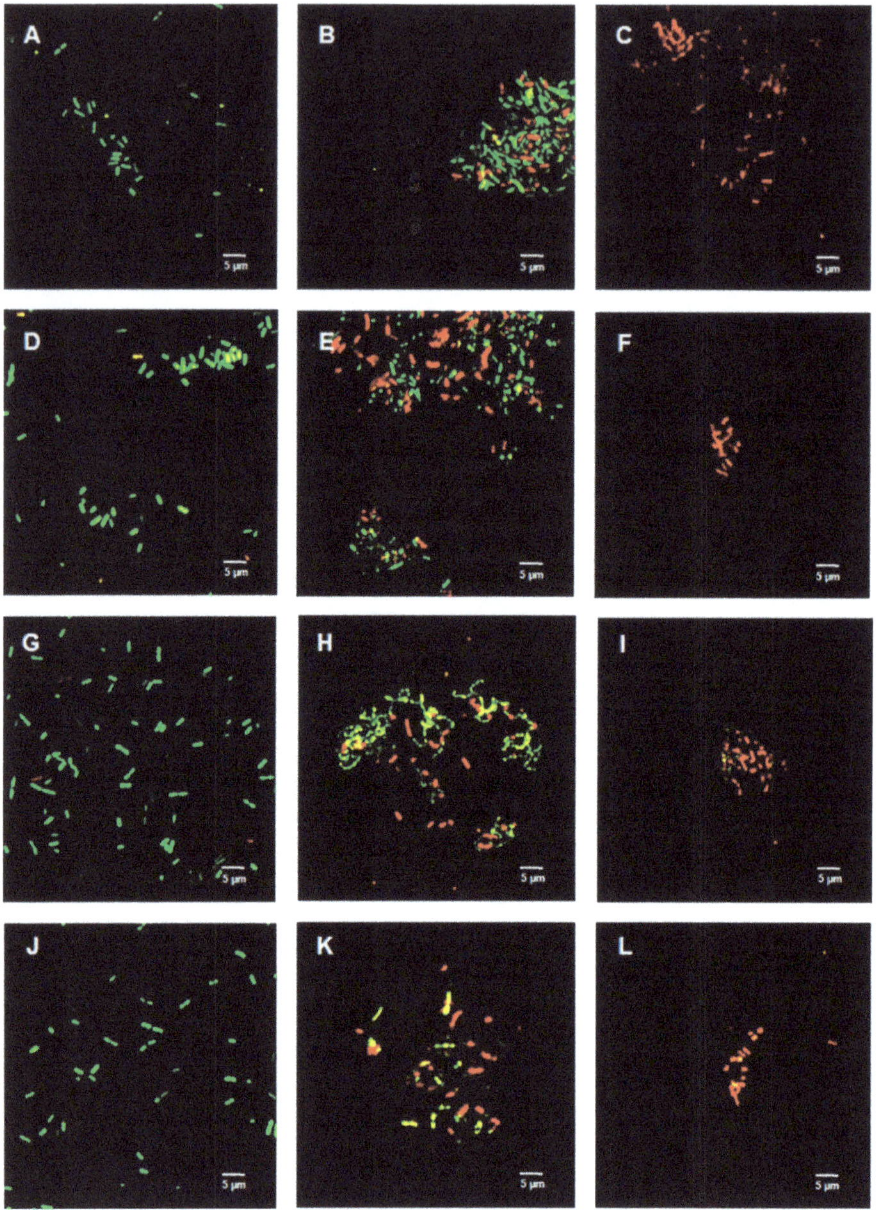

Figure 2. Live/Dead assay of Gram-negative species with various concentrations of TFDG at 6-h incubation. The samples were visualized using Olympus confocal microscope. The green indicates live bacteria, while the red indicates dead bacteria. (**A**) *K. aerogenes* control; (**B**) *K. aerogenes* with 62.5 µg/mL TFDG; (**C**) *K. aerogenes* with 250 µg/mL TFDG; (**D**) *E. coli* control; (**E**) *E. coli* with 62.5 µg/mL TFDG; (**F**) *E. coli* with 250 µg/mL TFDG; (**G**) *P. aeruginosa* control; (**H**) *P. aeruginosa* with 62.5 µg/mL TFDG; (**I**) *P. aeruginosa* with 250 µg/mL TFDG; (**J**) *P. mirabilis* control; (**K**) *P. mirabilis* with 62.5 µg/mL TFDG; and (**L**) *P. mirabilis* with 250 µg/mL TFDG.

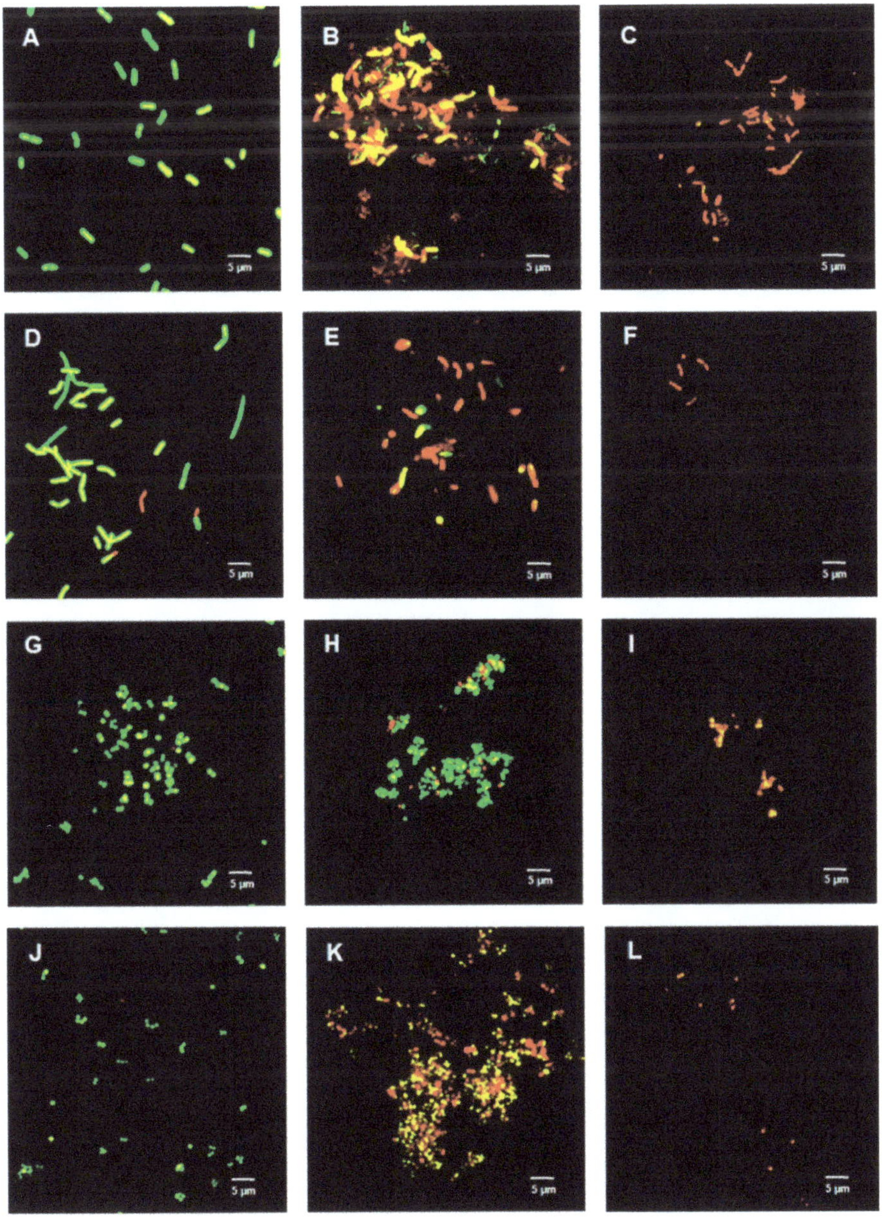

Figure 3. Live/Dead assay of Gram-positive species with various concentrations of TFDG at 6-h incubation. The samples were visualized using Olympus confocal microscope. The green indicates live bacteria, while the red indicates dead bacteria. (**A**) *B. cereus* control; (**B**) *B. cereus* with 62.5 μg/mL TFDG; (**C**) *B. cereus* with 250 μg/mL TFDG; (**D**) *B. subtilis* control; (**E**) *B. subtilis* with 62.5 μg/mL TFDG; (**F**) *B. subtilis* with 250 μg/mL TFDG; (**G**) *S. aureus* control; (**H**) *S. aureus* with 62.5 μg/mL TFDG; (**I**) *S. aureus* with 250 μg/mL TFDG; (**J**) *S. pyogenes* control; (**K**) *S. pyogenes* with 62.5 μg/mL TFDG; and (**L**) *S. pyogenes* with 250 μg/mL TFDG.

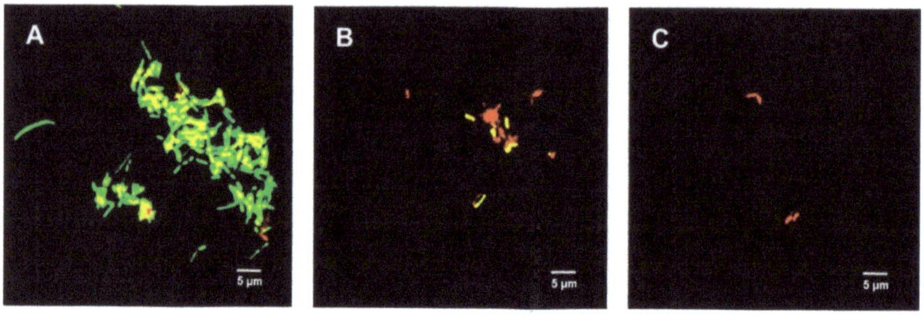

Figure 4. Live/Dead assay of *M. smegmatis* with various concentrations of TFDG at 6-h incubation. The samples were visualized using Olympus confocal microscope. The green indicates live bacteria, while the red indicates dead bacteria. (**A**) *M. smegmatis* control; (**B**) *M. smegmatis* with 62.5 µg/mL TFDG; and (**C**) *M. smegmatis* with 250 µg/mL TFDG.

2.5. Germination Inhibition via CFU Assay

The percent (%) inhibition was calculated from the CFU assay after a 60-min TFDG treatment. 312.5 µg/mL TFDG inhibited the *Bacillus* spores from germinating, ranging from 54.13% to 60.49%, while 625 µg/mL TFDG was able to inhibit germination ranging from 99.37% to 99.92% (Table 3).

Table 3. Germination inhibition assay of both *B. cereus* and *B. subtilis*.

		Bacteria	TFDG (µg/mL)	CFU/mL (Mean ± SD)	Log Reduction (Mean ± SD)	% Inhibition (Mean ± SD)
Gram-positive	Spore former	*B. cereus*	0	$(1.11 \pm 0.85) \times 10^{10}$	0	0
			312.5	$(4.79 \pm 3.55) \times 10^{9}$	0.34 ± 0.03	54. 13 ± 3.51%
			625	$(6.55 \pm 4.57) \times 10^{5}$	2.22 ± 0.12	99.37 ± 0.17%
		B. subtilis	0	$(7.24 \pm 4.90) \times 10^{9}$	0	0
			312.5	$(3.25 \pm 2.33) \times 10^{9}$	0.41 ± 0.09	60.49 ± 7.91%
			625	$(7.75 \pm 5.54) \times 10^{6}$	3.40 ± 0.64	99.92 ± 0.05%

2.6. Live/Dead Spore Viability Assay

Figure 5 shows the untreated (control) spores were primarily green. Samples treated with 312.5 µg/mL TFDG indicated the spores were impaired, while 625 µg/mL TFDG-treated spores were mainly non-viable.

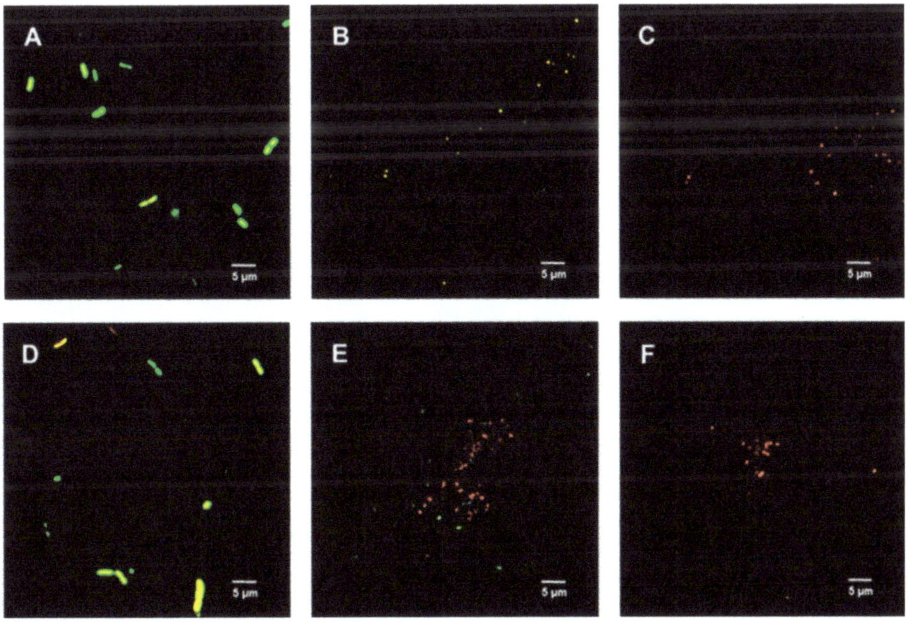

Figure 5. Live/Dead assay of *Bacillus* spp. spores with TFDG at 60-min incubation. The green indicates viable spores, while the red indicates non-viable spores. (**A**) *B. cereus* spores control; (**B**) *B. cereus* spores with 312.5 µg/mL TFDG; (**C**) *B. cereus* spores with 625 µg/mL TFDG; (**D**) *B. subtilis* spores control; (**E**) *B. subtilis* spores with 312.5 µg/mL TFDG; and (**F**) *B. subtilis* spores with 625 µg/mL TFDG.

2.7. Binding Pocket

The protein structures related to the four genes of interest were analyzed via CASTp to determine its binding pocket. Table 4 shows the binding pocket areas (Å^2) for GPR were 616.45 and 433.40 for *B. cereus* and *B. subtilis*, respectively. The binding pocket areas (Å^2) for Lgt were 1284.21 for *B. cereus* and 1565.20 for *B. subtilis*. The amino acid residues of each pocket were used as a guide to determine the location and size of the grid for *in silico* docking analysis.

Table 4. Binding pocket prediction and analysis of conserved germination protein via CASTp. The predicted binding pocket includes the pocket area, volume, and residues lining the pocket of conserved germination genes.

Bacteria	Protein	Pocket Area (Å^2)	Volume (Å^3)	Residue Lining Pocket
B. cereus	GPR	616.45	290.23	Arg196, Ser197, Ile198, Thr252, Ile253, Asp254, Phe255, Ile256, Leu257, Lys258, Phe260, Gly261, Arg262, Met264, Lys265, Ala304, Gly306, Glu309, Leu316, Leu319, Val320, Leu321, Ser322, Val330
	Lgt (GerF)	1284.21	1087.71	Trp3, Ile4, Val5, Arg6, Gln8, Pro9, Ser11, Leu12, Ile13, Gly15, Ser16, Gly19, Met23, Val41, Ala44, Phe45, 1le48, Ala49, Trp52, Lys53, Ile75, Lys79, His80, Val82, Cys85, Ile86, Ser89, Val90. Ile92, Leu107, Leu110, Pro111, Ile112, Ala113, Leu114, Cys115, Met116, Ser117, Ile118, Ile119, Phe120, Tyr 121, Glu154, Ala158, Leu159, Val162, Gly163, Leu165, Trp166, Ile178, Phe181, Leu182, Glu185, Gly186, His189, Phe203, Gly204, Met207, Gln208, Leu211, Ser212, Cys214, Val215, Leu218
B. subtilis	GPR	433.40	225.27	Arg44, His46, Lys50, Thr53, Asp55, Val56, Thr57, Glu59, Leu74, Ala76, Gln77, Gly78, Val90, Val93, Phe94, Glu96, Glu97, Ser99, Ala100, Phe101, Glu103, Asn104, Lys109, Ile206, Ile208, His355, Lys357, Val58, Ser359, Gln360, Asn362 Lys363, Gly364, Ser365, Tyr366,Asn367
	Lgt (GerF)	1565.20	1484.55	Leu18, Ala 19, His21, Tyr23, Gly24, Ile26, Ile27, Gly30, Ala31, Gly34, Ile37, Ala38, Arg40, Glu41, Lys44, Arg45, Gly46, Leu47, Phe52, Val56, Ala59, Ile60, Ala63, Ile64, Ala67, Ile89, Trp90, Gly93, Ile94, Gly99, Leu100, Ala103, Ile104, Thr106, Gly107, Leu116, Phe118, Lys120, Leu121, Ala122, Asp123, Ile124, Ala125, Ala126, Pro127, Ser128, Ile129, Leu 131, Gly132, Gln 133, Ile135, Gly136, Arg137, Gly139, Asn140, Glu145, Phe180, Glu183, Ser187, Ile192, Leu196, Arg198, Arg199, Ala200, Asn201, Leu202, Arg203, Arg204, Glu206, Met207, Phe208, Tyr211, Ile212, Tyr215, Arg219, Arg226, Thr233, Asp234, Ser235, Leu236

2.8. In Silico Docking Analysis

Table 5 details the molecular docking result of TFDG for both GPR and Lgt in *B. cereus* and *B. subtilis*. The *B. cereus* GPR docking score was −9.7 kcal/mol with five bonds, including conventional H-bond and Pi-Stacked. *B. cereus* Lgt binding score with TFDG was −7.6 kcal/mol with five different bonds that include conventional H-bond and pi-cation. Both GPR and Lgt of *B. subtilis* had the same binding score of −10.3 kcal/mol, but GPR has 12 bonds, including conventional H-bond, unfavorable donor-donor, and pi-donor H-bond. In contrast, Lgt has only seven bonds, including hydrophobic pi-sigma, conventional H bond, and carbon H bond. The binding pocket and the bond for each protein were observed using Discovery Studio, as seen in Figure 6.

Table 5. Docking analysis of conserved germination proteins. The molecular interaction of TFDG with various genes. The table shows the best binding probability.

Bacteria	Protein	Docking Score (kcal/mol)	Interacting Residue	Distance	Category
B. cereus	GPR	−9.7	Trp120	2.51	Conventional H-bond
			Trp120	3.98, 3.88	Pi-Pi Stacked
			Asn121	2.59	Conventional H-bond
			Val163	2.78	Conventional H-bond
			Glu340	2.37	Conventional H-bond
	Lgt (GerF)	−7.6	Lys26	1.85	Conventional H-bond
			Lys26	3.73	Pi-Cation
			Ser31	2.99	Conventional H-bond
			Lys168	2.00	Conventional H-bond
			Arg171	2.51	Conventional H-bond
B. subtilis	GPR	−10.3	Gly119	2.06, 2.94	Conventional H-bond
			ASN120	2.34	Conventional H-bond
			ASN120	2.92	Conventional H-bond
			ASN120	2.03	Conventional H-bond
			ASN120	1.97	Conventional H-bond
			ASN122	1.68	Unfavorable Donor-Donor
			ASP126	2.97	Conventional H-bond
			Ile170	1.93	Conventional H-bond
			Thr172	3.05	Pi Donor H-bond
			Lys222	1.22	Unfavorable Donor-Donor
			Asp336	2.49	Conventional H-bond
			Asp336	2.23	Conventional H-bond
	Lgt (GerF)	−10.3	Ala63	3.78	Hydrophobic Pi-Sigma
			Ala103	3.62	Hydrophobic Pi-Sigma
			Ala103	2.07	Conventional H-Bond
			Ile129	3.29	Carbon Hydrogen Bond
			Gly132	3.96	Hydrophobic Pi-Sigma
			Tyr215	1.92	Conventional H-bond
			Asp234	2.38	Conventional H-bond

Previous studies showed the −7.0 kcal/mol threshold as significant for AutoDock binding [48,49]. Since both proteins showed a higher negative value, it indicates these two are good candidates for TFDG anti-germination properties evaluation. Hydrogen bond regulates molecular interaction through donor-acceptor pairing, enhancing receptor-ligand interaction [50]. Instead, hydrophobic interaction is a major consideration for binding affinity as this interaction can be considered a weak hydrogen bond [50]. *B. cereus* GPR binding affinity consists of 4 hydrogen bond interactions, while Lgt (GerF) consists of four hydrogen interactions. *B. subtilis* GPR TFDG binding affinity consists of nine hydrogen bonds interactions, while Lgt (GerF) has four hydrogen bonds and three strengthening hydrophobic interactions.

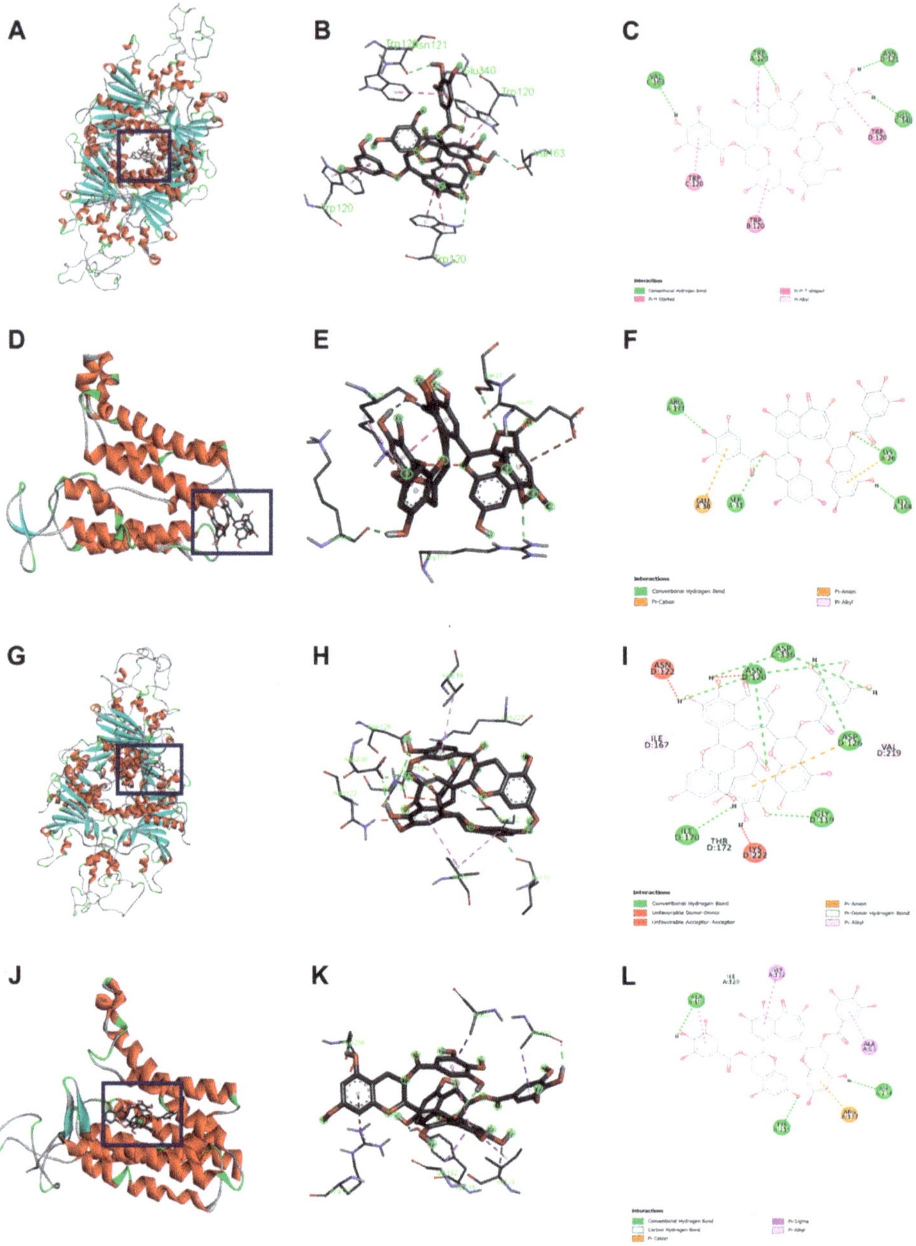

Figure 6. Docking visualization of TFDG with the germination protein using BIOVIA Discovery Studio Visualizer. (**A–C**) *B. cereus* GPR with TFDG; (**D–F**) *B. cereus* Lgt with TFDG; (**G–I**) *B. subtilis* GPR with TFDG; (**J–L**) *B. subtilis* Lgt with TFDG. For (**C**,**F**,**I**,**L**) the bright green line shows conventional hydrogen bond; bright pink shows the pi-pi interaction; light pink shows pi-alkyl interaction; orange shows pi cation, pi carbon, and pi-anion interaction; the red line shows unfavorable bond interaction; light green shows pi-donor hydrogen interaction and carbon-hydrogen interaction; and bright purple shows pi sigma interaction.

2.9. Semi-Quantitative RT-PCR

Figure 7 shows the relative expression of both *lgt* and *gpr* after a one-hour treatment of 625 µg/mL TFDG. In both *B. cereus* and *B. subtilis*, the expression of *gpr* dropped to 0.20 and 0.39, respectively, compared to the control (1.00). On the other hand, the expression of *lgt* was lower only in *B. cereus* (0.25) but not in *B. subtilis* (0.88) when compared to the control (1.00).

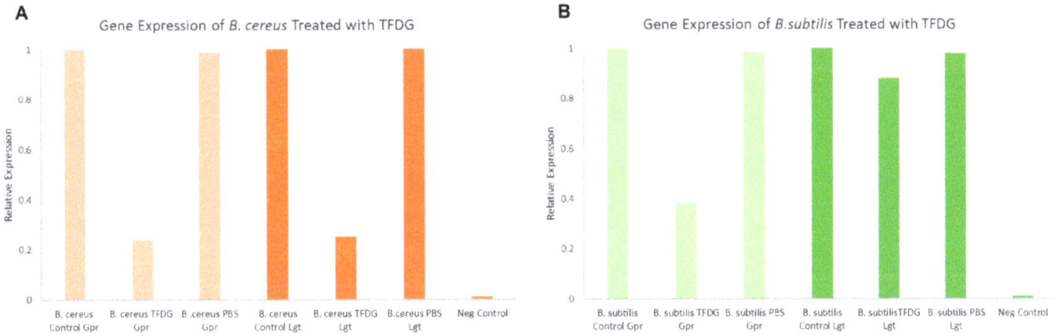

Figure 7. Semi-quantitative RT-PCR *lgt* and gpr gene expression analysis of *Bacillus* spore when treated with TFDG. (**A**) *B. cereus* spores; (**B**) *B. subtilis* spores.

3. Discussion

The urgency to find a novel antimicrobial agent has pushed researchers to look for either natural or synthetic alternatives. Currently, there are 42 new antibiotics under clinical development, but only 11 can treat pathogens that are considered critical by the World Health Organization (WHO) [51]. Antibiotic development projects from major pharmaceutical companies only account for four out of 42 studies, focusing on more profitable ventures like immune-oncology therapeutics [51]. For this reason, it is time for us to seek alternative solutions to ease the healthcare and economic burden of developing new antibiotics.

In this study, several methods were used to demonstrate the effectiveness of TFDG in inhibiting cell growth. As seen in Figures 2–4 and Tables 1 and 2, 250 µg/mL TFDG consistently inhibits $\geq$ 90% of cells compared to the control at 6-h incubation. BacTiter-Glo^{TM} measures the ATP level in the cell since extracellular ATP peaked at the end of the log phase but decreased during the stationary phase [52]. This test is more sensitive as it directly detects the presence of the ATP level in the sample, indicating the metabolically active viable cells, which do not discriminate between live and dead cells [53]. The Live/Dead assay measures the permeability of the cellular membrane. Red-colored cells indicate the cell membranes were damaged when treated with TFDG (Figures 2–4). These two assays provided further proof that TFDG could effectively inhibit bacterial growth. Ignasimuthu et al. [54] showed the MIC of EGCG for *B. subtilis*, *E. coli*, and *S. aureus* ranging from 130 to 580 µg/mL via broth dilution method. This suggests that TFDG might be comparable or even better as an antibacterial agent when compared to EGCG. Further studies of the effects of TFDG against clinically significant strains like ESKAPE (*Enterococcus faecium*, *S. aureus*, *K. pneumoniae*, *A. baumannii*, *P. aeruginosa*, and *Enterobacter* spp.) bacteria and other drug-resistant strains such as MRSA, VRSA, carbapenem-resistant Enterobacterales (CRE) will be carried out [55]. In terms of the antibacterial mechanism, TFDG decreased the eDNA and dextran production in *S. mutans* while decreasing the expression nucleoid synthesis in *Clostridium perfringens* (*C. perfringens*) [9,13]. A recent transcriptome study also shows that TFs (80% purity) could inhibit different virulence factors, including glucosyltransferases, gtfB, gtfC, and gtfD in *S. mutans*. The antimicrobial mechanism of TFDG on other species remains undetermined [56].

Bacterial spores are associated with foodborne diseases and food spoilage, and human diseases like gas gangrene, anthrax, and botulism [36]. Table 3 and Figure 5 show the successful inhibition of both *B. cereus* and *B. subtilis* from germinating. This is a promising observation, as TFDG could still prevent the spore from germinating above 99% for both species. The ability of EGCG to inhibit sporulation is well-documented across *Bacillus* spp. [16,57]. The findings in this study provide further evidence that tea polyphenols could serve as a potent antimicrobial agent. CASTp is an online tool that analytically predicts pocket cavities by utilizing the algorithmic and theoretical modeling that excludes shallow depression [58]. This binding pocket was utilized to determine the binding affinity of TFDG. Molecular docking in this study helps understand the mechanism of TFDG. Previous findings showed that compounds with binding energies of −7.0 kcal/mol or less are considered significant [48]. This threshold eliminates either weak or non-specific binding energies [49]. Chang et al. [49] showed that this threshold could detect 98% of known inhibitors of HIV therapeutics. This threshold has also been shown to eliminate 95% of non-inhibitor interaction [49]. This study uses AutoDock Vina for binding analysis. It is a freely accessible tool that best performed in predicting high-affinity ligands and showed the most consistent performance in a study by Kukol [59]. Table 4 and Figure 6 show that the binding affinity of TFDG for *B. cereus* GPR and Lgt were −9.7 and −7.6 kcal/mol, respectively. As for *B. subtilis*, TFDG affinity for GPR and Lgt were the same, at −10.3 kcal/mol. Based on the promising binding results, a semi-quantitative RT-PCR was carried out to investigate the relative expression of both genes when treated with TFDG. This method is sensitive and reliable in detecting limited transcripts from the samples [60]. The result in Figure 7 shows that the relative expression of *gpr* was significantly lower (0.20 to 0.39) than the control in both *B. cereus* and *B. subtilis*. The relative expression of *lgt* was higher in *B. subtilis* (0.88) than *B. cereus* (0.25) compared to the control. Overall, TFDG may affect both *lgt* and *gpr* expression in *B. cereus* while only *gpr* expression in *B. subtilis*. The GPR protease encoded by *gpr* is a germination protease in the spore coat, responsible for degrading the small acid-soluble protein (SASPs) [61]. This is a conserved gene in *Bacillus* spp. *Clostridium* spp. and *Clostridiodides* spp. involving in protein synthesis and energy metabolism for early spore outgrowth [61,62]. A conserved gene, *lgt* or *gerF* in *Bacillus* spp. and *Clostridium* spp. codes for prelipoprotein diacylglycerol transferase [62,63]. This enzyme acts as a catalyst for the transfer of diacylglycerol to a cysteine residue in bacterial membrane prelipoproteins [63]. Mutation in this gene results in a slower germination process even in a favorable environment [63,64]. The deletion of *lgt* in *B. anthracis* causes a decrease in surface hydrophobicity that eventually leads to lower virulence in the mutant strain [64]. In *B. subtilis*, the mixture of Ca^{2+} and dipicolinic acid (Ca-DPA) complex with GerF occurs during germination [63]. Li et al. [65] reported that the binding dissociation constant (Kd) between Ca-DPA and its native ligand SpoVAD was 0.8. To the best of our knowledge, this is the first study that investigates the binding affinity between Ca-DPA and GerF in *Bacillus* spp. Both GPR and GerF show favorable outcomes in inhibiting the germination process from *in silico* analysis. The favorable binding affinity, along with multiple numbers of hydrogen and hydrophobic bonds, suggests that these two proteins could be the potential targets of TFDG in inhibiting the germination process. Semi-quantitative results support that TFDG inhibits the expression of the conserved genes. Thus, TFDG should be further investigated as a natural food additive.

Figures 2–4 show the cells clumped together, the self-binding process known as auto-agglutination/auto-aggregation [66]. This is a widely observed phenomenon and is considered the first step in biofilm formation [66]. Auto-aggregation occurs under stressful conditions, such as temperature change, and protects the cells from external stressors [66]. Generally, auto-aggregation is mediated by surface proteins like the self-associating autotransporters (SAATs) in *Enterobacteriaceae* [66]. In *Actinobacillus pleuropneumoniae* (*A. pleuropneumoniae*), the adhesin gene *adh* was involved in the biofilm formation, and the deletion of this gene could decrease pathogenicity [67]. Similarly, the first steps of biofilm formation in *Helicobacter pylori*, *P. gingivalis*, and *Staphylococcus epidermidis* are also through auto-aggregation via their adhesin genes [68–70]. The effects of TFDG, especially pertaining to adhesion and biofilm formation, would be a pivotal step to better understanding the antimicrobial mechanism of TFDG.

4. Materials and Methods

4.1. Bacteria Culture

The bacterial cultures used in this study include Gram-negative: *Klebsiella aerogenes* (*K. aerogenes*) (155030A), *Escherichia coli* (*E. coli*) (155065A), *Pseudomonas aeruginosa* (*P. aeruginosa*) (155250A), and *Proteus mirabilis* (*P. mirabilis*) (155239A); Gram-positive: *Bacillus cereus* (*B. cereus*) (154870A), *Bacillus subtilis* (*B. subtilis*) (154921A), *Staphylococcus aureus* (*S. aureus*) (155554A), and *Streptococcus pyogenes* (*S. pyogenes*) (155630A); and acid-fast *Mycobacterium smegmatis* (*M. smegmatis*) (155180A). All cultures were obtained from Carolina Biological (Carolina Biological, Burlington, NC, USA).

4.2. Culture Maintenance

All cultures were maintained in tryptic soy broth (TSB) or tryptic soy agar (TSA) except for *S. pyogenes* and *M. smegmatis*, which were maintained in brain heart infusion broth (BHIB) (Bacto^{TM}, Sparks, MD, USA). The media were made with Milli-Q Integral 5 Water Purification System (Millipore Sigma, Billerica, MA, USA) based on the manufacturer's protocol. All experiments were performed using fresh overnight culture. The purity of the cultures was routinely checked.

4.3. Theaflavin Preparation

Theaflavins were obtained from a nutraceutical company (DH Nutraceuticals, LLC, Edison, NJ, USA). Theaflavin-3,3′-digallate (TFDG) was extracted and purified using ethyl acetate fraction, LH-20 column, 40% acetone solution elution then concentrated via rotary evaporator [71]. Purified 10 mg/mL TFDG stock solution was prepared with 200 proof ethanol (EtOH) (DLI, King of Prussia, PA, USA). The theaflavin stock was diluted in bacterial growth media to the desired concentrations accordingly.

4.4. Microplate Assay

The bacterial growth was monitored with different TFDG concentrations (0, 62.5, 125, and 250 μg/mL) over a 12-h period. In a 96-well plate, 10 μL of overnight culture (OD_{600nm} = 1.0) was added to each well along with various concentrations of TFDG and TSB to yield a final volume of 120 μL. The optical density was recorded hourly using a Varioskan^{TM} LUX multimode microplate reader and analyzed via SkanIt Software (Thermo Scientific^{TM}, Waltham, MA, USA). The positive control was 10% bleach, while bacterial growth media was used as the negative control. The highest solvent concentration (1% EtOH) was also tested. Erythromycin, a broad-spectrum antibiotic, has also been included as a reference molecule for antibacterial efficacy comparison. The experiments were performed in triplicate. The microplate assay results established the half-maximal inhibitory concentration (IC_{50}) and minimum inhibitory concentration (MIC). The lowest concentration with no bacterial growth was defined as MIC. The IC_{50} was calculated based on a dose-response curve with log (concentration) as the x-axis and percent inhibition as the y-axis based on 0, 62.5, 125, and 250 μg/mL. The concentration that correlates to the 50% inhibition is the IC_{50}.

4.5. Colony Forming Unit (CFU) Assay

Following the microplate assay, the cultures treated with 0, 62.5, and 250 μg/mL TFDG were collected after 6-h incubation, serially diluted (from 10^{-2} to 10^{-8}) plated on TSA. The plates were incubated for 12 h at 37 °C, and the experiments were done in triplicate. The CFUs were recorded, and the percent inhibition was calculated based on the following formula:

$$Percent\ Inhibition = \left[\frac{CFU_{untreated} - CFU_{treated}}{CFU_{untreated}}\right] \times 100 \quad (1)$$

The log reduction of the CFU was also calculated based on the following formula:

$$Log\ Reduction = Log10\left(\frac{CFU_{untreated}}{CFU_{treated}}\right) \quad (2)$$

4.6. BacTiter-Glo™ Microbial Cell Viability Assay

BacTiter-Glo™, the luciferase-based assay that quantifies the amount of ATP of metabolically active cells, was conducted according to the manufacturer's protocol (Promega, Madison, WI, USA) [54]. The reagent was prepared by mixing the BacTiter-Glo™ buffer with the BacTiter-Glo™ lyophilized substrate at room temperature. The mixture was then homogenized and incubated at room temperature for 15 min.

In a black 96-well plate, the bacteria were prepared based on the microplate assay (TFDG concentration of 0, 62.5, and 250 μg/mL) and placed in an IS-500 Incubator Shaker (Chemglass Life Sciences LLC, Vineland, NJ, USA) at 37 °C, 250 rpm for six hours. Then 120 μL of the BacTiter-Glo™ reagent was added to each well. The plate was wrapped in aluminum foil and placed in the incubator shaker for five minutes. The luminescence was read using a Varioskan™ LUX multimode microplate reader and analyzed via SkanIt Software (Thermo Scientific™, Waltham, MA, USA). The experiments were done in triplicate. The percent inhibition was calculated based on the following formula:

$$Percent\ Inhibition = \left[\frac{(RFU_{untreated} - RFU_{treated})}{RFU_{untreated}}\right] \times 100 \quad (3)$$

The log reduction of the RFU was also calculated based on the following formula:

$$Log\ Reduction = Log10\left(\frac{RFU_{untreated}}{RFU_{treated}}\right) \quad (4)$$

4.7. LIVE/DEAD™ BacLight™ Bacterial Viability Assay

The Live/Dead Viability is a two-dye system consisting of Syto9 green fluorescent dye and propidium iodide (PI) red fluorescent dye. Both nucleic acid dyes can be used to differentiate live from dead bacteria. PI penetrates damaged bacterial membranes while Syto9 stains bacteria with intact cell membranes. Thus, live cells will be stained in green, impaired cells in yellow, and dead cells in red.

The staining was done using the Invitrogen™ Live/Dead BacLight™ Bacterial Viability Kit. According to the manufacturer's recommendation, equal parts of the Syto9 and PI were combined (Thermo Fisher Scientific, Waltham, MA, USA).

Following the same experimental setup as the CFU assay mentioned above (0, 62.5, and 250 μg/mL TFDG), the dye mixture was added to each culture and incubated at room temperature in the dark for 15 min. The cells were then observed using Olympus IX81 FV1000 Confocal Microscope, and the images were analyzed using the FV10-ASW 4.2 viewer. This method was also utilized to visualize the germinated spores, except the spores were treated for 60 min.

4.8. Spore Preparation

This method was modified based on the previously published protocol [16,72]. *B. cereus* and *B. subtilis* are spore-forming bacteria. The spores were induced by adding 5 mL of fresh overnight culture (OD_{600nm} = 1.0) to 5 mL sterile diH_2O in a culture tube. The cultures were incubated at 37 °C and 250 rpm for 72 h (IS-500 Incubator Shaker, Chemglass Life Sciences LLC, Vineland, NJ, USA). After 72 h, the spores were heated for 20 min at 75 °C to inactivate the vegetative cells. The purity of the spores was confirmed through the Schaeffer Fulton differential stain method.

4.9. Spore Germination Inhibition Assay

100 µL of the 72-h spores were added to various concentrations of TFDG (312.5 µg/mL and 625 µg/mL) along with TSB to a final volume of 1 mL in a microcentrifuge tube. The tubes were incubated for 1 h at 37 °C and 250 rpm (IS-500 Incubator Shaker, Chemglass Life Sciences LLC, Vineland, NJ, USA). After the incubation period, the samples were serially diluted (from 10^{-2} to 10^{-9}), and 100 µL of the dilution was plated using the spread plate method with TSA. The plates were incubated for 12 h at 37 °C. The experiments were done in triplicate. The CFUs were recorded, and the percentage of inhibition and log reduction was calculated based on the formula above (1 and 2).

4.10. Ligand Preparation

The 2D structure of TFDG (structure ID: 135403795) was obtained from PubChem (https://pubchem.ncbi.nlm.nih.gov/, accessed on 27 August 2021). The structure was converted into 3D format using Vega ZZ software (http://www.vegazz.net, accessed on 27 August 2021) and .pdbqt file format using AutoDock Tools V1.5.6 [73].

4.11. Gene and Protein Selection

The germination genes for *in silico* modeling were selected based on conserveness in *Bacillus* spp. and *Clostridium* spp. [74]. The genes and their protein information were tabulated in Table 6. The protein structure of each gene was downloaded directly from PDB (https://www.rcsb.org/, accessed on 3 September 2021) for the binding analysis. If the protein structure was not yet crystalized, the protein sequence was used to construct a hypothetical structure using SwissModel (https://swissmodel.expasy.org/, accessed on 3 September 2021) [75]. The hypothetical structure with the highest sequence identity was chosen for the analysis. The binding pocket was then determined using the Computed Atlas of Surface Topography of Proteins (CASTp) (http://sts.bioe.uic.edu/castp/, accessed on 3 September 2021) [58].

Table 6. Genes and protein information of conserved germination genes of *B. cereus* and *B. subtilis*.

Bacteria	Gene	NCBI Gene ID	Crystal Structure	PDB Reference	% Sequence Identity
B. cereus	*gpr*	56320307	None	IC8B	71.47%
	lgt (gerF)	56322894	None	5AZC	16.74%
B. subtilis	*gpr*	937838	None	IC8B	68.68%
	lgt (gerF)	12085459	None	5AZC	35.21%

4.12. In Silico Docking Analysis and Visualization

In silico docking analysis was performed using AutoDock Vina. The size and search space of each protein were calculated using AutoDock Tools 1.5.6 based on the result from the CASTp analysis. Table 7 shows the grid box for each analysis. The spacing was left at the default value of 0.375 Å, as well as the exhaustiveness rate of 8 [73].

Table 7. Grid box information of conserved germination protein for binding analysis.

Bacteria	Protein	Center X	Center Y	Center Z	Size X	Size Y	Size Z
B. cereus	GPR	−2	10	110	126	126	126
	Lgt (GerF)	−20	0	0	92	120	104
B. subtilis	GPR	−20	40	50	126	126	126
	Lgt (GerF)	−15	0	−8	90	114	126

4.13. Total RNA Extraction, cDNA Synthesis, and Semi-Quantitative RT-PCR

The spore germination assay was carried out for control, PBS, and 625 μg/mL TFDG. After one hour of treatment, the RNA extraction was done using the Ambion® RiboPure™ Kit (Ambion Inc, Austin, TX, USA). Then 250 μL of the sample was mixed with the 1 mL TRI reagent. The mixture was sonicated 15 times at 3 s intervals (20% power) using the Branson Sonifier Cell Disruptor 200 (Emerson Industrial, St. Louis, MO, USA). The extraction process was carried out based on the manufacturer's protocol. The RNA was used as a template for the cDNA synthesis using the ABI High Capacity cDNA Reverse Transcription Kit (Applied Biosystems-Life Technologies, Camarillo, CA, USA). The cDNA synthesis was done according to the manufacturer's protocol. The cDNA synthesis was carried out in a Veriti 96-Well Thermocycler (Applied Biosystems, Camarillo, CA, USA). The cDNA purity and concentration were measured using a BioDrop uLite (Biochrom, Cambridge, United Kingdom). The samples were stored at −20 °C.

The oligonucleotides were designed based using NCBI Primer Design Tool (https://www.ncbi.nlm.nih.gov/tools/primer-blast/, accessed 3 November 2021). The following primers were generated: Bc_GPR_F2: 5′-ACACCAGATGCTCTTGGACC-3′ and Bc_GPR_R2: 5′-TCTGCTCTTTTCATCCGGCA-3′; Bc_Lgt_F2: 5′-CTGTATGGGCTTTTGGGGCA and Bc_Lgt_R2: 5′-TGAGCAAACCCCTCAACAAT-3′; Bs_GPR_F2: 5′-CCGATTTGGCAGTGG AAACG-3′ and Bs_GPR_R2: 5′-AACACCAAGCGTGTCTTTGC-3′; Bs_Lgt_F2: 5′-TTTGCT CGGGCTGTGGATAG-3′ and Bs_Lgt_R2 5′ CCCTTGACGCGTCTGAAGAT-3′; 16S ribosomal RNA 27F: 5′-AGAGTTTGATCCTGGCTCAG-3′ and 1492R: 5′-ACGGCTACCTTGTTAC GACTT-3′. The ~100 μg/mL cDNA was used, and the PCR was performed using the Applied Biosystems Veriti 96-Well Thermal Cycler (ThermoFisher Scientific, MA, USA): 95 °C for 60 s, 35 cycles of 95 °C for 10 s, 56 °C for 10 s and 72 °C for 90 s. A 2% agarose gel electrophoresis was carried out, and the amount of cDNA was determined [76]. The relative mRNA expression was then calculated.

4.14. Statistical Analysis

All experiments were performed in triplicate, and the mean and standard deviations (SD) were calculated. One-way Analysis of Variance (ANOVA) and Dunnett's post hoc analysis were used to analyze the data (GraphPad Prism 5, San Diego, CA, USA). A p-value less than 0.05 was considered statistically significant.

5. Conclusions

This study profiled the effects of TFDG on nine bacteria, including Gram-positive, Gram-negative, and acid-fast bacteria. Microplate assay and the CFU assay were carried out. The microplate assay results indicated the MIC was 250 μg/mL. BacTiter-Glo™ Microbial Cell Viability test was also performed to measure the level of ATP in the sample. The fluorescence-based Live/Dead Assay was utilized to visualize the morphological changes on individual cells to TFDG, thus precluding the possible antibacterial mechanism of TFDG. *In silico* modeling allowed us to analyze and propose the mechanism of TFDG on the bacterial spores at the molecular level. Semi-quantitative RT-PCR assays were carried out for gene expression analysis pre- and post-treatment. This study successfully shows the potential usage of TFDG as an antimicrobial agent for a wide selection of bacteria, ranging through Gram-negative, Gram-positive, and acid-fast species. This study also shows the anti-germination properties of TFDG as TFDG inhibits the expression of *gpr* and *lgt*, genes code for the conserved GPR and Lgt (GerF) germination proteins based on *in silico* modeling and semi-quantitative RT-PCR.

Supplementary Materials: The following supporting information can be downloaded at: https://www.mdpi.com/article/10.3390/ijms23042153/s1.

Author Contributions: Conceptualization, A.Y. and T.C.; methodology, A.Y. and T.C.; investigation, A.Y., B.C., O.F. and S.L.; formal analysis, A.Y. and T.C.; resources, T.C.; data curation, A.Y.; writing—original draft preparation, A.Y.; writing—review and editing, T.C.; visualization, A.Y. and T.C.;

supervision, T.C.; project administration, T.C.; funding acquisition, T.C. All authors have read and agreed to the published version of the manuscript.

Funding: A.Y. and S.L. were supported by the Seton Hall University (SHU) Graduate Teaching Assistantship. TC is supported by the SHU Biological Sciences Research Fund and the William and Doreen Wong Foundation.

Data Availability Statement: Data are contained within the article.

Conflicts of Interest: The authors declare no conflict of interest.

References

1. Piddock, L.J.V. The crisis of no new antibiotics—What is the way forward? *Lancet Infect. Dis.* **2012**, *12*, 249–253. [CrossRef]
2. Ventola, C.L. The Antibiotic Resistance Crisis Part 1: Causes and Threats. *Pharm. Ther.* **2015**, *40*, 277–283.
3. CDC. *Antibiotic Resistance Threats in the United States*; US Department of Health and Human Services, CDC: Atlanta, GA, USA, 2019. [CrossRef]
4. Martens, E.; Demain, A.L. The antibiotic resistance crisis, with a focus on the United States. *J. Antibiot.* **2017**, *70*, 520–526. [CrossRef]
5. Hilal, Y.; Engelhardt, U. Characterisation of white tea—Comparison to green and black tea. *J. Verbrauch. Lebensm.* **2007**, *2*, 414–421. [CrossRef]
6. Babich, H.; Gottesman, R.T.; Liebling, E.J.; Schuck, A.G. Theaflavin-3-gallate and theaflavin-3′-gallate, polyphenols in black tea with prooxidant properties. *Basic Clin. Pharmacol. Toxicol.* **2008**, *103*, 66–74. [CrossRef] [PubMed]
7. Pereira-Caro, G.; Moreno-Rojas, J.M.; Brindani, N.; Del Rio, D.; Lean, M.E.J.; Hara, Y.; Crozier, A. Bioavailability of Black Tea Theaflavins: Absorption, Metabolism, and Colonic Catabolism. *J. Agric. Food Chem.* **2017**, *65*, 5365–5374. [CrossRef] [PubMed]
8. de Oliveira, A.; Prince, D.; Lo, C.Y.; Lee, L.H.; Chu, T.C. Antiviral activity of theaflavin digallate against herpes simplex virus type 1. *Antivir. Res.* **2015**, *118*, 56–67. [CrossRef]
9. Wang, S.; Wang, Y.; Wang, Y.; Duan, Z.; Ling, Z.; Wu, W.; Tong, S.; Wang, H.; Deng, S. Theaflavin-3,3′-Digallate Suppresses Biofilm Formation, Acid Production, and Acid Tolerance in Streptococcus mutans by Targeting Virulence Factors. *Front. Microbiol.* **2019**, *10*, 1705. [CrossRef]
10. Engelhardt, U.H. Chemistry of Tea. In *Comprehensive Natural Products II*; Elsevier Science: Amsterdam, The Netherlands, 2010; pp. 999–1032.
11. Peterson, J.; Dwyer, J.; Jacques, P.; Rand, W.; Prior, R.; Chui, K. Tea variety and brewing techniques influence flavonoid content of black tea. *J. Food Compos. Anal.* **2004**, *17*, 397–405. [CrossRef]
12. Leung, L.K.; Su, Y.; Chen, R.; Zhang, Z.; Huang, Y.; Chen, Z.-Y. Theaflavins in Black Tea and Catechins in Green Tea Are Equally Effective Antioxidants. *J. Nutr.* **2001**, *131*, 2248–2251. [CrossRef]
13. Noor Mohammadi, T.; Maung, A.T.; Sato, J.; Sonoda, T.; Masuda, Y.; Honjoh, K.; Miyamoto, T. Mechanism for antibacterial action of epigallocatechin gallate and theaflavin-3,3′-digallate on Clostridium perfringens. *J. Appl. Microbiol.* **2019**, *126*, 633–640. [CrossRef] [PubMed]
14. Hui, X.; Yue, Q.; Zhang, D.D.; Li, H.; Yang, S.Q.; Gao, W.Y. Antimicrobial mechanism of theaflavins: They target 1-deoxy-D-xylulose 5-phosphate reductoisomerase, the key enzyme of the MEP terpenoid biosynthetic pathway. *Sci. Rep.* **2016**, *6*, 38945. [CrossRef] [PubMed]
15. Teng, Z.; Guo, Y.; Liu, X.; Zhang, J.; Niu, X.; Yu, Q.; Deng, X.; Wang, J. Theaflavin-3,3-digallate increases the antibacterial activity of β-lactam antibiotics by inhibiting metallo-beta-lactamase activity. *J. Cell Mol. Med.* **2019**, *23*, 6955–6964. [CrossRef] [PubMed]
16. Ali, B.; Lee, L.H.; Laskar, N.; Shaikh, N.; Tahir, H.; Hsu, S.D.; Newby, R., Jr.; Valsechi-Diaz, J.; Chu, T. Modified Green Tea Polyphenols, EGCG-S and LTP, Inhibit Endospore in Three *Bacillus* spp. *Adv. Microbiol.* **2017**, *7*, 175–187. [CrossRef]
17. Renzetti, A.; Betts, J.W.; Fukumoto, K.; Rutherford, R.N. Antibacterial green tea catechins from a molecular perspective: Mechanisms of action and structure-activity relationships. *Food Funct.* **2020**, *11*, 9370–9396. [CrossRef]
18. Ben Lagha, A.; Grenier, D. Black tea theaflavins attenuate Porphyromonas gingivalis virulence properties, modulate gingival keratinocyte tight junction integrity and exert anti-inflammatory activity. *J. Periodontal Res.* **2017**, *52*, 458–470. [CrossRef]
19. Chowdhury, P.; Sahuc, M.E.; Rouille, Y.; Riviere, C.; Bonneau, N.; Vandeputte, A.; Brodin, P.; Goswami, M.; Bandyopadhyay, T.; Dubuisson, J.; et al. Theaflavins, polyphenols of black tea, inhibit entry of hepatitis C virus in cell culture. *PLoS ONE* **2018**, *13*, e0198226. [CrossRef]
20. Kong, J.; Zhang, G.; Xia, K.; Diao, C.; Yang, X.; Zuo, X.; Li, Y.; Liang, X. Tooth brushing using toothpaste containing theaflavins reduces the oral pathogenic bacteria in healthy adults. *3 Biotech* **2021**, *11*, 150. [CrossRef]
21. Wang, M.; Li, J.; Hu, T.; Zhao, H. Metabolic fate of tea polyphenols and their crosstalk with gut microbiota. *Food Sci. Hum. Wellness* **2022**, *11*, 455–466. [CrossRef]
22. Passarelli-Araujo, H.; Palmeiro, J.K.; Moharana, K.C.; Pedrosa-Silva, F.; Dalla-Costa, L.M.; Venancio, T.M. Genomic analysis unveils important aspects of population structure, virulence, and antimicrobial resistance in *Klebsiella aerogenes*. *FEBS J.* **2019**, *286*, 3797–3810. [CrossRef]
23. Kaper, J.B.; Nataro, J.P.; Mobley, H.L. Pathogenic Escherichia coli. *Nat. Rev. Microbiol.* **2004**, *2*, 123–140. [CrossRef] [PubMed]

24. Sondi, I.; Salopek-Sondi, B. Silver nanoparticles as antimicrobial agent: A case study on E. coli as a model for Gram-negative bacteria. *J. Colloid Interface Sci.* **2004**, *275*, 177–182. [CrossRef] [PubMed]
25. Blount, Z.D. The Natural History of Model Organisms: The unexhausted potential of *E. coli*. *elife* **2015**, *4*, e05826. [CrossRef] [PubMed]
26. Iakovides, I.C.; Michael-Kordatou, I.; Moreira, N.F.F.; Ribeiro, A.R.; Fernandes, T.; Pereira, M.F.R.; Nunes, O.C.; Manaia, C.M.; Silva, A.M.T.; Fatta-Kassinos, D. Continuous ozonation of urban wastewater: Removal of antibiotics, antibiotic-resistant Escherichia coli and antibiotic resistance genes and phytotoxicity. *Water Res.* **2019**, *159*, 333–347. [CrossRef] [PubMed]
27. Zhang, C.M.; Xu, L.M.; Wang, X.C.; Zhuang, K.; Liu, Q.Q. Effects of ultraviolet disinfection on antibiotic-resistant *Escherichia coli* from wastewater: Inactivation, antibiotic resistance profiles and antibiotic resistance genes. *J. Appl. Microbiol.* **2017**, *123*, 295–306. [CrossRef] [PubMed]
28. Roth, N.; Kasbohrer, A.; Mayrhofer, S.; Zitz, U.; Hofacre, C.; Domig, K.J. The application of antibiotics in broiler production and the resulting antibiotic resistance in *Escherichia coli*: A global overview. *Poult. Sci.* **2019**, *98*, 1791–1804. [CrossRef]
29. Davis, G.S.; Waits, K.; Nordstrom, L.; Grande, H.; Weaver, B.; Papp, K.; Horwinski, J.; Koch, B.; Hungate, B.A.; Liu, C.M.; et al. Antibiotic-resistant Escherichia coli from retail poultry meat with different antibiotic use claims. *BMC Microbiol.* **2018**, *18*, 174. [CrossRef]
30. Poole, K. Pseudomonas aeruginosa: Resistance to the max. *Front. Microbiol.* **2011**, *2*, 65. [CrossRef]
31. Hamilton, A.L.; Kamm, M.A.; Ng, S.C.; Morrison, M. *Proteus* spp. as Putative Gastrointestinal Pathogens. *Clin. Microbiol. Rev.* **2018**, *31*, e00085-17. [CrossRef]
32. Cohen-Nahum, K.; Saidel-Odes, L.; Riesenberg, K.; Schlaeffer, F.; Borer, A. Urinary tract infections caused by multi-drug resistant Proteus mirabilis: Risk factors and clinical outcomes. *Infection* **2010**, *38*, 41–46. [CrossRef]
33. Ehling-Schulz, M.; Lereclus, D.; Koehler, T.M. The Bacillus cereus Group: Bacillus Species with Pathogenic Potential. *Microbiol. Spectr.* **2019**, *7*. [CrossRef] [PubMed]
34. Errington, J.; Aart, L.T.V. Microbe Profile: Bacillus subtilis: Model organism for cellular development, and industrial workhorse. *Microbiology* **2020**, *166*, 425–427. [CrossRef] [PubMed]
35. Pogmore, A.R.; Seistrup, K.H.; Strahl, H. The Gram-positive model organism Bacillus subtilis does not form microscopically detectable cardiolipin-specific lipid domains. *Microbiology* **2018**, *164*, 475–482. [CrossRef] [PubMed]
36. Setlow, P. Germination of Spores of Bacillus Species: What We Know and Do Not Know. *J. Bacteriol.* **2014**, *196*, 1297–1305. [CrossRef]
37. Keijser, B.J.; Ter Beek, A.; Rauwerda, H.; Schuren, F.; Montijn, R.; van der Spek, H.; Brul, S. Analysis of temporal gene expression during Bacillus subtilis spore germination and outgrowth. *J. Bacteriol.* **2007**, *189*, 3624–3634. [CrossRef]
38. Levinson, H.S.; Hyatt, M. Effects of Temperature on Activation, Germination, and Outgrowth of Bacillus megaterium Spores. *J. Bacteriol.* **1970**, *101*, 56–64. [CrossRef]
39. Hornstra, L.M.; de Vries, Y.P.; Wells-Bennik, M.H.; de Vos, W.M.; Abee, T. Characterization of germination receptors of Bacillus cereus ATCC 14579. *Appl. Environ. Microbiol.* **2006**, *72*, 44–53. [CrossRef]
40. Traag, B.A.; Pugliese, A.; Eisen, J.A.; Losick, R. Gene Conservation among Endospore-Forming Bacteria Reveals Additional Sporulation Genes in Bacillus subtilis. *J. Bacteriol.* **2013**, *195*, 253–260. [CrossRef]
41. Seo, Y.S.; Lee, D.Y.; Rayamahji, N.; Kang, M.L.; Yoo, H.S. Biofilm-forming associated genotypic and phenotypic characteristics of Staphylococcus spp. isolated from animals and air. *Res. Vet. Sci.* **2008**, *85*, 433–438. [CrossRef]
42. Sriskandan, S.; Faulkner, L.; Hopkins, P. Streptococcus pyogenes: Insight into the function of the streptococcal superantigens. *Int. J. Biochem. Cell Biol.* **2007**, *39*, 12–19. [CrossRef]
43. Zhu, L.; Olsen, R.J.; Horstmann, N.; Shelburne, S.A.; Fan, J.; Hu, Y.; Musser, J.M. Intergenic Variable-Number Tandem-Repeat Polymorphism Upstream of rocA Alters Toxin Production and Enhances Virulence in Streptococcus pyogenes. *Infect. Immun.* **2016**, *84*, 2086–2093. [CrossRef] [PubMed]
44. Forbes, B.A. Mycobacterial Taxonomy. *J. Clin. Microbiol.* **2017**, *55*, 380–383. [CrossRef] [PubMed]
45. WHO. *W.H.O. Global Tuberculosis Report*; World Health Organization: Geneva, Switzerland, 2020; pp. 1–232.
46. Lelovic, N.; Mitachi, K.; Yang, J.; Lemieux, M.R.; Ji, Y.; Kurosu, M. Application of Mycobacterium smegmatis as a surrogate to evaluate drug leads against Mycobacterium tuberculosis. *J. Antibiot.* **2020**, *73*, 780–789. [CrossRef] [PubMed]
47. Altaf, M.; Miller, C.H.; Bellows, D.S.; O'Toole, R. Evaluation of the Mycobacterium smegmatis and BCG models for the discovery of Mycobacterium tuberculosis inhibitors. *Tuberculosis* **2010**, *90*, 333–337. [CrossRef]
48. Kwofie, S.K.; Broni, E.; Asiedu, S.O.; Kwarko, G.B.; Dankwa, B.; Enninful, K.S.; Tiburu, E.K.; Wilson, M.D. Cheminformatics-Based Identification of Potential Novel Anti-SARS-CoV-2 Natural Compounds of African Origin. *Molecules* **2021**, *26*, 406. [CrossRef]
49. Chang, M.W.; Lindstrom, W.; Olson, A.J.; Belew, R.K. Analysis of HIV Wild-Type and Mutant Structures via in Silico Docking against Diverse Ligand Libraries. *J. Chem. Inf. Model.* **2007**, *47*, 1258–1262. [CrossRef]
50. Chen, D.; Oezguen, N.; Urvil, P.; Ferguson, C.; Dann, S.M.; Savidge, T.C. Regulation of protein-ligand binding affinity by hydrogen bond pairing. *Sci. Adv.* **2016**, *2*, e1501240. [CrossRef]
51. Ardal, C.; Balasegaram, M.; Laxminarayan, R.; McAdams, D.; Outterson, K.; Rex, J.H.; Sumpradit, N. Antibiotic development—Economic, regulatory and societal challenges. *Nat. Rev. Microbiol.* **2020**, *18*, 267–274. [CrossRef]
52. Mempin, R.; Tran, H.; Chen, C.; Gong, H.; Kim Ho, K.; Lu, S. Release of extracellular ATP by bacteria during growth. *BMC Microbiol.* **2013**, *13*, 301. [CrossRef]

53. Reyneke, B.; Dobrowsky, P.H.; Ndlovu, T.; Khan, S.; Khan, W. EMA-qPCR to monitor the efficiency of a closed-coupled solar pasteurization system in reducing Legionella contamination of roof-harvested rainwater. *Sci. Total Environ.* **2016**, *553*, 662–670. [CrossRef]
54. Ignasimuthu, K.; Prakash, R.; Murthy, P.S.; Subban, N. Enhanced bioaccessibility of green tea polyphenols and lipophilic activity of EGCG octaacetate on gram-negative bacteria. *LWT* **2019**, *105*, 103–109. [CrossRef]
55. Santajit, S.; Indrawattana, N. Mechanisms of Antimicrobial Resistance in ESKAPE Pathogens. *Biomed. Res. Int.* **2016**, *2016*, 2475067. [CrossRef]
56. Feng, S.; Eucker, T.P.; Holly, M.K.; Konkel, M.E.; Lu, X.; Wang, S. Investigating the responses of Cronobacter sakazakii to garlic-drived organosulfur compounds: A systematic study of pathogenic-bacterium injury by use of high-throughput whole-transcriptome sequencing and confocal micro-raman spectroscopy. *Appl. Environ. Microbiol.* **2014**, *80*, 959–971. [CrossRef]
57. Shigemune, N.; Nakayama, M.; Tsugukuni, T.; Hitomi, J.; Yoshizawa, C.; Mekada, Y.; Kurahachi, M.; Miyamoto, T. The mechanisms and effect of epigallocatechin gallate (EGCg) on the germination and proliferation of bacterial spores. *Food Control* **2012**, *27*, 269–274. [CrossRef]
58. Tian, W.; Chen, C.; Lei, X.; Zhao, J.; Liang, J. CASTp 3.0: Computed atlas of surface topography of proteins. *Nucleic Acids Res.* **2018**, *46*, W363–W367. [CrossRef] [PubMed]
59. Kukol, A. Consensus virtual screening approaches to predict protein ligands. *Eur. J. Med. Chem.* **2011**, *46*, 4661–4664. [CrossRef] [PubMed]
60. Marone, M.; Mozzetti, S.; Ritis, D.D.; Pierelli, L.; Scambia, G. Semiquantitative RT-PCR analysis to assess the expression levels of multiple transcripts from the same sample. *Biol. Proced. Online* **2001**, *3*, 19–25. [CrossRef] [PubMed]
61. Xiao, Y.; Francke, C.; Abee, T.; Wells-Bennik, M.H. Clostridial spore germination versus bacilli: Genome mining and current insights. *Food Microbiol.* **2011**, *28*, 266–274. [CrossRef]
62. Norsigian, C.J.; Danhof, H.A.; Brand, C.K.; Oezguen, N.; Midani, F.S.; Palsson, B.O.; Savidge, T.C.; Britton, R.A.; Spinler, J.K.; Monk, J.M. Systems biology analysis of the Clostridioides difficile core-genome contextualizes microenvironmental evolutionary pressures leading to genotypic and phenotypic divergence. *NPJ Syst. Biol. Appl.* **2020**, *6*, 31. [CrossRef]
63. Igarashi, T.; Setlow, B.; Paidhungat, M.; Setlow, P. Effects of a gerF (lgt) mutation on the germination of spores of Bacillus subtilis. *J. Bacteriol.* **2004**, *186*, 2984–2991. [CrossRef]
64. Okugawa, S.; Moayeri, M.; Pomerantsev, A.P.; Sastalla, I.; Crown, D.; Gupta, P.K.; Leppla, S.H. Lipoprotein biosynthesis by prolipoprotein diacylglyceryl transferase is required for efficient spore germination and full virulence of Bacillus anthracis. *Mol. Microbiol.* **2012**, *83*, 96–109. [CrossRef] [PubMed]
65. Li, Y.; Davis, A.; Korza, G.; Zhang, P.; Li, Y.Q.; Setlow, B.; Setlow, P.; Hao, B. Role of a SpoVA protein in dipicolinic acid uptake into developing spores of Bacillus subtilis. *J. Bacteriol.* **2012**, *194*, 1875–1884. [CrossRef] [PubMed]
66. Trunk, T.; Khalil, H.S.; Leo, J.C. Bacterial autoaggregation. *AIMS Microbiol.* **2018**, *4*, 140–164. [CrossRef]
67. Wang, L.; Qin, W.; Yang, S.; Zhai, R.; Zhou, L.; Sun, C.; Pan, F.; Ji, Q.; Wang, Y.; Gu, J.; et al. The Adh adhesin domain is required for trimeric autotransporter Apa1-mediated Actinobacillus pleuropneumoniae adhesion, autoaggregation, biofilm formation and pathogenicity. *Vet. Microbiol.* **2015**, *177*, 175–183. [CrossRef]
68. Yonezawa, H.; Osaki, T.; Kurata, S.; Zaman, C.; Hanawa, T.; Kamiya, S. Assessment of in vitro biofilm formation by Helicobacter pylori. *J. Gastroenterol. Hepatol.* **2010**, *25* (Suppl. 1), S90–S94. [CrossRef]
69. Yamaguchi, M.; Sato, K.; Yukitake, H.; Noiri, Y.; Ebisu, S.; Nakayama, K. A Porphyromonas gingivalis mutant defective in a putative glycosyltransferase exhibits defective biosynthesis of the polysaccharide portions of lipopolysaccharide, decreased gingipain activities, strong autoaggregation, and increased biofilm formation. *Infect. Immun.* **2010**, *78*, 3801–3812. [CrossRef] [PubMed]
70. Ziebuhr, W.; Heilmann, C.; Götz, F.; Meyer, P.; Wilms, K.; Straube, E.; Hacker, J. Detection of the intercellular adhesion gene cluster (ica) and phase variation in Staphylococcus epidermidis blood culture strains and mucosal isolates. *Infect. Immun.* **1997**, *65*, 890–896. [CrossRef]
71. Lo, C.Y.; Li, S.; Tan, D.; Pan, M.H.; Sang, S.; Ho, C.T. Trapping reactions of reactive carbonyl species with tea polyphenols in simulated physiological conditions. *Mol. Nutr. Food Res.* **2006**, *50*, 1118–1128. [CrossRef]
72. Gray, D.A.; Dugar, G.; Gamba, P.; Strahl, H.; Jonker, M.J.; Hamoen, L.W. Extreme slow growth as alternative strategy to survive deep starvation in bacteria. *Nat. Commun.* **2019**, *10*, 890. [CrossRef]
73. Trott, O.; Olson, A.J. AutoDock Vina: Improving the speed and accuracy of docking with a new scoring function, efficient optimization, and multithreading. *J. Comput. Chem.* **2010**, *31*, 455–461. [CrossRef]
74. Galperin, M.Y.; Mekhedov, S.L.; Puigbo, P.; Smirnov, S.; Wolf, Y.I.; Rigden, D.J. Genomic determinants of sporulation in Bacilli and Clostridia: Towards the minimal set of sporulation-specific genes. *Environ. Microbiol.* **2012**, *14*, 2870–2890. [CrossRef] [PubMed]
75. Waterhouse, A.; Bertoni, M.; Bienert, S.; Studer, G.; Tauriello, G.; Gumienny, R.; Heer, F.T.; de Beer, T.A.P.; Rempfer, C.; Bordoli, L.; et al. SWISS-MODEL: Homology modelling of protein structures and complexes. *Nucleic Acids Res.* **2018**, *46*, W296–W303. [CrossRef] [PubMed]
76. Alambra, J.R.; Alenton, R.R.R.; Gulpeo, P.C.R.; Mecenas, C.L.; Miranda, A.P.; Thomas, R.C.; Velando, M.K.S.; Vitug, L.D.; Maningas, M.B.B. Immunomodulatory effects of turmeric, Curcuma longa (Magnoliophyta, Zingiberaceae) on Macrobrachium rosenbergii (Crustacea, Palaemonidae) against Vibrio alginolyticus (Proteobacteria, Vibrionaceae). *Aquac. Aquar. Conserv. Legis. Int. J. Bioflux Soc.* **2012**, *5*, 13–17.

International Journal of
Molecular Sciences

MDPI

Article

The Antimicrobial Peptides Human β-Defensins Induce the Secretion of Angiogenin in Human Dermal Fibroblasts

Yoshie Umehara [1], Miho Takahashi [1,2], Hainan Yue [1], Juan Valentin Trujillo-Paez [1], Ge Peng [1], Hai Le Thanh Nguyen [1], Ko Okumura [1], Hideoki Ogawa [1] and François Niyonsaba [1,3,*]

1 Atopy (Allergy) Research Center, Juntendo University Graduate School of Medicine, Tokyo 113-8421, Japan
2 Department of Dermatology and Allergology, Juntendo University Graduate School of Medicine, Tokyo 113-8421, Japan
3 Faculty of International Liberal Arts, Juntendo University, Tokyo 113-8421, Japan
* Correspondence: francois@juntendo.ac.jp; Tel.: +81-3-5802-1591; Fax: +81-3-3813-5512

Abstract: The skin produces a plethora of antimicrobial peptides that not only show antimicrobial activities against pathogens but also exhibit various immunomodulatory functions. Human β-defensins (hBDs) are the most well-characterized skin-derived antimicrobial peptides and contribute to diverse biological processes, including cytokine production and the migration, proliferation, and differentiation of host cells. Additionally, hBD-3 was recently reported to promote wound healing and angiogenesis, by inducing the expression of various angiogenic factors and the migration and proliferation of fibroblasts. Angiogenin is one of the most potent angiogenic factors; however, the effects of hBDs on angiogenin production in fibroblasts remain unclear. Here, we investigated the effects of hBDs on the secretion of angiogenin by human dermal fibroblasts. Both in vitro and ex vivo studies demonstrated that hBD-1, hBD-2, hBD-3, and hBD-4 dose-dependently increased angiogenin production by fibroblasts. hBD-mediated angiogenin secretion involved the epidermal growth factor receptor (EGFR), Src family kinase, c-Jun N-terminal kinase (JNK), p38, and nuclear factor-kappa B (NF-κB) pathways, as evidenced by the inhibitory effects of specific inhibitors for these pathways. Indeed, we confirmed that hBDs induced the activation of the EGFR, Src, JNK, p38, and NF-κB pathways. This study identified a novel role of hBDs in angiogenesis, through the production of angiogenin, in addition to their antimicrobial activities and other immunomodulatory properties.

Keywords: human β-defensin (hBD); dermal fibroblast; angiogenin; angiogenesis

Citation: Umehara, Y.; Takahashi, M.; Yue, H.; Trujillo-Paez, J.V.; Peng, G.; Nguyen, H.L.T.; Okumura, K.; Ogawa, H.; Niyonsaba, F. The Antimicrobial Peptides Human β-Defensins Induce the Secretion of Angiogenin in Human Dermal Fibroblasts. *Int. J. Mol. Sci.* **2022**, *23*, 8800. https://doi.org/10.3390/ijms23158800

Academic Editor: Helena Felgueiras

Received: 28 January 2022
Accepted: 6 August 2022
Published: 8 August 2022

1. Introduction

The skin is the primary interface between the body and the surrounding environment. To defend against pathogens, skin produces hundreds of antimicrobial peptides that exhibit antimicrobial activity against bacteria, fungi, and viruses. In addition to their antimicrobial activity, antimicrobial peptides regulate inflammatory responses, cytokine/chemokine secretion, and cell migration and proliferation, and improve skin barrier function [1,2]. Two major groups of antimicrobial peptides, defensins and cathelicidins, have been well characterized in human skin [3]. Based on sequence homology and the connectivity of conserved cysteine (Cys) residues, human defensins are classified into α-defensins and β-defensins. The characteristic connection of disulfide bridges in human α-defensins is Cys^1–Cys^6, Cys^2–Cys^4, and Cys^3–Cys^5, while that in human β-defensins (hBDs) is Cys^1–Cys^5, Cys^2–Cys^4, and Cys^3–Cys^6 [4]. Human α-defensin-1, -2, -3, and -4 are also termed human neutrophil peptides (HNPs), because they are mainly expressed in neutrophils. HNP-1, -2, and -3 differ only in the first amino acid, whereas HNP-4 has a distinct amino acid sequence [5,6]. hBDs are some of the most important skin-derived antimicrobial peptides and are well known for their wide range of microbicidal activities and immunomodulatory properties [7]. Six hBDs have been identified, among which hBD-1, hBD-2, hBD-3, and hBD-4 are primarily found in the epithelium of the skin, eyes, and oral, respiratory, and urogenital tracts, while hBD-5 and hBD-6 are exclusively expressed in the epididymis [7]. In normal skin, hBD-1 is constitutively expressed, whereas the expression of hBD-2, hBD-3, and hBD-4 is induced in lesional skin by injury, infection, or inflammation [7]. As hBDs activate various types of host cells, such as keratinocytes, fibroblasts, mast cells, neutrophils, and macrophages, hBDs greatly contribute to biological processes. It has been reported that hBDs are involved in pro- and anti-inflammatory responses, neutralization of lipopolysaccharides, chemoattraction, activation of autophagy, maintenance of the skin barrier, and promotion of wound healing [1,3,7–9]. In cutaneous wound healing, which occurs in healthy subjects, hBD-2 and hBD-3 are especially expressed by keratinocytes at wound sites [8]. hBD-3 was recently reported to promote wound healing by modulating inflammatory responses, angiogenesis, and cell proliferation and migration in dermal fibroblasts [10]. Angiogenesis, which is the formation of new blood vessels, is orchestrated by angiogenic factors and is an important process in development, as well as wound healing [11]. A recent study showed that hBD-3 induced the production of angiogenic factors, including vascular endothelial growth factor (VEGF), platelet-derived growth factors (PDGF), and fibroblast growth factor (FGF), by dermal fibroblasts [10]. Angiogenin (ANG), a member of the RNase family that was initially discovered to be a tumor angiogenesis factor, is one of the most potent angiogenic factors and promotes the growth, survival, migration, and invasion of endothelial cells [12].

Although antimicrobial peptide derived from insulin-like growth factor-binding protein 5 (AMP-IBP5) was recently reported to increase ANG production by human epidermal keratinocytes [13], there have been no reports on hBD-induced secretion of ANG. Therefore, this study investigated the effects of the antimicrobial peptides hBD-1, hBD-2, hBD-3, and hBD-4 on the production of ANG in human dermal fibroblasts, with both in vitro and ex vivo models. The secretion of angiogenin was dose-dependently increased by hBD-1, hBD-2, hBD-3, and hBD-4, and this secretion was mediated by activation of the epidermal growth factor receptor (EGFR), Src family kinase, c-Jun N-terminal kinase (JNK), p38, and nuclear factor-kappa B (NF-κB) signaling pathways. These findings identified a novel role of hBDs in angiogenesis, through the production of ANG in dermal fibroblasts.

2. Results

2.1. hBDs Induce ANG Production by Human Dermal Fibroblasts in Both In Vitro and Ex Vivo Models

Normal human dermal fibroblasts were incubated with 10–20 μg/mL hBD-1, hBD-2, hBD-3, and hBD-4, and both the mRNA expression and extracellular secretion of ANG at different time points were examined. The mRNA expression of *ANG* and the amounts of ANG secreted in the cell-free culture supernatants were evaluated by quantitative real-time polymerase chain reaction (PCR) and enzyme-linked immunosorbent assay (ELISA), respectively. We observed that incubation with hBDs had little effect on the mRNA expression of *ANG* (Supplementary Figure S1), whereas all hBDs dose- and time-dependently enhanced the secretion of ANG by fibroblasts (Figure 1a). A five-fold increase in ANG levels was observed at 6 h poststimulation, whereas a 10-fold increase was observed at 12 h. hBD-1, hBD-3, and hBD-4 significantly induced the production of ANG as early as 3 h, and hBD-3 displayed the strongest effect at concentrations as low as 10 μg/mL (Figure 1a).

Fibroblasts in vivo reside in a three-dimensional context. The three-dimensional matrix culture allows fibroblasts to grow into tissues that closely resemble their in vivo counterparts [14]. To determine whether hBDs induce ANG production under physiological conditions, normal human dermal fibroblasts were cultured in an ex vivo model for two days using type I collagen gels as scaffolds [15–17]. Fibroblasts were then stimulated with 20 μg/mL hBD-1, hBD-2, hBD-3, and hBD-4, and the amounts of ANG in the cell-free culture supernatants were evaluated using ELISA. The secretion of ANG by ex vivo-cultured fibroblasts was significantly increased following the addition of hBD-1, hBD-2, hBD-3, and hBD-4 (Figure 1b). The hBD-1-mediated stimulatory effect was only observed at 6 h poststimulation, whereas stimulation with hBD-2, hBD-3, and hBD-4 resulted in a time-dependent secretion of large amounts of ANG as early as 3 h after stimulation (Figure 1b). These findings suggested that hBDs are potent inducers of ANG secretion by human dermal fibroblasts, both in vitro and ex vivo.

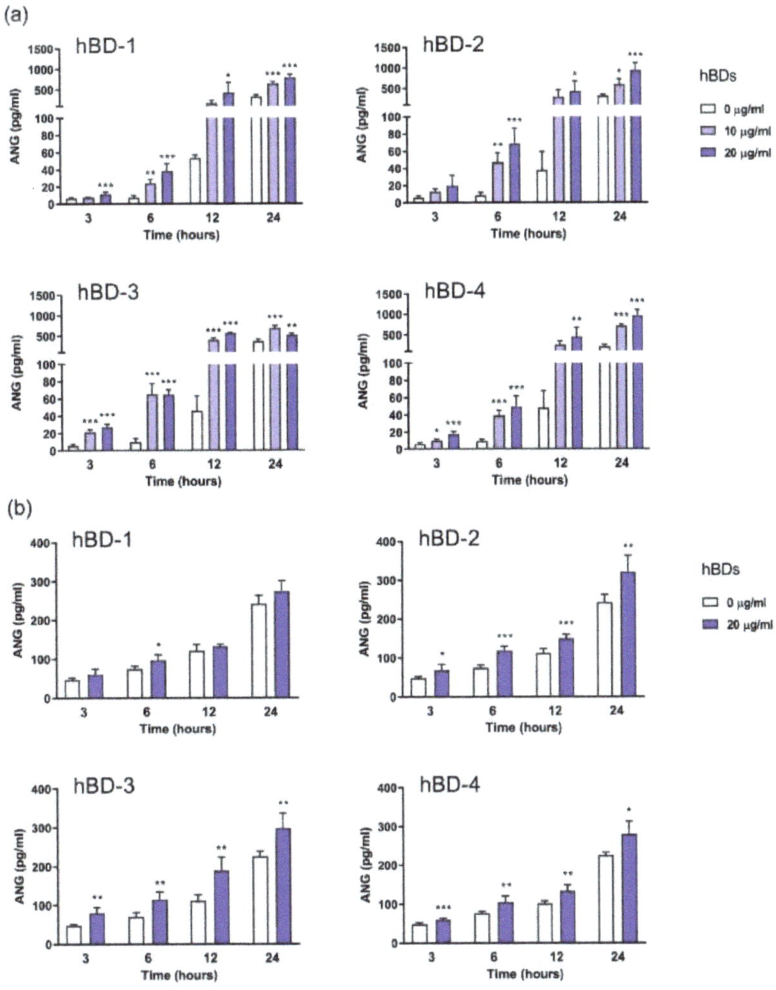

Figure 1. hBDs induce the secretion of the angiogenic factor ANG by human dermal fibroblasts. (**a**) Normal human dermal fibroblasts were stimulated with 10–20 µg/mL hBDs or vehicle (0 µg/mL hBDs) for 3–24 h, and the amounts of ANG in the culture supernatant were determined by ELISA. (**b**) Normal human dermal fibroblasts were cultured in a three-dimensional context using type I collagen gels and then stimulated with 20 µg/mL hBDs or vehicle (0 µg/mL hBDs) for 3–24 h. The amounts of ANG in the culture supernatant were determined by ELISA. The data represent the means ± SDs of 4–5 separate experiments. * $p < 0.05$, ** $p < 0.01$, and *** $p < 0.001$ compared with the vehicle at each time point by one-way ANOVA with Tukey's multiple comparisons test.

The observation that all hBDs displayed an ANG-inducing effect prompted us to examine whether the ANG production was limited to hBDs. Therefore, we treated human fibroblasts with human α-defensins, whose disulfide linkages are different from those in hBDs. Among the human α-defensins tested, only HNP-4 induced ANG production. The effect of HNP-4 was dose- and time-dependent and was observed as early as 3 h after stimulation (Figure 2a). Other α-defensins, such as HNP-1, -2, and -3, did not show any effect (data not shown). In addition to defensins, we examined the ANG-inducing effect of cathelicidin LL-37, which does not contain disulfide linkages in its sequence. We found that LL-37 also significantly induced ANG secretion. Therefore, it appears that hBD-mediated ANG production is not dependent on the presence of disulfide bridges in hBDs, and that among antimicrobial peptides, ANG production is not limited to hBDs.

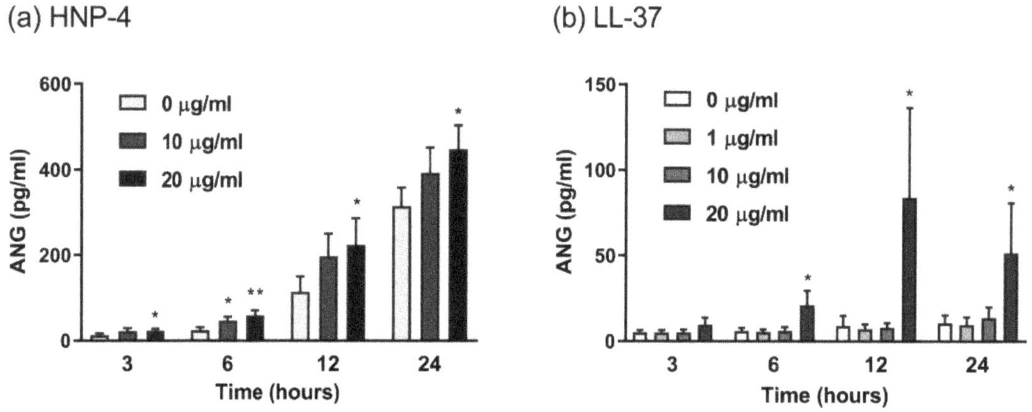

Figure 2. The production of ANG is promoted by HNP-4 and LL-37. Normal human dermal fibroblasts were cultured with 10–20 μg/mL HNP-4 (**a**) or 1–20 μg/mL LL-37 (**b**) for 3–24 h. The concentration of ANG in the culture supernatant was determined by ELISA. The data represent the means ± SDs of 3–4 separate experiments. * $p < 0.05$ and ** $p < 0.01$ compared with the vehicle at each time point by one-way ANOVA with Tukey's multiple comparisons test.

2.2. EGFR and Src Family Kinase Activation Is Necessary for the hBD-Mediated Production of ANG in Dermal Fibroblasts

The EGFR signaling pathway regulates fundamental cellular functions, including cell survival, proliferation, and migration [18]. Since hBDs have been shown to activate hu man keratinocytes via EGFR [19], we examined the role of EGFR signaling in the hBD-mediated ANG production by human dermal fibroblasts. First, we confirmed that hBDs activate EGFR. As shown in Figure 3a, the phosphorylation of EGFR increased between 30 and 120 min after stimulation with hBD-1, hBD-2, hBD-3, and hBD-4. To examine whether increased EGFR activation was indeed necessary for hBD-mediated ANG production, fibroblasts were preincubated with an EGFR-specific inhibitor, AG1478, for 2 h before stimulation with each hBD. As shown in Figure 3a, the ANG secretion induced by hBDs was suppressed by pretreatment with AG1478, confirming that hBDs enhanced ANG production via the EGFR pathway.

It has been reported that the Src family tyrosine kinases are activated by tyrosine kinase receptors and promote signaling through various growth factor receptors, including EGFR [20–22]. As hBDs promoted the activation of EGFR, we examined the effects of hBDs on the Src signaling pathway in fibroblasts. Figure 4a shows that all hBDs induced Src phosphorylation. This activation was first observed at 30 min poststimulation and peaked at 120 min. Moreover, pretreating fibroblasts with the Src family tyrosine kinase inhibitor PP2 significantly suppressed hBD-induced ANG production (Figure 4b), indicating the involvement of the Src signaling pathway in hBD-mediated ANG secretion. The observation that treatment of fibroblasts with either EGFR inhibitor (AG1478) or Src inhibitor (PP2) only partially inhibited hBD-induced ANG production suggests that pathways other than EGFR and Src may be involved in hBD-induced secretion of ANG by human fibroblasts. We confirmed that both AG1478 (Supplementary Figure S2) and PP2 (Supplementary Figure S3) completely inhibited EGFR and Src phosphorylation, respectively, indicating that the incubation time and doses of inhibitors used in this study were sufficient to inhibit the EGFR and Src pathways.

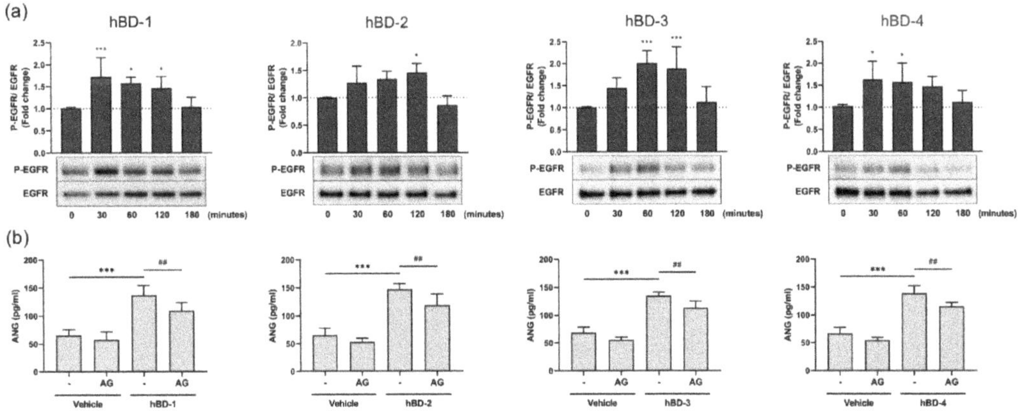

Figure 3. hBDs induce ANG production by activating the EGFR pathway. (**a**) Human dermal fibroblasts were stimulated with 20 μg/mL hBD-1, 20 μg/mL hBD-2, 10 μg/mL hBD-3, or 20 μg/mL hBD-4 for 30–120 min, and the levels of phosphorylated and unphosphorylated EGFR in whole cell lysates were analyzed by Western blotting. * $p < 0.05$ and *** $p < 0.001$ compared between the unstimulated (0 min) and the hBD-stimulated groups by one-way ANOVA with Tukey's multiple comparisons test. (**b**) Fibroblasts were preincubated with 100 nM AG1478 (AG, EGFR inhibitor) or solvent (-) for 2 h. Cells were then stimulated for 6 h with 20 μg/mL hBD-1, 20 μg/mL hBD-2, 10 μg/mL hBD-3, or 20 μg/mL hBD-4. The concentrations of ANG in cell-free supernatants were determined by ELISA. *** $p < 0.001$ compared between the presence and absence of hBDs without inhibitors; ## $p < 0.01$ compared between the inhibitor-treated and untreated group with hBD stimulation by one-way ANOVA with Tukey's multiple comparisons test. All results are the means ± SDs of 5–6 independent experiments.

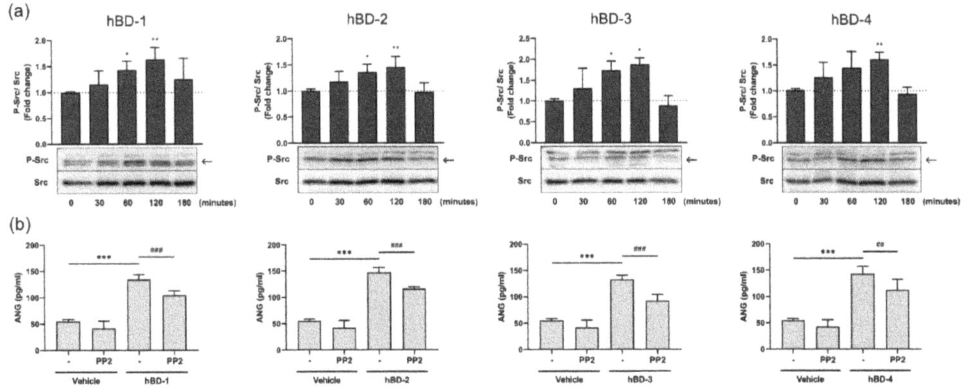

Figure 4. hBDs induce ANG production by activating the Src pathway. (**a**) Human dermal fibroblasts were stimulated with 20 μg/mL hBD-1, 20 μg/mL hBD-2, 10 μg/mL hBD-3, or 20 μg/mL hBD-4 for 30–120 min, and the levels of phosphorylated and unphosphorylated Src in whole cell lysates were analyzed by Western blotting. * $p < 0.05$ and ** $p < 0.01$ compared between the unstimulated (0 min) and the hBD-stimulated groups by one-way ANOVA with Tukey's multiple comparisons test. (**b**) Fibroblasts were preincubated with 20 μM PP2 (Src inhibitor) or solvent (-) for 2 h. Cells were then stimulated for 6 h with 20 μg/mL hBD-1, 20 μg/mL hBD-2, 10 μg/mL hBD-3, or 20 μg/mL hBD-4.

The concentrations of ANG in cell-free supernatants were determined by ELISA. *** $p < 0.001$ compared between the presence and absence of hBDs without inhibitors; ## $p < 0.01$ and ### $p < 0.001$ compared between the inhibitor-treated and untreated groups with hBD stimulation using one-way ANOVA with Tukey's multiple comparisons test. All results are the means ± SDs of 3–6 independent experiments.

2.3. hBD-Mediated ANG Production Requires the Activation of the Mitogen-Activated Protein Kinase (MAPK) and Nuclear Factor-Kappa B (NF-κB) Pathways

The MAPK pathways play key roles in many biological activities, including cell survival and metabolism, and have been reported to be activated by hBDs in keratinocytes and mast cells [23–25]. To evaluate whether hBDs could also activate MAPKs in fibroblasts, cells were incubated with hBD-1, hBD-2, hBD-3, and hBD-4 for 5–60 min, and the phosphorylation of MAPK p38, JNK, and extracellular signal-regulated kinase (ERK) 1/2 was examined using Western blotting. hBD-1, hBD-2, hBD-3, and hBD-4 increased the phosphorylation of p38 at 5 min, and this phosphorylation was still remarkable at 60 min after stimulation with hBD-1 and hBD-3. All hBDs also enhanced JNK and ERK1/2 phosphorylation, which peaked at 5 min, before decreasing (Figure 5a). The requirement for MAPK pathways in hBD-mediated ANG production was evaluated by treating fibroblasts with MAPK inhibitors for 2 h, before stimulation with hBDs. SB203580 (p38 inhibitor) and JNK inhibitor II markedly decreased hBD-mediated ANG production, while U0126 (ERK inhibitor) had no effect on ANG secretion (Figure 5b). The failure of U0126 to inhibit hBD-induced ANG production by fibroblasts was not due to the inactivity of this inhibitor, because treatment of fibroblasts with U0126 completely suppressed both hBD-induced and spontaneous ERK phosphorylation. Other inhibitors, SB203580 and JNK inhibitor II, also abolished p38 and JNK phosphorylation (Supplementary Figure S4).

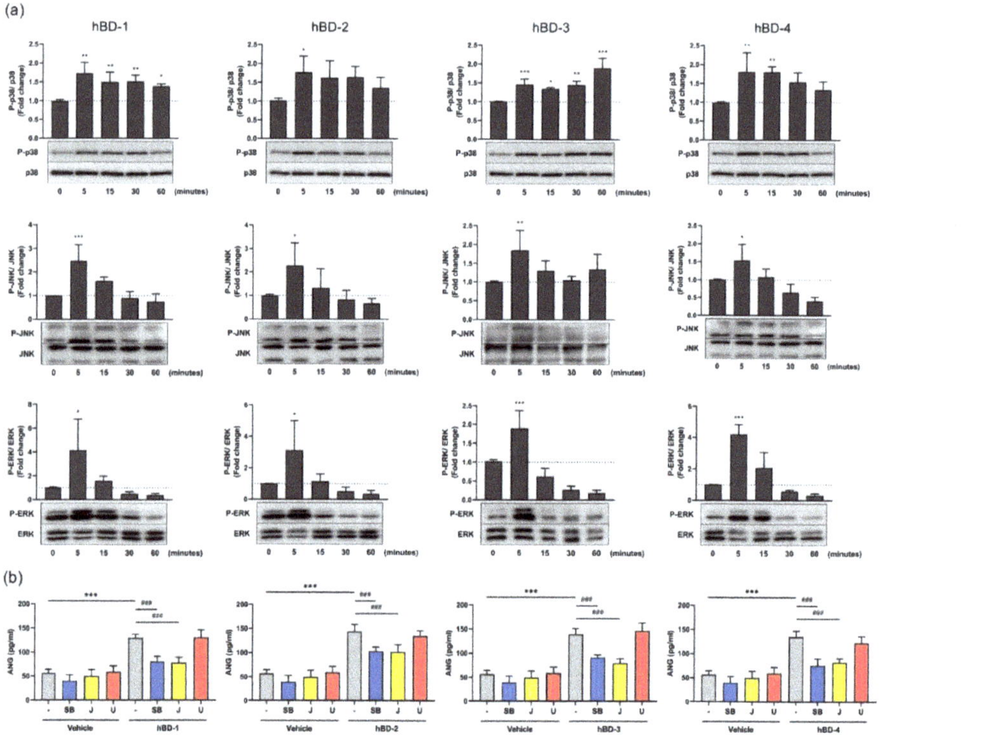

Figure 5. hBDs induce ANG production by activating the p38 and JNK signaling. (**a**) Human dermal

fibroblasts were stimulated with 20 μg/mL hBD-1, 20 μg/mL hBD-2, 10 μg/mL hBD-3, or 20 μg/mL hBD-4 for 5–60 min, and the levels of phosphorylated and unphosphorylated MAPKs (p38, JNK and ERK1/2) in whole cell lysates were analyzed by Western blotting. * $p < 0.05$, ** $p < 0.01$ and *** $p < 0.001$ compared between the unstimulated (0 min) and the hBD-stimulated groups by one-way ANOVA with Tukey's multiple comparisons test. (**b**) Fibroblasts were preincubated with 10 μM SB203580 (SB, p38 inhibitor), 10 μM JNK inhibitor II (J), 10 μM U0126 (U, ERK inhibitor), or solvent (-) for 2 h. Cells were then stimulated for 6 h with 20 μg/mL hBD-1, 20 μg/mL hBD-2, 10 μg/mL hBD-3, or 20 μg/mL hBD-4. The concentrations of ANG in cell-free supernatants were determined by ELISA. *** $p < 0.001$ compared between the presence and absence of hBDs without inhibitor; ### $p < 0.001$ compared between the inhibitor-treated and untreated group with hBD stimulation by one-way ANOVA with Tukey's multiple comparisons test. All results are the means ± SDs of 3–6 independent experiments.

In addition, we focused on the NF-κB pathway, because this pathway has been implicated in antimicrobial peptide-mediated cell activation [26,27], and hBDs have been demonstrated to activate the NF-κB signaling pathway in human epidermal keratinocytes and cervical cancer cells [28,29]. To determine whether hBDs activated NF-κB signaling in fibroblasts and thereby promoted the nuclear translocation of NF-κB, NF-κB expression in the nucleus was analyzed after hBD stimulation of fibroblasts. hBD-1, hBD-2, hBD-3, and hBD-4 significantly increased the levels of NF-κB in the nucleus at 60 min poststimulation (Figure 6a). The observation that hBD-mediated ANG secretion was suppressed by pretreatment with NF-κB activation inhibitor II suggests that the NF-κB signaling pathway is necessary for hBD-mediated ANG secretion (Figure 6b). We confirmed that the nuclear translocation of NF-κB was suppressed in fibroblasts following treatment of cells with NF-κB activation inhibitor II (Supplementary Figure S5). Collectively, these data demonstrated that the MAPK JNK and p38 and NF-κB signaling pathways are necessary for the hBD-mediated production of ANG by fibroblasts.

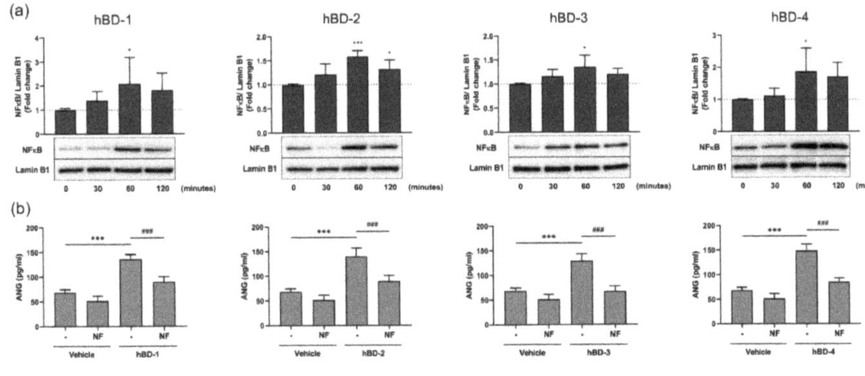

Figure 6. hBDs induce ANG production by activating NF-κB signaling. (**a**) Human dermal fibroblasts were stimulated with 20 μg/mL hBD-1, 20 μg/mL hBD-2, 10 μg/mL hBD-3, or 20 μg/mL hBD-4 for 5–60 min, and the levels of NF-κB in nuclear lysates were analyzed by Western blotting. The expression of Lamin B1 is shown as a loading control. * $p < 0.05$ and *** $p < 0.001$ compared between the unstimulated (0 min) and the hBD-stimulated groups by one-way ANOVA with Tukey's multiple comparisons test. (**b**) Fibroblasts were preincubated with 40 μM NF-κB activation inhibitor II (NF) or solvent (-) for 2 h. Cells were then stimulated for 6 h with 20 μg/mL hBD-1, 10 μg/mL hBD-2, 10 μg/mL hBD-3, or 20 μg/mL hBD-4. The concentrations of ANG in cell-free supernatants were determined by ELISA. *** $p < 0.001$ compared between the presence and absence of hBDs without inhibitor; ### $p < 0.001$ compared between the inhibitor-treated and untreated groups with hBD stimulation by one-way ANOVA with Tukey's multiple comparisons test. All results are the means ± SDs of 4–6 independent experiments.

3. Discussion

A recent study indicated that the skin-derived antimicrobial peptide hBD-3 promoted wound healing, angiogenesis, proliferation, and migration in fibroblasts in an in vivo mouse model and in cultured primary human dermal fibroblasts. Furthermore, hBD-3 promoted angiogenesis by enhancing the dermal fibroblast production of angiogenic factors, such as VEGF, PDGF, and FGF [10]. In this study, we demonstrate that the secretion of another angiogenic factor ANG by fibroblasts was increased not only by hBD-hBD-1, hBD-2, hBD-3, and hBD-4. hBD-mediated ANG production involved the EGFR, Src, p38, JNK, and NF-κB signaling pathways.

As a first line of defense against microbial invasion, human skin produces antimicrobial peptides, which play crucial roles in both innate and adaptive immune responses during injury and inflammation. In addition to antimicrobial properties, hBDs exhibit diverse bioactivities and regulate cell proliferation and migration, skin barrier function, wound healing, and angiogenesis [7]. It has been reported that hBDs also induce the production of various cytokines, growth factors, and angiogenic factors and induce autophagy in epidermal keratinocytes [9,10,19,23,24]. Angiogenesis plays a critical role in many biological processes, such as development, tissue remodeling, reproduction, wound healing, and carcinogenesis. Although ANG is one of the most potent angiogenic factors, it has not been investigated whether hBDs regulate the production of ANG in human dermal fibroblasts. Here, we demonstrated that ANG production was greatly induced by hBD-1, hBD-2, hBD-3, and hBD-4 in fibroblasts cultured in both in vitro and ex vivo models.

As hBDs are induced in skin tissues following injury, infection, or inflammation, there may be an interaction between various resident skin cells, due to impairment of the skin structure and infiltration of inflammatory cells [8]. During the wound healing process, cellular interactions become dominated by the interplay between keratinocytes and fibro blasts, which gradually shift the microenvironment away from an inflammatory site toward synthesis-driven granulation tissue [30]. Of note, the effect of hBDs on fibroblasts has been investigated, to develop a potential agent for wound healing [31,32]. Moreover, the possibility that hBDs may be expressed in the dermis has been reported in lesional skin of acne vulgaris [33,34], and hBDs are upregulated in the dermis of chronic wounds [35], where they may directly interact with fibroblasts.

Although the exact physiological concentrations of hBDs are not well known, the doses of hBD-2 have been estimated to be 3.5–16 μM (15–70 μg/mL) in IL-1α-stimulated epidermal cultures [36] and approximately 20 μM (87 μg/mL) in skin tissues from patients with psoriasis [37]. Furthermore, high doses of hBDs have been detected in wound healing [38], where ANG plays a critical role [12]. Therefore, we assume that the doses of hBDs (20 μg/mL, equivalent to 4–5 μM) used in this study are physiologically relevant.

As all hBDs increased ANG secretion, one could speculate that hBD-mediated ANG production is dependent on hBD structure. In fact, the presence of disulfide bridges has been shown to be important in hBD-mediated immunomodulatory activities, although it is not indispensable for hBD-induced antimicrobial activities [39]. To investigate the importance of disulfide bridges in hBD-induced ANG secretion, fibroblasts were treated with α-defensins, whose disulfide linkages are different from those in hBDs. Only HNP-4, but not HNP-1, HNP-2, or HNP-3, induced ANG production. HNP-4 has also been previously reported to be more effective than other HNPs in protecting peripheral blood mononuclear cells from HIV-1 infection [40]. In addition, because LL-37, which is unable to form disulfide bonds, also induced ANG secretion by fibroblasts, it is assumed that hBD-mediated ANG production is independent of the presence of disulfide bridges in hBDs.

hBDs have been reported to activate the EGFR and MAPK pathways in human keratinocytes [19,23,28]. Accordingly, in this study, we observed that hBDs induced the phosphorylation of EGFR, Src and MAPK p38, JNK, and ERK1/2. Although the phosphorylation of ERK was strongly increased by hBDs, it seems that ERK activation was not involved in ANG production, because an ERK-specific inhibitor failed to suppress ANG production. In addition to EGFR, Src, and MAPK, hBD-induced ANG production was also mediated by the NF-κB signaling pathway. This finding is consistent with previous studies reporting that antimicrobial peptides activate the NF-κB signaling pathway [26–28,41]. However, the observation that EGFR and Src inhibitors partially suppress hBD-induced ANG suggests the possibility of other pathways with hBD-driven activities. In fact, hBDs have been reported to activate various physiological regulators of intracellular signaling pathways, such as reactive oxygen species, which are involved in ANG secretion [42,43]. Further studies are needed to clarify whether these pathways are involved in hBD-mediated ANG secretion.

The levels of angiogenic factors have been shown to be downregulated in nonhealing chronic wounds [44]. As a recent study indicated that hBD-3 induced the production of angiogenic factors, such as VEGF, PDGF, and FGF2, by dermal fibroblasts [10], and because this report demonstrated that hBDs promote ANG secretion by fibroblasts, these findings indicate that hBDs may contribute to angiogenesis, in addition to their antimicrobial and other immunomodulatory activities. Therefore, it is hypothesized that promoting the production or receptor activation of angiogenic factors may be a useful treatment strategy for chronic wounds. In conclusion, hBD treatment may be effective in promoting angiogenesis and wound healing through angiogenin secretion by fibroblasts.

4. Materials and Methods

4.1. Reagents

The antimicrobial peptides hBD-1, hBD-2, hBD-3, hBD-4, and HNP-4 were obtained from the Peptide Institute (Osaka, Japan) and dissolved in 0.01% acetic acid. LL-37 (L^1LGDFFRKSKEKIGKEFKRIVQRIKDFLRNLVPRTES^{37}) was synthesized by the solid-phase method, as previously reported [24]. AG1478 was purchased from Selleck (Houston, TX). PP2, JNK inhibitor II, U0126, SB203580, and NF-κB activation inhibitor II were obtained from Calbiochem (La Jolla, CA, USA). Can Get Signal® Immunoreaction Enhancer Solution (TOYOBO Co., Ltd., Osaka, Japan) was used as the diluent for the antibodies.

The primary antibodies anti-EGFR (1:2000 dilution), anti-phospho-EGFR (1:1000 dilution), anti-SAPK/JNK (1:500 dilution), anti-phospho-SAPK/JNK (1:1000 dilution), anti-p38 (1:1000 dilution), anti-phospho-p38 (1:2000 dilution), anti-p44/42 (ERK1/2) (1:2000 dilution), anti-phospho-p44/42 (ERK1/2) (1:2000 dilution), and anti-NF-κB p65 (1:1000 dilution) were purchased from Cell Signaling Technology (Beverly, MA, USA), and anti-Lamin B1 (1:20,000 dilution) was obtained from Proteintech (Rosemont, IL, USA). Horseradish peroxidase (HRP)-linked anti-rabbit IgG and HRP-linked anti-mouse IgG secondary antibodies were purchased from Cytiva (Tokyo, Japan) and diluted at 1:2000.

4.2. Cell Culture and Stimulation

Primary human dermal fibroblasts isolated from neonatal foreskin were purchased from Lifeline Cell Technology (Osaka, Japan) and cultured in FibroLife Basal Medium (Lifeline Cell Technology) containing L-glutamine (7.5 mM), human FGF-basic (5 ng/mL), insulin (5 μg/mL), ascorbic acid (50 μg/mL), hydrocortisone (1 μg/mL), gentamycin (30 μg/mL), amphotericin B (15 ng/mL), and fetal bovine serum (2% vol/vol) at 37 °C with 5% CO_2 and used within 3 passages. All experiments were performed using subconfluent cells grown in FibroLife Basal Medium without supplements, but with antibiotics, in a 12-well cell culture plate (Greiner Bio-One, Frickenhausen, Germany).

For the ex vivo model, primary human dermal fibroblasts were suspended in Dulbecco's modified Eagle medium (DMEM, Sigma–Aldrich, St Louis, MO, USA) containing 0.15% atelocollagen (KOKEN, Tokyo, Japan) at a density of 5×10^5 cells/mL, and 100 μL of cell suspension was seeded in a 96 well cell culture plate (Greiner Bio-One). After 1 h, DMEM supplemented with 10% fetal bovine serum (Biosera, Boussens, France) was added to the collagen gels. Two days later, the cells were used for studies to mimic ex vivo physiological conditions, as reported previously [14–17].

4.3. Preparation of Total RNA and Quantitative Real-Time PCR

Total RNA was extracted from cultured fibroblasts using a RNeasy Plus Micro Kit (Qiagen, Tokyo, Japan), according to the manufacturer's guidelines. Samples were reverse-transcribed with ReverTra Ace qPCR RT Master Mix (TOYOBO, Osaka, Japan), according to the manufacturer's protocol. Quantitative real-time PCR was performed on a StepOne Plus Real-time PCR System (Applied Biosystems, Foster City, CA, USA) using a QuantiNova SYBR Green PCR kit (Qiagen). Each sample was analyzed in duplicate; the amounts of ANG mRNA in each sample were normalized to those of ribosomal protein S18 (RPS18), and the expression of ANG mRNA was expressed relative to its expression in untreated control cells. The pairs of specific primers for ANG (forward primer: 5′-GTGCTGGGTCTGGGTCTGAC-3′; reverse primer: 5′-GGCCTTGATGCTGCGCTTG-3′), and RPS18 (forward primer: 5′-TTTGCGAGTACTCAACACCAACATC-3′; reverse primer: 5′-GAGCATATCTTCGGCCCACAC-3′).

4.4. ELISA

Fibroblasts were stimulated with 10–20 μg/mL hBDs for 3–24 h, and cell-free supernatants were collected. In some experiments, fibroblasts were pretreated for 2 h with 100 nM AG1478 (EGFR inhibitor), 20 μM PP2 (Src inhibitor), 10 μM SB203580 (p38 inhibitor), 10 μM JNK inhibitor II, 10 μM U0126 (ERK inhibitor), and 40 μM NF-κB activation inhibitor II, before stimulation with 20 μg/mL hBD-1, 20 μg/mL hBD-2, 10 μg/mL hBD-3, and 20 μg/mL hBD-4 for 6 h. In the preliminary dose-dependent experiments, the abovementioned concentrations were the most effective and less toxic (data not shown). ANG was quantified using DuoSet ELISA kits obtained from R&D Systems (Minneapolis, MN, USA).

4.5. Western Blotting

Following stimulation, fibroblasts were lysed with RIPA buffer (Cell Signaling Technology) containing phosphatase inhibitor cocktails 2 and 3 (Sigma-Aldrich, St. Louis, MO, USA). Nuclear lysates were prepared using a LysoPure™ Nuclear and Cytoplasmic Extractor Kit (FUJIFILM Wako Pure Chemical Corporation, Tokyo, Japan) containing protease inhibitor cocktail Set III (FUJIFILM Wako Pure Chemical Corporation). Protein levels were quantified using precision red advanced protein assay reagent #2 (Cytoskeleton, Denver, CO, USA). Equal amounts of total protein were separated on 10% SDS-polyacrylamide gels. After electrophoresis, the proteins were transferred onto an immobilon-P transfer membrane (Millipore, Billerica, MA, USA) by a PoweredBLOT 2M system (ATTO, Tokyo, Japan). The membranes were blocked with ImmunoBlock (KAC, Hyogo, Japan) for 1 h at room temperature and incubated with primary antibodies at 4 °C overnight. The membranes were washed with Tris-buffered saline with 0.1% Tween 20 and incubated with HRP-conjugated secondary antibodies. After being washed, the membranes were developed with Luminata Western HRP substrate (Millipore, Billerica, MA, USA), and the bands were detected with ImageQuant™ LAS 4000 (FUJIFILM Wako Pure Chemical Corporation). The intensity of the bands was quantified using ImageJ software (NIH, Bethesda, MD, USA).

4.6. Statistical Analysis

The data were analyzed using GraphPad Prism 8 (GraphPad Software Inc., San Diego, CA, USA). The differences between means were analyzed by one-way ANOVA with Tukey's multiple comparison tests. In all analyses, $p < 0.05$ was considered statistically significant.

Supplementary Materials: The following supporting information can be downloaded at: https://www.mdpi.com/article/10.3390/ijms23158800/s1.

Author Contributions: Y.U. and F.N. designed the study and wrote the manuscript. Y.U. and M.T. performed the experiments and data analysis. H.Y., J.V.T.-P., G.P. and H.L.T.N. assisted with data acquisition and analysis. K.O. and H.O. contributed to conceptualization and procurement of reagents and materials. All authors have read and agreed to the published version of the manuscript.

Funding: Parts of this research were supported by a Grant-in-Aid for Scientific Research from the Ministry of Education, Culture, Sports, Science and Technology, Japan (Grant numbers 26461703 and 21K08309 to F.N.) and by the Atopy (Allergy) Research Center, Juntendo University, Tokyo, Japan.

Institutional Review Board Statement: Ethics approval was obtained from the Institutional Review Committee of Juntendo University (no: 1387-2021255).

Informed Consent Statement: Not applicable.

Data Availability Statement: The data presented in this study are available upon request from the corresponding author.

Acknowledgments: The authors wish to thank Michiyo Matsumoto for secretarial assistance and the members of the Atopy (Allergy) Research Center for discussion.

Conflicts of Interest: The authors declare no conflict of interest.

References

1. Niyonsaba, F.; Kiatsurayanon, C.; Chieosilapatham, P.; Ogawa, H. Friends or Foes? Host defense (antimicrobial) peptides and proteins in human skin diseases. *Exp. Dermatol.* **2017**, *26*, 989–998. [CrossRef] [PubMed]
2. Rademacher, F.; Glaser, R.; Harder, J. Antimicrobial peptides and proteins: Interaction with the skin microbiota. *Exp. Dermatol.* **2021**, *30*, 1496–1508. [CrossRef] [PubMed]
3. Hancock, R.E.; Haney, E.F.; Gill, E.E. The immunology of host defence peptides: Beyond antimicrobial activity. *Nat. Rev. Immunol.* **2016**, *16*, 321–334. [CrossRef] [PubMed]
4. Niyonsaba, F.; Nagaoka, I.; Ogawa, H.; Okumura, K. Multifunctional antimicrobial proteins and peptides: Natural activators of immune systems. *Curr. Pharm. Des.* **2009**, *15*, 2393–2413. [CrossRef] [PubMed]
5. Pundir, P.; Kulka, M. The role of G protein-coupled receptors in mast cell activation by antimicrobial peptides: Is there a connection? *Immunol. Cell Biol.* **2010**, *88*, 632–640. [CrossRef]
6. Holly, M.K.; Diaz, K.; Smith, J.G. Defensins in viral infection and pathogenesis. *Annu. Rev. Virol.* **2017**, *4*, 369–391. [CrossRef]
7. Niyonsaba, F.; Kiatsurayanon, C.; Ogawa, H. The role of human β-defensins in allergic diseases. *Clin. Exp. Allergy* **2016**, *46*, 1522–1530. [CrossRef]
8. Mangoni, M.L.; McDermott, A.M.; Zasloff, M. Antimicrobial peptides and wound healing: Biological and therapeutic considerations. *Exp. Dermatol.* **2016**, *25*, 167–173. [CrossRef]
9. Peng, G.; Tsukamoto, S.; Ikutama, R.; Le Thanh Nguyen, H.; Umehara, Y.; Trujillo-Paez, J.V.; Yue, H.; Takahashi, M.; Ogawa, T.; Kishi, R.; et al. Human-β-defensin-3 attenuates atopic dermatitis-like inflammation through autophagy activation and the aryl hydrocarbon receptor signaling pathway. *J. Clin. Investig.* **2022**. [CrossRef]
10. Takahashi, M.; Umehara, Y.; Yue, H.; Trujillo-Paez, J.V.; Peng, G.; Nguyen, H.L.T.; Ikutama, R.; Okumura, K.; Ogawa, H.; Ikeda, S.; et al. The Antimicrobial Peptide Human beta-Defensin-3 Accelerates Wound Healing by Promoting Angiogenesis, Cell Migration, and Proliferation through the FGFR/JAK2/STAT3 Signaling Pathway. *Front. Immunol.* **2021**, *12*, 712781. [CrossRef]
11. Lee, H.J.; Hong, Y.J.; Kim, M. Angiogenesis in chronic inflammatory skin disorders. *Int. J. Mol. Sci.* **2021**, *22*, 12035. [CrossRef] [PubMed]
12. Cucci, L.M.; Satriano, C.; Marzo, T.; La Mendola, D. Angiogenin and copper crossing in wound healing. *Int. J. Mol. Sci.* **2021**, *22*, 10704. [CrossRef] [PubMed]
13. Yue, H.; Song, P.; Sutthammikorn, N.; Umehara, Y.; Trujillo-Paez, J.V.; Nguyen, H.L.T.; Takahashi, M.; Peng, G.; Ikutama, R.; Okumura, K.; et al. Antimicrobial peptide derived from insulin-like growth factor-binding protein 5 improves diabetic wound healing. *Wound Repair Regen.* **2022**, *30*, 232–244. [CrossRef] [PubMed]
14. Franco-Barraza, J.; Raghavan, K.S.; Luong, T.; Cukierman, E. Engineering clinically-relevant human fibroblastic cell-derived extracellular matrices. *Cell-Deriv. Matrices Part A* **2020**, *156*, 109–160. [CrossRef]
15. Kanke, M.; Fujii, M.; Kameyama, K.; Kanzaki, J.; Tokumaru, Y.; Imanishi, Y.; Tomita, T.; Matsumura, Y. Role of CD44 variant exon 6 in invasion of head and neck squamous cell carcinoma. *Arch. Otolaryngol. Head Neck Surg.* **2000**, *126*, 1217–1223. [CrossRef]
16. Hirabayashi, S.; Tajima, M.; Yao, I.; Nishimura, W.; Mori, H.; Hata, Y. JAM4, a junctional cell adhesion molecule interacting with a tight junction protein, MAGI-1. *Mol. Cell Biol.* **2003**, *23*, 4267–4282. [CrossRef]
17. Li, F.J.; Surolia, R.; Li, H.; Wang, Z.; Liu, G.; Kulkarni, T.; Massicano, A.V.F.; Mobley, J.A.; Mondal, S.; de Andrade, J.A.; et al. Citrullinated vimentin mediates development and progression of lung fibrosis. *Sci. Transl. Med.* **2021**, *13*, eaba2927. [CrossRef]
18. Pastore, S.; Mascia, F.; Mariani, V.; Girolomoni, G. The epidermal growth factor receptor system in skin repair and inflammation. *J. Investig. Dermatol.* **2008**, *128*, 1365–1374. [CrossRef]
19. Niyonsaba, F.; Ushio, H.; Nakano, N.; Ng, W.; Sayama, K.; Hashimoto, K.; Nagaoka, I.; Okumura, K.; Ogawa, H. Antimicrobial peptides human beta-defensins stimulate epidermal keratinocyte migration, proliferation and production of proinflammatory cytokines and chemokines. *J. Investig. Dermatol.* **2007**, *127*, 594–604. [CrossRef]
20. Bromann, P.A.; Korkaya, H.; Courtneidge, S.A. The interplay between Src family kinases and receptor tyrosine kinases. *Oncogene* **2004**, *23*, 7957–7968. [CrossRef]

21. Zhang, S.; Yu, D. Targeting Src family kinases in anti-cancer therapies: Turning promise into triumph. *Trends Pharmacol. Sci.* **2012**, *33*, 122–128. [CrossRef] [PubMed]
22. Zheng, K.; Kitazato, K.; Wang, Y. Viruses exploit the function of epidermal growth factor receptor. *Rev. Med. Virol.* **2014**, *24*, 274–286. [CrossRef] [PubMed]
23. Niyonsaba, F.; Ushio, H.; Nagaoka, I.; Okumura, K.; Ogawa, H. The human beta-defensins (−1, −2, −3, −4) and cathelicidin LL-37 induce IL-18 secretion through p38 and ERK MAPK activation in primary human keratinocytes. *J. Immunol.* **2005**, *175*, 1776–1784. [CrossRef] [PubMed]
24. Niyonsaba, F.; Ushio, H.; Hara, M.; Yokoi, H.; Tominaga, M.; Takamori, K.; Kajiwara, N.; Saito, H.; Nagaoka, I.; Ogawa, H.; et al. Antimicrobial peptides human beta-defensins and cathelicidin LL-37 induce the secretion of a pruritogenic cytokine IL-31 by human mast cells. *J. Immunol.* **2010**, *184*, 3526–3534. [CrossRef] [PubMed]
25. Chen, X.; Niyonsaba, F.; Ushio, H.; Hara, M.; Yokoi, H.; Matsumoto, K.; Saito, H.; Nagaoka, I.; Ikeda, S.; Okumura, K.; et al. Antimicrobial peptides human β-defensin (hBD)-3 and hBD-4 activate mast cells and increase skin vascular permeability. *Eur. J. Immunol.* **2007**, *37*, 434–444. [CrossRef] [PubMed]
26. Yanashima, K.; Chieosilapatham, P.; Yoshimoto, E.; Okumura, K.; Ogawa, H.; Niyonsaba, F. Innate defense regulator IDR-1018 activates human mast cells through G protein-, phospholipase C-, MAPK- and NF-kB-sensitive pathways. *Immunol. Res.* **2017**, *65*, 920–931. [CrossRef] [PubMed]
27. Niyonsaba, F.; Song, P.; Yue, H.; Sutthammikorn, N.; Umehara, Y.; Okumura, K.; Ogawa, H. Antimicrobial peptide derived from insulin-like growth factor-binding protein 5 activates mast cells via Mas-related G protein-coupled receptor X2. *Allergy* **2019**, *75*, 203–207. [CrossRef]
28. Smithrithee, R.; Niyonsaba, F.; Kiatsurayanon, C.; Ushio, H.; Ikeda, S.; Okumura, K.; Ogawa, H. Human β-defensin-3 increases the expression of interleukin-37 through CCR6 in human keratinocytes. *J. Dermatol. Sci.* **2015**, *77*, 46–53. [CrossRef]
29. Xu, D.; Zhang, B.; Liao, C.; Zhang, W.; Wang, W.; Chang, Y.; Shao, Y. Human beta-defensin 3 contributes to the carcinogenesis of cervical cancer via activation of NF-κB signaling. *Oncotarget* **2016**, *7*, 75902–75913. [CrossRef]
30. Bickenbach, J.R.; Kulesz-Martin, M.F. Signaling to structures: Skin appendages, development and diseases–meeting report of the 55th annual Montagna Symposium on the Biology of Skin. *J. Investig. Dermatol.* **2007**, *127*, 988–990. [CrossRef] [PubMed]
31. Gomes, A.P.; Mano, J.F.; Queiroz, J.A.; Gouveia, I.C. Incorporation of antimicrobial peptides on functionalized cotton gauzes for medical applications. *Carbohydr. Polym.* **2015**, *127*, 451–461. [CrossRef] [PubMed]
32. Van Kilsdonk, J.W.J.; Jansen, P.A.M.; van den Bogaard, E.H.; Bos, C.; Bergers, M.; Zeeuwen, P.L.J.M.; Schalkwijk, J. The effects of human beta-defensins on skin cells in vitro. *Dermatology* **2017**, *233*, 155–163. [CrossRef]
33. Chronnell, C.M.T.; Ghali, L.R.; Quinn, A.G.; Bull, J.J.; McKay, I.A.; Philpott, M.P.; Müller-Röver, S.; Ali, R.S.; Holland, D.B.; Cunliffe, W.J. Human β defensin-1 and -2 expression in human pilosebaceous units: Upregulation in acne uulgaris lesions. *J. Investig. Dermatol.* **2001**, *117*, 1120–1125. [CrossRef]
34. Harder, J.; Tsuruta, D.; Murakami, M.; Kurokawa, I. What is the role of antimicrobial peptides (AMP) in acne vulgaris? *Exp. Dermatol.* **2013**, *22*, 386–391. [CrossRef] [PubMed]
35. Butmarc, J.; Yufit, T.; Carson, P.; Falanga, V. Human beta-defensin-2 expression is increased in chronic wounds. *Wound Repair Regen.* **2004**, *12*, 439–443. [CrossRef] [PubMed]
36. Liu, A.Y.; Destoumieux, D.; Wong, A.V.; Park, C.H.; Valore, E.V.; Liu, L.; Ganz, T. Human β-Defensin-2 Production in Keratinocytes is Regulated by Interleukin-1, Bacteria, and the State of Differentiation. *J. Investig. Dermatol.* **2002**, *118*, 275–281. [CrossRef] [PubMed]
37. Ong, P.Y.; Ohtake, T.; Brandt, C.; Strickland, I.; Boguniewicz, M.; Ganz, T.; Gallo, R.L.; Leung, D.Y.M. Endogenous Antimicrobial Peptides and Skin Infections in Atopic Dermatitis. *N. Engl. J. Med.* **2002**, *347*, 1151–1160. [CrossRef]
38. Sorensen, O.E. Injury-induced innate immune response in human skin mediated by transactivation of the epidermal growth factor receptor. *J. Clin. Investig.* **2006**, *116*, 1878–1885. [CrossRef]
39. Wu, Z.; Hoover, D.M.; Yang, D.; Boulègue, C.; Santamaria, F.; Oppenheim, J.J.; Lubkowski, J.; Lu, W. Engineering disulfide bridges to dissect antimicrobial and chemotactic activities of human β-defensin 3. *Proc. Natl. Acad. Sci. USA* **2003**, *100*, 8880–8885. [CrossRef]
40. Wu, Z.; Cocchi, F.; Gentles, D.; Ericksen, B.; Lubkowski, J.; Devico, A.; Lehrer, R.I.; Lu, W. Human neutrophil alpha-defensin 4 inhibits HIV-1 infection in vitro. *FEBS Lett.* **2005**, *579*, 162–166. [CrossRef] [PubMed]
41. Kiatsurayanon, C.; Niyonsaba, F.; Chieosilapatham, P.; Okumura, K.; Ikeda, S.; Ogawa, H. Angiogenic peptide (AG)-30/5C activates human keratinocytes to produce cytokines/chemokines and to migrate and proliferate via MrgX receptors. *J. Dermatol. Sci.* **2016**, *83*, 190–199. [CrossRef]
42. Wang, W.; Qu, X.; Dang, X.; Shang, D.; Yang, L.; Li, Y.; Xu, D.; Martin, J.G.; Hamid, Q.; Liu, J.; et al. Human β-defensin-3 induces IL-8 release and apoptosis in airway smooth muscle cells. *Clin. Exp. Allergy* **2017**, *47*, 1138–1149. [CrossRef]
43. Schaafhausen, M.K.; Yang, W.-J.; Centanin, L.; Wittbrodt, J.; Bosserhoff, A.; Fischer, A.; Schartl, M.; Meierjohann, S. Tumor angiogenesis is caused by single melanoma cells in a reactive oxygen species and NF-κB dependent manner. *J. Cell Sci.* **2013**, *126*, 3862–3872. [CrossRef]
44. Dinh, T.; Braunagel, S.; Rosenblum, B.I. Growth factors in wound healing: The present and the future? *Clin. Podiatr. Med. Surg.* **2015**, *32*, 109–119. [CrossRef] [PubMed]

International Journal of
Molecular Sciences

MDPI

Article

A Novel Antimicrobial Peptide Sparanegtin Identified in *Scylla paramamosain* Showing Antimicrobial Activity and Immunoprotective Role In Vitro and Vivo

Xuewu Zhu [1], Fangyi Chen [1,2,3], Shuang Li [1], Hui Peng [1,2,3] and Ke-Jian Wang [1,2,3,*]

1 State Key Laboratory of Marine Environmental Science, College of Ocean & Earth Sciences, Xiamen University, Xiamen 361005, China; zhuxuewu@stu.xmu.edu.cn (X.Z.); chenfangyi@xmu.edu.cn (F.C.); 22320170154929@stu.xmu.edu.cn (S.L.); penghui@xmu.edu.cn (H.P.)
2 State-Province Joint Engineering Laboratory of Marine Bioproducts and Technology, College of Ocean & Earth Sciences, Xiamen University, Xiamen 361005, China
3 Fujian Innovation Research Institute for Marine Biological Antimicrobial Peptide Industrial Technology, College of Ocean & Earth Sciences, Xiamen University, Xiamen 361005, China
* Correspondence: wkjian@xmu.edu.cn

Abstract: The abuse of antibiotics in aquaculture and livestock no doubt has exacerbated the increase in antibiotic-resistant bacteria, which imposes serious threats to animal and human health. The exploration of substitutes for antibiotics from marine animals has become a promising area of research, and antimicrobial peptides (AMPs) are worth investigating and considering as potential alternatives to antibiotics. In the study, we identified a novel AMP gene from the mud crab *Scylla paramamosain* and named it Sparanegtin. *Sparanegtin* transcripts were most abundant in the testis of male crabs and significantly expressed with the challenge of lipopolysaccharide (LPS) or *Vibrio alginolyticus*. The recombinant Sparanegtin (rSparanegtin) was expressed in *Escherichia coli* and purified. rSparanegtin exhibited activity against Gram-positive and Gram-negative bacteria and had potent binding affinity with several polysaccharides. In addition, rSparanegtin exerted damaging activity on the cell walls and surfaces of *P. aeruginosa* with rougher and fragmented appearance. Interestingly, although rSparanegtin did not show activity against *V. alginolyticus* in vitro, it played an immunoprotective role in *S. paramamosain* and exerted an immunomodulatory effect by modulating several immune-related genes against *V. alginolyticus* infection through significantly reducing the bacterial load in the gills and hepatopancreas and increasing the survival rate of crabs.

Keywords: *Scylla paramamosain*; antimicrobial peptide; Sparanegtin; antimicrobial activity; immunoprotective role

Citation: Zhu, X.; Chen, F.; Li, S.; Peng, H.; Wang, K.-J. A Novel Antimicrobial Peptide Sparanegtin Identified in *Scylla paramamosain* Showing Antimicrobial Activity and Immunoprotective Role In Vitro and Vivo. *Int. J. Mol. Sci.* **2022**, *23*, 15. https://doi.org/10.3390/ijms23010015

Academic Editor: Helena Felgueiras

Received: 15 November 2021
Accepted: 17 December 2021
Published: 21 December 2021

1. Introduction

It is estimated that China accounts for over 60% of the global aquaculture production under the accelerated development of aquaculture industry [1]. Accordingly, various diseases often occur in the process of aquaculture, especially the bacterial infectious diseases, which cause the antibiotics widely used in aquaculture, either as pharmaceuticals in control diseases or routinely used in feedstuff as additives. The abuse of antibiotics leads to antibiotic residual problems in aquatic products. Through the consumption of aquatic products tainted by antibiotics, humans may acquire adverse drug reactions [2]. In particular, the abuse of antibiotics increased numbers of antibiotic-resistant pathogenic microorganisms in the aquatic environment, which poses a challenge to the development and use of antibiotic strategies to control fish diseases [3,4]. As it is known that antibiotic medications have been widely used not only in clinical treatment and the prevention of microbial infections, but also in feedstuffs [5], the wide spread of antimicrobial resistance (AMR) seriously affects animal and human health [6]. To control the antibiotic-resistant pathogens, a variety of effective first-line drug treatments (such as chloramphenicol, erythromycin, and terramycin) have recently been developed to control aquatic bacteria; however, these drugs often negatively affect many organisms, including fish and humans [3,7]. Therefore, the exploration and development of effective alternatives to substitute for antibiotics becomes a promising research hotspot.

It is well known that marine invertebrates including crustaceans mainly depend on innate immune defense to protect themselves against invading pathogens. Of various effective immune-related components, the antimicrobial peptides (AMPs) are the most concerned because they play a significant role in innate immunity and serve as effective defense weapons against bacterial, fungal, and viral infections [8,9]. The antimicrobial mechanism of most AMPs is to disrupt the membrane integrity of invading microorganisms [10,11]. Compared with antibiotics, AMPs can offer multiple advantages as candidates for the development of antimicrobial agents, as their uses may include acting alone or in synergy with other antimicrobial agents to reduce the effective bactericidal concentration and thereby reduce cytotoxicity, and it is not easy to induce drug resistance in bacteria [12]. In addition to direct antibacterial functions, AMPs have an important capability to regulate the innate immune system [13]. Therefore, AMPs can not only improve the immune resistance of aquatic animals but also alleviate the problems of bacterial resistance and antibiotic contamination of aquatic products in aquaculture.

AMPs can also produce immunological protection against bacterial challenge in vivo. Epinecidin-1, a synthetic 21-mer antimicrobial peptide originally identified from grouper (*Epinephelus coioides*), significantly improves the survival rate of zebrafish infected with *Vibrio vulnificus* [14]. LcLEAP-2C from large yellow croaker (*Larimichthys crocea*) can reduce the mortality of large yellow croaker after *V. alginolyticus* challenge [15], and white spot syndrome virus (WSSV) pre-incubated with anti-lipopolysaccharide factor (ALF) results in an increased survival rate of red claw crayfish (*Cherax quadricarinatus*) [16]. Similarly, in our laboratory, the recombinant product of one AMP SpHyastatin, which is identified in *S. paramamosain* can enhance the protection of the host against *Vibrio parahaemolyticus* infection in crabs [17]; there are two other AMPs: rSpALF7 could obviously improve the survival of crabs infected by *V. alginolyticus* [18] and rScyreprocin significantly decreased the mortality of *Vibrio harveyi*-infected marine medaka [19]. The action mechanism of antimicrobial peptides in vivo has been also investigated. Several recent studies have found that the administration of AMPs to fish can lead to a decrease in the number of bacteria in tissues, showing a direct antibacterial activity in vivo [20]. Some AMPs could be attributed to their ability to enhance immune response by modulating host gene expression [13], inducing or inhibiting cytokine production [20], and promoting the production of antimicrobial substances such as lysozymes and antioxidant enzymes [21].

In the study, based on the transcriptome database of *S. paramamosain* established by our laboratory, we identified an uncharacterized gene for the first time and named it Sparanegtin. The expression profiles of *Sparanegtin* in *S. paramamosain* with the challenge of LPS or *V. alginolyticus* were investigated. The recombinant product of Sparanegtin (rSparanegtin) in a prokaryotic expression system *Escherichia coli* was obtained. The antimicrobial activity assay, scanning electron microscopy (SEM), observation, and microbial surface components binding assays were performed to analyze the antimicrobial features of rSparanegtin against various microorganisms in vitro. In addition, the effect of rSparanegtin in vivo was evaluated by detecting the bacterial clearance ability in the gills and hepatopancreas of *S. paramamosain* infected with *V. alginolyticus*, as well as any effect on the expression patterns of some immune-related genes after the in vivo administration of rSparanegtin. This study aims to preliminarily study the function, immune-protective effect, and related mechanism of Sparanegtin, providing effective strategies for mud crab aquaculture disease control. This study aims to characterize the new AMP Sparanegtin, elucidating its immune-protective effect and the underlying mechanism and thus developing a potential effective antimicrobial agent that could be substituted for antibiotics to be used in animal husbandry or medicine in the future.

2. Results

2.1. Cloning and Sequence Analysis of Sparanegtin

The full-length cDNA sequence of *Sparanegtin* was obtained, which is 525 bp, including a 252-bp open reading frame (GenBank accession number: MN612064). It had a predicted signal peptide of 23aa, and the cleavage position is between Gly-23 and Ala-24. The mature peptide contained 60 amino acid residues, and its calculated mass is 5.818 kDa with an estimated isoelectric point (pI) of 5.2, the total net charge of -1 (Figure 1A). The predicted tertiary structure of Sparanegtin contains three α-helices (Figure 1B).

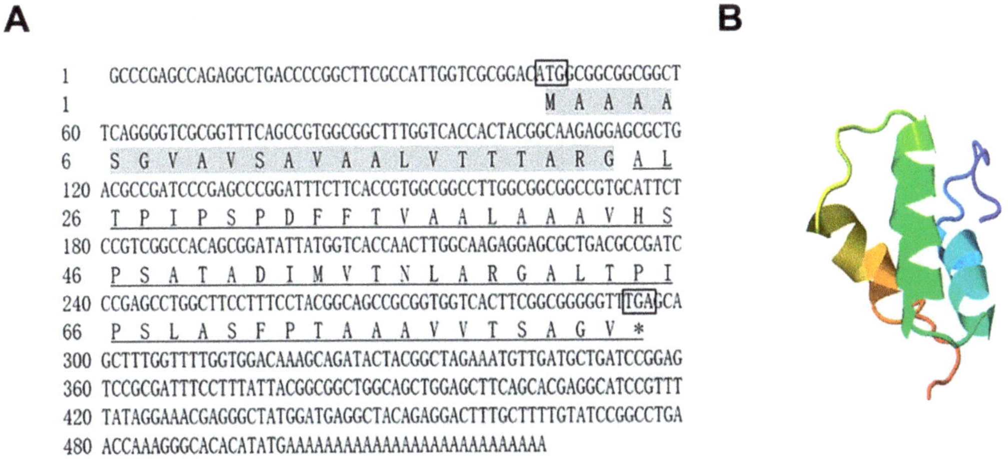

Figure 1. Bioinformatics analysis of Sparanegtin. The cDNA and deduced amino acid sequences of Sparanegtin: the boxed sequence represents the initiation codons; the boxed sequence and "*" represents the stop codons; the predicted signal peptide is shaded; underline regions indicate the mature peptide (**A**). The protein structure of Sparanegtin mature peptide was predicted by I-TASSER server (**B**).

2.2. Gene Expression Profiles of Sparanegtin

The qPCR results showed that *Sparanegtin* was widely distributed in different tissues (Figure 2A,B). In male adult crabs, *Sparanegtin* was dominantly expressed in the testis (Figure 2A), and the highest expression level of *Sparanegtin* was found in the hemocytes of female adult crabs (Figure 2B). We further investigated the expression profiles of *Sparanegtin* in the testis and hemocytes of male crabs after LPS or *V. alginolyticus* challenge (Figure 2C–F). In the testis, the expression of *Sparanegtin* was significantly down-regulated by LPS challenge at 3 hpi (Figure 2C), while it showed significant up-regulation at 3 hpi and 72 hpi under *V. alginolyticus* challenge (Figure 2D). In the hemocytes, *Sparanegtin* gene was significantly up-regulated at 3 hpi under both LPS and bacterial challenge (Figure 2E,F).

2.3. rSparanegtin Shows Antimicrobial Activity

The recombinant product of Sparanegtin (rSparanegtin) was successfully expressed in *E. coli*. SDS-PAGE analysis showed that the purity of rTrx and rSparanegtin was high, as shown in Figure 3A. In addition, the results from the mass spectrometry also confirmed that the purified protein was the target protein rSparanegtin (Figure S1). The antimicrobial activity of rSparanegtin was determined. As shown in Table 1, rSparanegtin displayed good antimicrobial activities against several Gram-negative (*E. coli*, *P. aeruginosa*, *P. stutzeri*, *P. fluorescens*, *S. flexneri*), Gram-positive (*B. subtilis*, *C. glutamicum*, *S. aureus*) bacteria (MICs ranging from 12 to 48 μM and MBCs ranging from 24 to 48 μM), and yeast (*C. neoformans* and *P. pastoris* GS115) (MICs ranging from 24 to 48 μM).

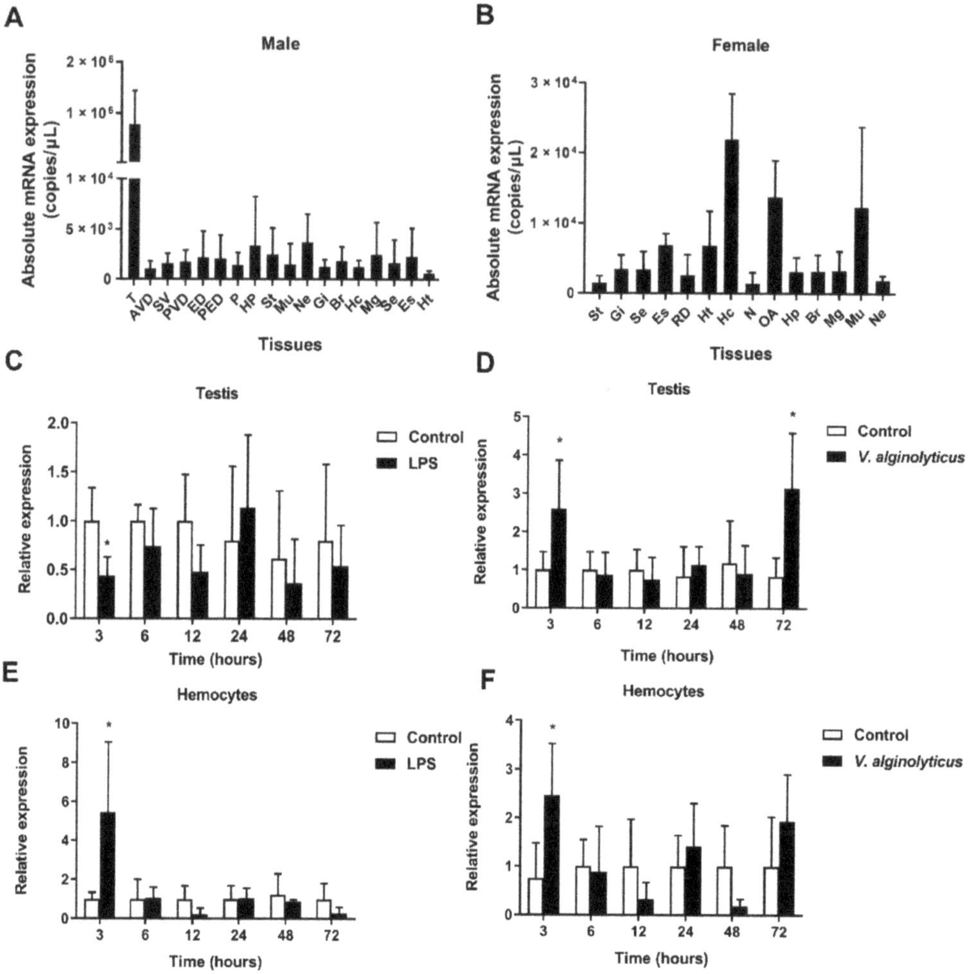

Figure 2. Gene expression profiles of *Sparanegtin* in *S. paramamosain*. The expression profile of *Sparanegtin* in adult male (**A**) and female (**B**) crabs under natural status was determined by absolute qPCR. Data are presented as mean ± standard deviation (SD). The relative expression of *Sparanegtin* in male testes after LPS (**C**) and *V. alginolyticus* (**D**) challenges, and in male hepatopancreas after LPS (**E**) and *V. alginolyticus* (**F**) challenges was examined. In panel (**C–F**), data are presented as mean ± SD. * $p < 0.05$, one-way analysis of variance (ANOVA) and Bonferroni post-test. Abbreviations: T, testis; AVD, anterior vas deferens; SV, seminal vesicle; PVD, posterior vas deferens; ED, ejaculatory duct; PED, posterior ejaculatory duct; P, penis; OA, ovary; N, spermathecae; RD, reproductive duct; Mu, muscle; Ne, thoracic ganglion; Gi, gills; Br, brain; Hc, hemocytes; Mg, midgut; Se, subcuticular epidermis; Es, eye stalk; Ht, heart; Hp, hepatopancreas; St, stomach.

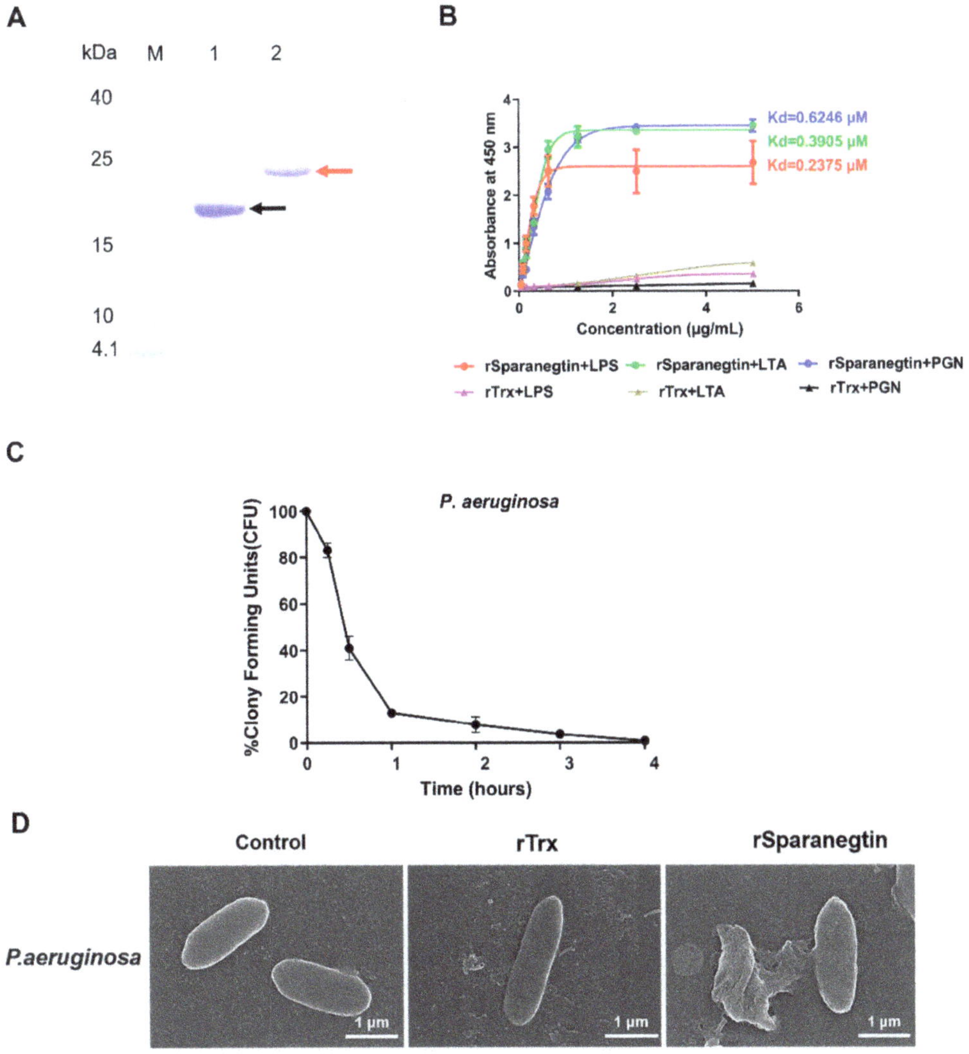

Figure 3. Binding activity and antibacterial mechanism of rSparanegtin. Expression and purification of recombinant Sparanegtin. Lane M: protein molecular standard; lane 1: purified rTrx; lane 2: purified rSparanegtin; the arrow indicates the size of the protein (**A**). Binding activity of rSparanegtin and rTrx to PAMPs (LTA for lipoteichoic acid, LPS for lipopolysaccharide, PGN for peptidoglycan) (**B**). Time-killing curves of *P. aeruginosa* treated with rSparanegtin (**C**). *P. aeruginosa* was suspended in culture media supplemented with PBS, rTrx, or rSparanegtin and observed by a scanning electron microscopy (SEM) (**D**).

Table 1. Antimicrobial activity of rSparanegtin.

Microorganisms.	CGMCC No. [a]	MIC (μM) [b]	MBC (μM) [b]
Gram-negative bacteria			
Escherichia coli	1.2389	24–48	24–48
Pseudomonas aeruginosa	1.2421	12–24	24–48
Pseudomonas fluorescens	1.1802	12–24	>48
Aeromonas hydrophila	1.2017	12–24	>48
Shigella flexneri	1.1868	12–24	>48
Gram-positive bacteria			
Bacillus subtilis	1.3358	24–48	>48
Staphylococcus epidermidis	1.4260	24–48	>48
Staphylococcus aureus	1.2465	12–24	>48
Fungi			
Cryptococcus neoformans	2.1563	24–48	>48
Pichia pastoris (GS115)	Invitrogen	24–48	>48

[a] CGMCC No., China General Microbiological Culture Collection Number. [b] The MIC and MBC values are presented as the interval (A)–(B): (A) is the highest concentration tested with visible microbial growth, while (B) is the lowest concentration without visible microbial growth ($n = 3$).

2.4. Preliminary Study on the Antibacterial Mechanism of rSparanegtin

2.4.1. Binding Properties

ELISA assay was used to investigate the binding properties of rSparanegtin to different microbial surface molecules and bacteria. In order to evaluate whether the label protein Trx would have any effect on the following results, rTrx was selected as the control group. Compared with the rTrx group, rSparanegtin had strong binding affinity with LPS, LTA, and PGN in a concentration-dependent manner, and their calculated apparent dissociation constants (K_d) were 0.2375, 0.3905, and 0.6246 μM, respectively (Figure 3B).

2.4.2. Killing Kinetic

The results of the time-killing kinetic assay were applied to further evaluate the bactericidal activity of rSparanegtin. When rSparanegtin was incubated with *P. aeruginosa* at a concentration of 48 μM, all bacteria could be killed after 4 h of incubation (Figure 3C).

2.4.3. rSparanegtin Induces Morphological Changes in Microorganisms

In order to study the antibacterial mechanism of rSparanegtin against *P. aeruginosa*, SEM was employed to observe the morphological changes of the microbial membrane after rSparanegtin and rTrx treatment. After incubating with rSparanegtin and rTrx for a certain period of time, the SEM images of *P. aeruginosa* showed a significant destruction of membrane integrity and even leakage of cell contents compared with the control group and rTrx group (Figure 3D).

2.5. rSparanegtin Shows No Cytotoxicity and Could Reduce the V. alginolyticus Endotoxin Level In Vitro

The cytotoxicity of rSparanegtin was analyzed using primarily cultured crab hemocytes, HEK-293T and NCI-H460. As shown in Figure 4A–C, rSparanegtin showed no cytotoxicity.

In addition, it was found that rSparanegtin treatment could significantly reduce the endotoxin level of *V. alginolyticus*, which also showed a dose-dependent manner. Under the treatment of 48 μM, the endotoxin level was reduced by about 70% (Figure 4D).

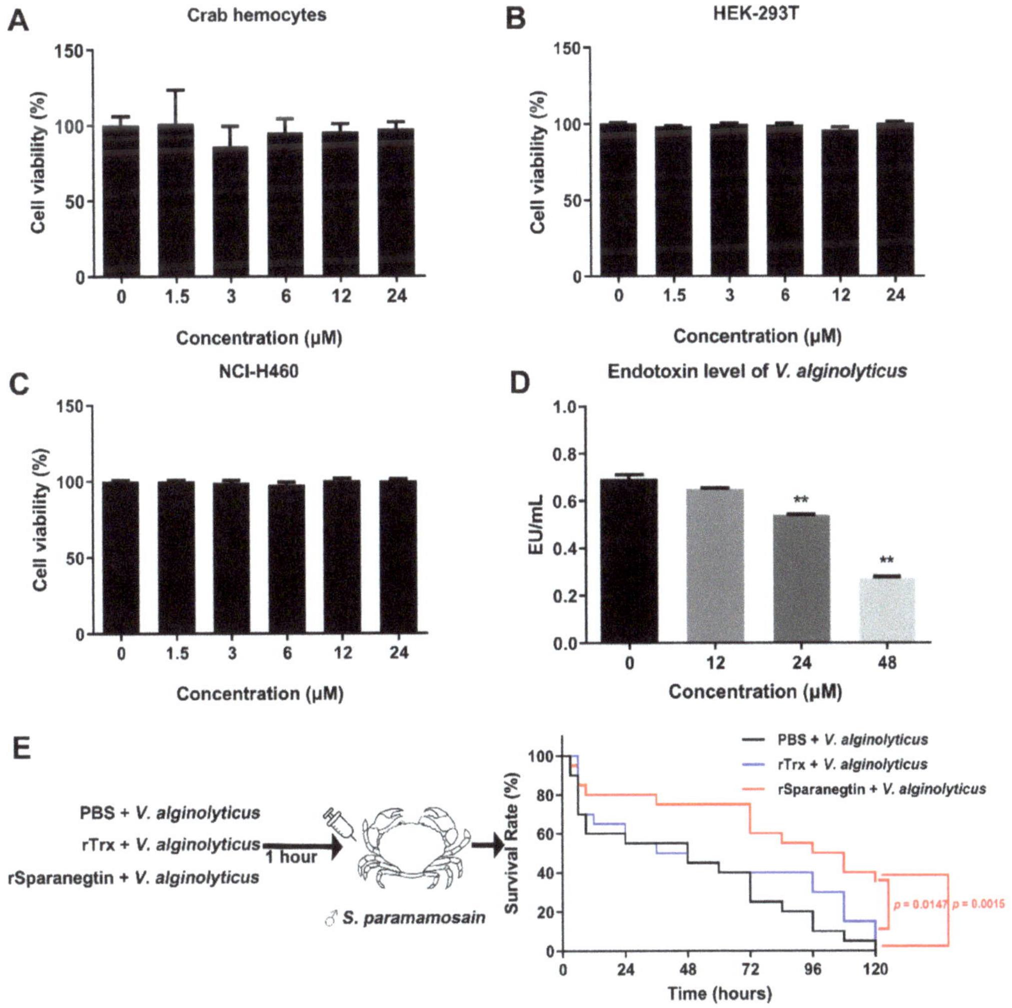

Figure 4. In vivo protective effect of rSparanegtin on *V. alginolyticus*-infected *S. paramamosain*. The cytotoxic effect of rSparanegtin on crab hemocytes (**A**), HEK-293T (**B**), and NCI-H460 (**C**) was determined by the MTS method; data are presented as mean ± standard deviation (SD) ($n = 3$). **: $p < 0.01$, one-way analysis of variance (ANOVA) and Dunnett post-test. Endotoxin level of *V. alginolyticus* after rSparanegtin treatment in vitro (**D**). In vivo protective effect of rSparanegti was evaluated (**E**). The rSparanegtin (20 μg/crab), rTrx (20 μg/crab), and PBS was incubated with *V. alginolyticus* (1×10^6 CFU/crab) at room temperature for 60 min and then injected into the male crabs ($n = 20$ for each group). The survival curves were analyzed using the Kaplan–Meier Log rank test.

2.6. The Immunoprotective Effect of rSparanegtin on S. paramamosain

2.6.1. Survival Rate Comparison

To investigate the in vivo protective effect of rSparanegtin, male mud crabs were challenged with different groups, including the PBS and *V. alginolyticus* pre-incubation group (short as PBS group), rTrx and *V. alginolyticus* pre-incubation group (short as rTrx group), and rSparanegtin and *V. alginolyticus* pre-incubation group (short as rSparanegtin group). As shown in Figure 4E, 48 h after different treatments, the survival rate of the crab

PBS and rTrx groups dropped to 50%, while the survival rate of the rSparanegtin group was around 75%. Crabs in the PBS and rTrx groups died faster, and none of them survived 120 h after injection, while the survival rate of the rSparanegtin group was still about 40% ($p < 0.05$) (Figure 4E).

2.6.2. Pre-Incubation of rSparanegtin and *V. alginolyticus* Reduces Bacterial Load in the Tissues

Bacterial clearance represents a major endpoint of innate host immunity in response to infection. As we all know, AMPs are important components of the innate immune system. We evaluated the ability of rSparanegtin to eliminate bacteria in the tissues of mud crabs under different treatments as mentioned above. As shown in Figure 5A, compared with the PBS and rTrx groups, the rSparanegtin group showed a significant reduction in *V. alginolyticus* load in the gills at the 3, 6, 12, and 24 hpi (Figure 5A). In the hepatopancreas, the *V. alginolyticus* load significantly decreased at 6, 12, and 24 hpi (Figure 5B).

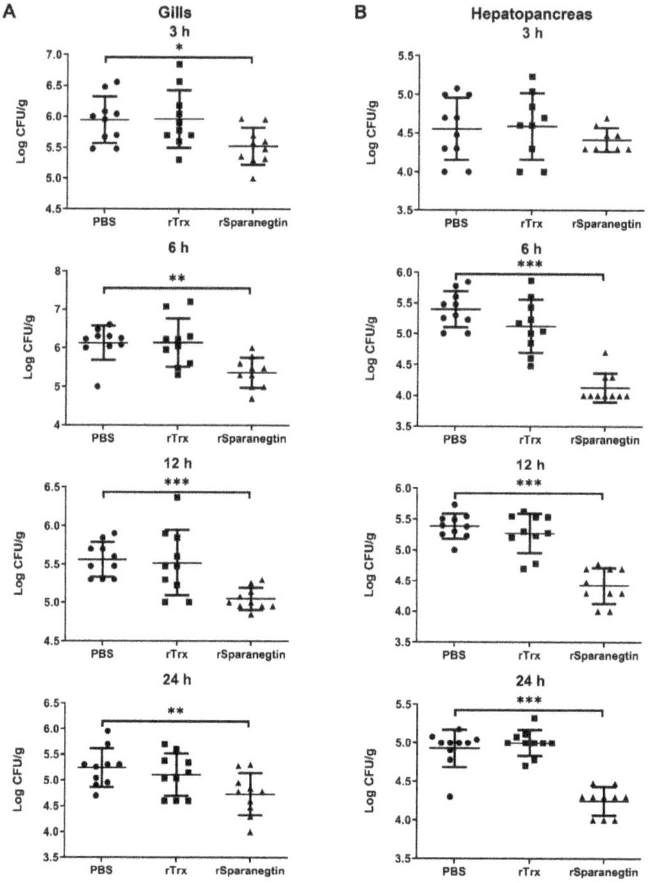

Figure 5. In vivo antimicrobial effect of rSparanegtin on *V. alginolyticus* growth in *S. paramamosain*. The rSparanegtin (20 μg/crab), rTrx (20 μg/crab), and PBS were incubated with *V. alginolyticus* (1×10^6 CFU/crab) at room temperature for 60 min and then injected into the base of the right fourth leg of crabs. Infected crabs were dissected, and tissues including gills (**A**), midgut, and hepatopancreas (**B**) were collected at different time points (3, 6, 12, and 24 h). Homogenates were cultured onto marine broth 2216E plates. Colony numbers were normalized to tissue weight. Data represent the bacterial load in gills, midgut, and hepatopancreas. * $p < 0.05$, ** $p < 0.01$; *** $p < 0.001$.

2.6.3. Pre-Incubation of rSparanegtin and *V. alginolyticus* Modulate Immune-Related Gene Expression Profiles

The results of qPCR showed the effect of pre-incubation of rSparanegtin and *V. alginolyticus* on the immune response of *S. paramomosain* (Figure 6). Compared with the PBS group and the rTrx group, the transcription levels of the canonical components of the immune pathway (including *Sp*Toll2, *Sp*Myd88, and *Sp*STAT), two AMPs (SpHyastatin and *Sp*ALF2), and antioxidant enzyme genes (including *Sp*CAT, *Sp*SOD, and *Sp*GPx) were increased significantly at 6 h in the rSparanegtin group.

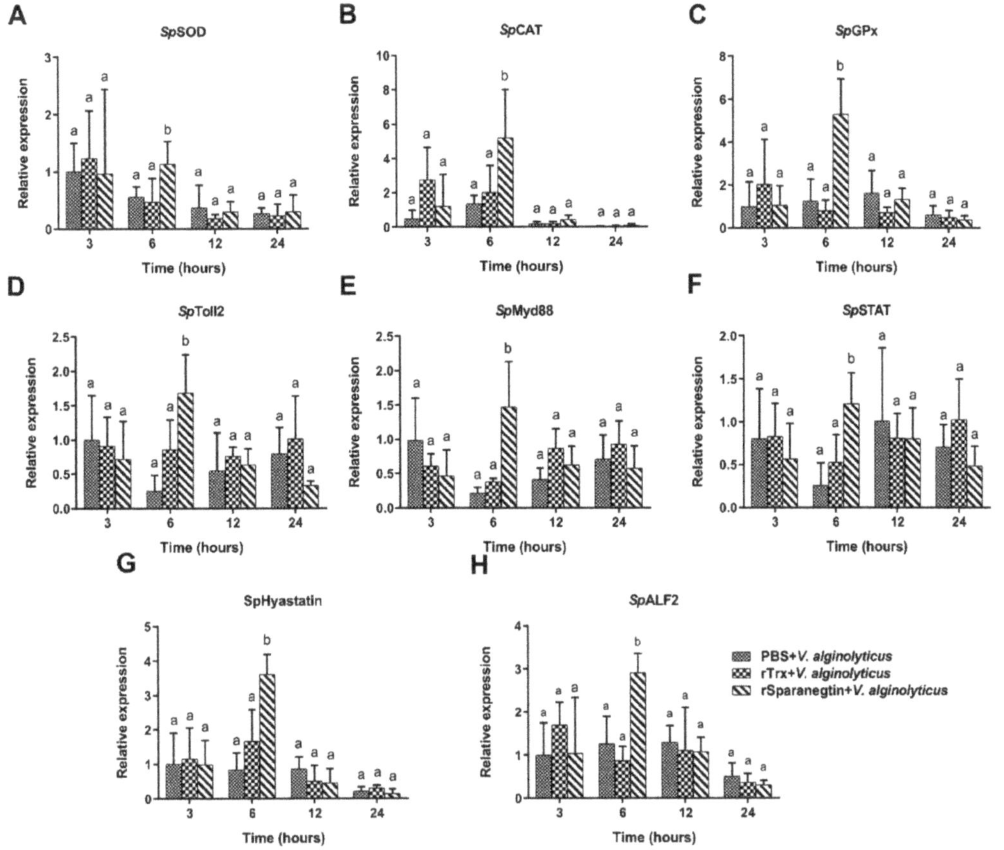

Figure 6. rSparanegtin effects on the *V. alginolyticus* infection-mediated immune gene expression profiles in *S. paramamosain.* Crabs were divided into PBS + *V. alginolyticus*, rTrx + *V. alginolyticus*, and rSparanegtin + *V. alginolyticus* groups. The expression levels of *Sp*SOD, *Sp*CAT, *Sp*GPx, *Sp*Toll2, *Sp*Myd88, *Sp*STAT, *Sp*ALF2, and SpHyastain (**A–H**) were evaluated using qPCR at 3, 6, 12, and 24 h post-injection. Each bar represents the means ± SD (n = 5). The same letters (a–b) indicate no significant difference between groups, and different letters indicate statistically significant differences between groups ($p < 0.05$) as calculated by one-way ANOVA followed by Tukey's test. It was noted that only the means at each time point were compared for the denotation with the letters, whereas the means at different time points could not be compared with one another.

3. Discussion

In the study, based on the transcriptome database of *S. paramamosain* established by our laboratory, we identified a novel AMP and named it Sparanegtin. According to the theoretical pI 5.2 of its mature peptide, Sparanegtin is an anionic AMP. As it is known, most reported AMPs are cationic peptides; however, more anionic AMPs have been gradually identified in different species in recent years and also have a potent antimicrobial activity. Dermcidin is a novel human antibiotic peptide secreted by sweat glands and has a net negative charge of −5 that shows antimicrobial activity in response to a variety of pathogenic microorganisms [22]. The three antifungal peptides from the *Litopenaeus stylirostris* and *Litopenaeus vannamei* have a negative net charge at physiological pH with a pI and a broad spectrum of antifungal activity [23]. Our previous studies report that two novel AMPs, Scygonadin [24] and its homologous SCY2 [25], are anionic peptides and both have antimicrobial activity. In the present study, it was found that rSparanegtin displayed a potent activity against several Gram-negative bacteria (*E. coli*, *P. aeruginosa*, *P. stutzeri*, *P. fluorescens*, and *S. flexneri*) (MICs ranging from 12 to 48 μM), Gram-positive bacteria (*B. subtilis*, *C. glutamicum*, and *S. aureus*), and yeast (*C. neoformans* and *P. pastoris GS115*) (MICs ranging from 24 to 48 μM) (Table 1). The in vivo expression pattern of the Sparanegtin gene was tissue-specific. The mRNA transcripts of Sparanegtin were highly expressed in the testis of male crabs. In addition, some known AMPs are sex-specifically expressed; for instance, Adropin is specifically expressed in the ejaculatory duct of *Drosophila melanogaster* [26], as observed in our early study on Scygonadin that is dominantly expressed in the ejaculatory duct of male mud crabs and is involved in the reproductive immunity [24]. A recently reported AMP, scyreprocin, is identified as an interacting partner of SCY2 from the reproductive system of male *S. paramamosain* and highly expressed in the testis [19]. It is known that testes are organs of the male reproductive system of decapod crustaceans and harbor germ cells and produces spermatozoa [27], as well as being functional either at the beginning or during the entire spermatogenesis process [28]. Therefore, Sparanegtin that is highly present in testes may play an immune defense role in spermatogenesis and the reproduction process of male crabs.

Binding to the surface of microorganisms is the first step for AMP to exert its antimicrobial effect. In order to better understand the underlying antimicrobial mechanism of AMPs, microbial cell wall polysaccharides binding assays were conducted in this study. The present study revealed that rSparanegtin had a strong binding ability to LPS, PGN, and LTA in a concentration-dependent manner and exhibited a higher binding ability to LPS than to PGN and LTA. Many AMPs are reported with similar activities via binding to microbial cell wall polysaccharides. rPcALF1 from red swamp crayfish (*Procambarus clarkii*) could bind with different amounts of microbial polysaccharides, mostly with LPS, followed by glucan, and the least with LTA, and then find that it has stronger antibacterial activity against Gram-negative bacteria [29]. In *Marsupenaeus japonicus*, MjCru I-1 could agglutinate bacteria and bind to bacteria by binding to the bacterial cell wall molecules including LPS, LTA, and PGN. MjCru I-1 had antibacterial activity against some bacteria by destroying the membrane of bacteria [30]. rLvCrustinB from Pacific white shrimp *Litopenaeus vannamei* directly binds to polysaccharides, including PGN, LTA, and LPS, indicating that LvCrustinB may be involved in the defense against Gram-positive and Gram-negative bacteria [31]. In the study, the SEM images of *P. aeruginosa* showed a significantly destruction of membrane integrity and even leakage of cell contents, suggesting that the activities of rSparanegtin may be via the interaction with the specific components of bacterial cell wall. This is consistent with the fact that rSparanegtin has high antimicrobial activity against *P. aeruginosa*. The antimicrobial mechanism of rSparanegtin may be similar to that of most AMPs that destroy the integrity of the microbial membrane, which leads to the leakage of the cytoplasmic contents and ultimately kills them [32].

It was interesting to note in the study that the survival rate of *S. paramamosain* challenged with *V. alginolyticus* was increased when rSparanegtin was given to crabs; correspondingly, there was a significant reduction in *V. alginolyticus* load in the gills and hepatopancreas at 6, 12, and 24 h. The results suggested that rSparanegtin might exert an immunological defense against the invading *V. alginolyticus* by which the survival rate of crabs was enhanced. Analysis of the *Sparanegtin* gene in vivo demonstrated that this peptide was significantly expressed in the testis at 3 h and 72 h or hemocytes at 3 h with the *V. alginolyticus* challenge; meanwhile, other AMPs such as SpHyastatin and *Sp*ALF2 as well as signal pathway associated genes such as *Sp*Toll2, *Sp*Myd88, and *Sp*STAT were up-regulated at 6 h. All of these findings suggested that Sparanegtin may directly participate in the immune response or indirectly play a role by inducing the expression of other immune-associated genes with the injection of rSparanegtin when bacterial infection occurred in crabs; that means that Sparanegtin may generate immunoprotective and immunomodulatory activities. AMPs as products of immune response are testified to play important roles in killing or cleaning the infected pathogens directly. The significant expression of SpHyastatin and *Sp*ALF2 at 6 h after *V. alginolyticus* challenge might be due to the immunomodulatory effect of rSparanegtin. In a previous study on SpHyastatin, this peptide is down-regulated at 24 h and then up-regulated at 96 h but does not show any change in expression at 6 h after bacterial challenge [33], suggesting that the expression of SpHyastatin might be directly induced by the injection of rSparanegtin. The significant expression of *Sp*Toll2, *Sp*Myd88, and *Sp*STAT implied that the immune-associated signal pathways participated in the defense against the *V. alginolyticus* challenge and may induce the activation of downstream effectors such as AMPs.

In addition to resistance to a variety of pathogenic microorganisms, AMPs are also reported to regulate the expression of other immune genes [34]. We found that the pre-incubation of rSparanegtin and *V. alginolyticus* could induce the transcription levels of several immune-related genes, including immune signaling pathway-related genes (*Sp*Toll2, *Sp*Myd88, *Sp*STAT), AMPs (SpHyastatin and *Sp*ALF2), and antioxidant-associated genes (*Sp*SOD, *Sp*CAT, and *Sp*GPx). Such immunoenhancing properties are demonstrated in several other marine-derived AMPs, for example, shrimp and *limulus* anti-lipopolysaccharide factor [35–37]. The innate humoral immune response is mainly mediated by three immune signaling pathways, namely, the Toll pathway, IMD pathway, and JAK/STAT pathway [38]. By regulating or stimulating the Toll signaling pathway, the production of some immune factors related to its downstream pathway, such as antimicrobial peptides (AMPs), can be activated against microbial infection [39]. The JAK/STAT signaling pathway positively regulates AMP gene expression that plays an important role in immune response [40]. In this study, the expression trend of both AMPs (SpHyastatin and *Sp*ALF2) genes was consistent with the expression of *Sp*Toll2, *Sp*MyD88, and *Sp*STAT, suggesting that the expression of both AMPs might be regulated through the Toll and JAK/STAT pathways. The up-regulation of SpHyastatin and *Sp*ALF2 may participate in eliminating the infected bacteria. In addition, bacterial infection can prompt the body to produce ROS, and excessive ROS will cause tissue damage and inflammation [41,42]. The up-regulated expression of antioxidant enzymes (*Sp*SOD, *Sp*CAT, and *Sp*GPx) might be associated with the action of removing ROS in vivo. These results suggested that Sparanegtin was likely generating an immunomodulatory effect that helps eliminate the invading bacteria.

The interactions among the induced expression of AMPs, clear degree of infected bacterial numbers, and survival rate of marine animals have been much reported in previous studies. For example, MjALF-E2 were upregulated by bacterial challenge and could promote the clearance of bacteria in vivo. After knockdown of MjALF-E2 and infection with *Vibrio anguillarum*, shrimp showed high and rapid mortality compared with GFPi shrimp, suggesting that MjALF-E2 serves a protective function against bacterial infection in shrimp [43]. A crustin gene PcCru isolated from red swamp crayfish *Procambarus clarkia* is significantly induced by bacterial stimulations at both the translational and transcriptional levels and could protect crayfish from infection by the pathogenic bacteria *Aeromonas hydrophila* in vivo [44]. In a bacteria challenge test, As-CATH4 and 5 (two vertebrate-derived cathelicidins family HDPs) could significantly decrease the bacterial numbers in crabs and increase the survival rates of crabs in both pre-stimulation and co-stimulation groups [45]. Similarly, the expression level of PcALF1 is induced by bacteria, and the injection of PcALF1 in crayfish (*Procambarus clarkii*) enhances the elimination of bacteria in vivo [29]. Our previous studies on other two AMPs, SCY2 and SpHyastatin, also show an immunoprotective effect on *S. paramamosain*, although both have differential antimicrobial activity and in vivo expression patterns. rSpHyastatin, a peptide that is highly expressed in hemolymphs with bacterial challenge, could confer immune-protective resistance against pathogenic challenge in *S. paramamosain*, causing less significant change in level of the mRNA expression of all tested immune and antioxidant-associated genes [17]. For SCY2, even though its gene expression is uniquely expressed during the mating of crabs and could not be directly induced by the injection of bacteria, rSCY2 could significantly increase the survival rate of *S. paramamosain* [46]. It is worth noting that rSparanegtin had no inhibitory or killing effect on cultured *V. alginolyticus* in vitro; however, it could be significantly expressed at some timepoints with the *V. alginolyticus* challenge in vivo and could significantly improve the survival rate of *S. paramamosain* after *V. alginolyticus* challenge as well as reduce *V. alginolyticus* load in the gills and hepatopancreas. The similar phenomenon is also found in our early study on an AMP SpHyastatin that is also identified in *S. paramamosain* [17].

4. Materials and Methods

4.1. Microorganism Strains

All strains were purchased from the China General Microbiological Culture Collection Center (CGMCC), including *Staphylococcus aureus* (CGMCC No. 1.2465), *Staphylococcus epidermidis* (CGMCC No. 1.4260), *Escherichia coli* (CGMCC No. 1.2389), *Pseudomonas aeruginosa* (CGMCC No. 1.2421), *Pseudomonas fluorescens* (CGMCC No. 1.1802), *Shigella flexneri* (CGMCC No. 1.1868), *Bacillus subtilis* (CGMCC No. 1.3358), *Cryptococcus neoformans* (CGMCC No. 2.1563), and *Vibrio alginolyticus* (CGMCC No. 1.1833). *Pichia pastoris* (GS115) was purchased from Invitrogen (Thermo Fisher Scientific, Waltham, MA, USA).

4.2. Animals, Challenge and Tissue Collection

Mud crabs (*S. paramamosain*) were purchased from the Zhangzhou Crab Farm (Fujian, China). Healthy male and female adult mud crabs (body weight 300 $\pm$ 30 g, n = 5) were dissected, and the tissues including testis, anterior vas deferens, seminal vesicle, posterior vas deferens, ejaculatory duct, posterior ejaculatory duct, penis, ovary, spermathecae, reproductive duct, muscle, thoracic ganglion, gills, brain, midgut, subcuticular epidermis, eye stalk, heart, hepatopancreas, and stomach were collected. Hemocytes were isolated from the hemolymph as described previously [47]. For the challenge experiment, adult male crabs (body weight 300 $\pm$ 30 g, n = 5) were injected with LPS at a dosage of 0.5 mg kg^{-1} or *V. alginolyticus* (1×10^6 CFU $crab^{-1}$). Crabs injected with crab saline (NaCl, 496 mM; KCl, 9.52 mM; $MgSO_4$, 12.8 mM; $CaCl_2$, 16.2 mM; $MgCl_2$, 0.84 mM; $NaHCO_3$, 5.95 mM; HEPES, 20 mM; pH 7.4) were set up as the control group. Tissue samples (testes and hemocytes) were collected at 3, 6, 12, 24, 48, and 72 h post-injection (hpi). All tissues were stored at −80 °C until use. All animal procedures were carried out in strict accordance with the National Institute of Health Guidelines for the Care and Use of Laboratory Animals and were approved by the Animal Welfare and Ethics Committee of Xiamen University.

4.3. Cloning, Expression, Purification, and Analysis of Recombinant Proteins

Total RNA of testis was extracted using TRIzol™ reagent (Invitrogen, Carlsbad, CA, USA) and cDNA was generated using PrimeScript™ RT reagent Kit with gDNA Eraser Kit (Takara, China). The cDNA templates for 5′- and 3′-random amplification of cDNA ends (RACE) PCR were synthesized using a SMARTer® RACE 5′/3′ Kit (Takara, Dalian, China). Gene-specific primers were designed based on the partial sequences obtained from the transcriptome database established by our laboratory (Table 2). The amplified fragments were cloned into the pMD18-T vector (Takara, Dalian, China) and sequenced by Borui Biotechnology Ltd. (Xiamen, China).

Table 2. Primer sequences.

Primers	Sequence (5′–3′)
Sparanegtin-ORF-F	ATGGCGGCGGCGGCTTCAGG
Sparanegtin-ORF-R	TCAAACCCCCGCCGAAGTGA
Sparanegtin-5′-R1	CGGCTGCCGTAGGAAAGGAA
Sparanegtin-5′-R2	AATATCCGCTGTGGCCGACG
Sparanegtin-3′-F1	CGTCGGCCACAGCGGATATT
Sparanegtin-3′-F2	ACCAACTTGGCAAGAGGAGCG
Long primer	CTAATACGACTCACTATAGGGCAAGCAGTGGTATCAACGCAGAGT
Short primer	CTAATACGACTCACTATAGGGC
NUP	AAGCAGTGGTATCAACGCAGAGT
M13–47F	CGCCAGGGTTTTCCCAGTCACGAC
M13–48R	AGCGGATAACAATTTCACACAGGA
Sparanegtin-qPCR-F	TCCCCGGTTTCCCGACCCAG
Sparanegtin-qPCR-R	ACCAGGAGGCAGCACCGTCT
GAPDH-qPCR-F	CTCCACTGGTGCCGCTAAGGCTGTA
GAPDH-qPCR-R	CAAGTCAGGTCAACCACGGACACAT

The open reading frame of Sparanegtin was constructed into the pET-32a (+) vector (with 6× His tag and thioredoxin (Trx) tag) and transformed into *E. coli* BL21 (DE3) and further expressed (the specific primer sequences were listed in Table 2). A pET32a (+) vector with only 6× His tag and Trx (thioredoxin) tag was constructed, and the expressed product was used as a control. Isopropyl β-D-Thiogalactoside (IPTG) was added to a final concentration of 0.5 mM to induce protein expression at 28 °C for 8 h. The recombinant Sparanegtin (rSparanegtin) was expressed and purified through HisTrap TM FF crude (GE Healthcare, Chicago, IL, USA) on the ÄKTA Pure system (GE Healthcare, Chicago, IL, USA) according to the standard protocol. The purified proteins were dialyzed and concentrated, and the protein concentration was determined by Bradford assay. The purified proteins were confirmed by sodium dodecyl sulfate-polyacrylamide gel electrophoresis (SDS-PAGE), Western blotting, and mass spectrometry identification. All recombinant proteins were stored at −80 °C

4.4. Quantitative Real-Time PCR

The total RNA of all samples was extracted and cDNA was synthesized as described above. Quantitative reverse transcription PCR (qRT-PCR) was performed using the cDNA as the template to detect the expression level of Sparanegtin in a real-time thermal cycler (ABI 7500, Waltham, MA, USA) using FastStart DNA Master SYBR Green I (Roche Diagnostics, Mannheim, Germany). The expression profiles of Sparanegtin gene in various adult crab tissues were determined by absolute quantitative real-time PCR (qPCR) and the expression changes of Sparanegtin during the response patterns of Sparanegtin gene to LPS and *V. alginolyticus* challenge were analyzed by relative qPCR. The specific primer sequences (Sparanegtin-qPCR-F/Sparanegtin-qPCR-R, GADPH-qPCR-F/GADPH-qPCR-R) are listed in Table 1. The qPCR cycle conditions were set as follows: an initial denaturing step at 95 °C for 10 min, 40 cycles at 95 °C for 15 s, 60 °C for 30 s, and 72 °C for 1 min. The $2^{-\Delta\Delta Ct}$ algorithm was applied to the expression profile analysis [48].

4.5. Antimicrobial Assay

Microorganisms in the logarithmic growth phase were harvested and used to evaluate the antimicrobial activity of rSparanegtin. The minimum inhibitory concentration (MIC) and the minimum bactericidal concentration (MBC) were determined according to the previously described liquid growth inhibition assay, which were performed three times independently [19]. Compared with the negative control, the MIC value is defined as the lowest protein concentration that does not induce visible bacterial growth. Then, we spread the culture without visible bacterial growth on a solid medium plate. The MBC is the concentration that kills more than 99.9% of the microorganisms after incubation at 28 or 37 °C for 24 h.

4.6. Binding Assays

In order to determine the binding properties of rSparanegtin with lipopolysaccharides (LPS B5, Sigma, St. Louis, MO, USA), lipoteichoic acid (LTA, L2515, Sigma, St. Louis, MO, USA), and peptidoglycan (PGN from *Bacillus subtilis*, Sigma, St. Louis, MO, USA), a modified ELISA assay was performed as described previously [19]. Briefly, a 96-well ELISA plate was coated overnight with LPS, LTA, and PGN at 4 °C; then, it was blocked with 5% skimmed milk and incubated with a serial dilution of rSparanegtin and rTrx (0 to 5 μg mL^{-1}) for 2 h at 37 °C. Bound peptides were detected by incubation with mouse anti-His antibody (1:3000, prepared in 1% skimmed milk) followed by adding goat anti-mouse HRP antibody (1:5000, prepared in 1% skim milk). After the colorimetric reaction, the absorbance at 450 nm was measured using a microplate reader (TECAN GENios, GMI, Brooklyn Park, MN, USA). The independent assays were performed three times. The binding parameters, apparent dissociation constant (Kd), and maximum binding (Amax) were determined using non-linear fitting as A = Amax [L] / (Kd + [L]), where A is the absorbance at 450 nm and [L] is the protein concentration [17].

4.7. Time-Killing Kinetic Assay

The Gram-negative bacteria *P. aeruginosa* were subjected for time-killing kinetic assay according to the previous description. rSparanegtin was incubated with bacteria at a concentration of 48 μM. The cultures were sampled and plated at different time points (n = 3). The plates were incubated at 37 °C for 24 h, and the total viable count (TVC) was determined. The independent experiments were performed three times.

4.8. SEM Observation

SEM was used to further study the antibacterial mechanism of rSparanegtin. *P. aeruginosa* (5×10^7 CFU mL^{-1}) was prepared as described in the antimicrobial assay. PBS, rTrx, and rSparanegtin were separately added into each individual culture medium and incubated at a concentration of 48 μM for 30 min. The microbial cells were collected and fixed with pre-cooled 2.5% glutaraldehyde at 4 °C for 2 h. Then, the samples were dehydrated with a graded series of ethanol (30%, 50%, 70%, 80%, 95%, and 100%) and further dehydrated in a critical point dryer (EM CPD300, Leica, Wetzlar, Germany) and gold coated [50]. Finally, the change in morphology of the bacteria was observed by SEM (SUPRA 55 SAPPHIRE, Carl Zeiss, Oberkochen, Germany).

4.9. Cytotoxicity Assay

The cytotoxicity of rSparanegtin was evaluated using hemocytes from *S. paramamosain*. The hemocytes of *S. paramamosain* were isolated as previously described [51]. Briefly, the hemocytes were maintained in L-15 medium prepared in crab saline and supplemented with 5% fetal bovine serum, inoculated on a 96-well cell culture plate with approximately 10^4 cells $well^{-1}$, and incubated overnight at 26 °C. HEK-293T cells were maintained in Dulbecco's Modified Eagle Medium supplemented with 10% fetal bovine serum, and NCI-H460 cells were maintained in Roswell Park Memorial Institute 1640 supplemented with 10% fetal bovine serum. HEK-293T and NCI-H460 cells were inoculated on a 96-well cell culture plate and incubated at 37 °C with 5% CO_2 overnight. Finally, all the cells were incubated with culture medium supplemented with various concentrations of rSparanegtin (3, 6, 12, 24 and 48 μM, n = 3). After 24 h of incubation, cell viability was assessed using a CellTiter 96 R ® Aqueous Kit (Promega, Madison, WI, USA). The independent experiments were carried out three times.

4.10. Endotoxin Assay

The endotoxin level of *V. alginolyticus* after rSparanegtin treatment was detected by the Toxin Sensor™ Chromogenic LAL Endotoxin Assay Kit (GenScript, Piscataway, NJ, USA) following the manufacturer's instructions [52]. When *V. alginolyticus* reached the logarithmic growth phase, they were collected and adjusted to a concentration of

10^7 CFU/mL. Then, they were incubated with different concentrations of rSparanegtin (0, 12, 24, 48 μM, $n = 3$) at room temperature for 1 h and analyzed by a spectrophotometer at an absorbance of 545 nm (Agilent Technologies, Bayan Lepas, Malaysia). Each sample had three biological parallels. The independent experiments were carried out three times.

4.11. Evaluation of the In Vivo Activity of rSparanegtin on S. paramamosain Infected with V. alginolyticus

In order to investigate the in vivo protective effect of rSparanegtin, we performed a mortality comparison assay using male *S. paramamosain* (average weight 40 ± 5 g) infected with *V. alginolyticus*. rSparanegtin, rTrx, and *V. alginolyticus* were prepared in PBS. First, the recombinant protein (20 μg/crab) was incubated with *V. alginolyticus* (1 × 10^6 CFU/crab) at room temperature for 1 h, and then, the mixture was injected into the base of the right fourth leg of crabs. The control group received an equal volume of *V. alginolyticus* diluted in PBS. Sixty crabs were divided into three groups (including PBS and *V. alginolyticus* pre-incubation group, rTrx and *V. alginolyticus* pre-incubation group, and rSparanegtin and *V. alginolyticus* pre-incubation group) with 20 crabs in each group. The survival rates of crabs in each group were recorded at different time points (3, 6, 9, 12, 24, 36, 48, 60, 72, 96, and 120 h).

4.12. Bacterial Load Assay and Quantification of Immune-Related Gene Expression after Different Treatment

In order to investigate the bacterial load in tissues, male *S. paramamosain* (average weight 40 ± 5 g each) was performed different treatments as described above. The crabs were dissected, and tissues including hemocytes, gills, and hepatopancreas were collected at different time points (3, 6, 12, and 24 h, $n = 5$). Gills and hepatopancreas (0.1–0.2 g fresh weight per tissue) were homogenized in PBS. Then, the tissue homogenates were spread on marine broth 2216E plates, and the plates were incubated at 28 °C for 24 h. The colonies were counted separately for each sample at each time point.

The total RNA of the collected tissues was extracted, and the cDNA was synthesized as described above. The expression profiles of several immune-related genes were analyzed by qRT-PCR. The GenBank accession numbers for those genes are listed as follows: *Sp*Toll2: SLM84439.1; *Sp*Myd88: KC342028.1; *Sp*STAT: KC711050.1; *Sp*SOD: FJ774661.1; *Sp*CAT: FJ774660.1; *Sp*GPx: JN565286.1; *Sp*ALF2: JQ069031.1 and SpHyastatin: AFY10070.1. The specific primers for these genes are summarized in Table S1.

4.13. Statistical Analysis

The results are presented as the mean ± standard deviation (SD). For the absolute qPCR assays, statistical analyses were performed by one-way analysis of variance (ANOVA) following a Tukey post-test. For the relative qPCR assays, statistical analyses were performed by two-way ANOVA following a Bonferroni post-test. For cytotoxicity assays, statistical analysis was performed by one-way ANOVA following Dunnett's post-test. For the mortality comparison assay, data were analyzed using the Kaplan–Meier log rank test. For the immune-related gene expression, one-way analysis of variance (ANOVA) was used for statistical analysis using SPSS 18.0 (IBM, Armonk, NY, USA) to determine the expression difference within groups. Significant levels were accepted at $p < 0.05$.

5. Conclusions

In summary, a new antimicrobial peptide named Sparanegtin was identified in *S. paramamosain*, and its transcripts were specifically distributed in tissues and significantly expressed with bacterial challenge. rSparanegtin had antimicrobial activity, and the antimicrobial mechanism involved initial damage to the outer membrane of bacteria, eventually resulting in the loss of cellular components and the complete collapse of the cell architecture. rSparanegtin showed no cytotoxicity and could reduce the *V. alginolyticus* endotoxin level in vitro. This AMP had an in vivo protective and immunomodulatory effect in *S. paramamosain* that could reduce the bacterial load in tissues and enhance the survival rate of crabs challenged with *V. alginolyticus*. Taken together, Sparanegtin might be a potential effective antimicrobial agent to be used in aquaculture or animal husbandry.

Supplementary Materials: The following are available online at https://www.mdpi.com/article/10.3390/ijms23010015/s1.

Author Contributions: K.-J.W. and F.C.: Conceptualization; Funding acquisition; Project administration; Supervision; Writing—review and editing. X.Z.: Data curation; Formal analysis; Investigation; Methodology; Writing—original draft. S.L. and H.P.: Investigation; Methodology. All authors have read and agreed to the published version of the manuscript.

Funding: This study was supported by the National Natural Science Foundation of China (U1805233); the Fujian Marine Economic Development Subsidy Fund Project (grant #FJHJF-L-2019-1) from the Fujian Ocean and Fisheries Department, the Xiamen Ocean and Fishery Development Special Fund Project (grant #20CZP011HJ06) from the Xiamen Municipal Bureau of Ocean Development, a grant (grant #3502Z20203012) from the Xiamen Science and Technology Planning Project, and the Fundamental Research Funds from Central Universities (grant #20720190109).

Acknowledgments: We thank laboratory engineers Huiyun Chen, Zhiyong Lin and Ming Xiong for providing technical assistance.

Conflicts of Interest: The authors declare no conflict of interest.

References

1. Wenning, R. The State of World Fisheries and Aquaculture (Sofia) 2020 Report. *Integr. Environ. Asses.* **2020**, *16*, 800–801.
2. Liu, X.; Steele, J.C.; Meng, X.Z. Usage, residue, and human health risk of antibiotics in Chinese aquaculture: A review. *Environ. Pollut.* **2017**, *223*, 161–169. [CrossRef]
3. Shah, S.Q.; Cabello, F.C.; L'Abee-Lund, T.M.; Tomova, A.; Godfrey, H.P.; Buschmann, A.H.; Sorum, H. Antimicrobial resistance and antimicrobial resistance genes in marine bacteria from salmon aquaculture and non-aquaculture sites. *Environ. Microbiol.* **2014**, *16*, 1310–1320. [CrossRef]
4. Verraes, C.; Van Boxstael, S.; Van Meervenne, E.; Van Coillie, E.; Butaye, P.; Catry, B.; de Schaetzen, M.A.; Van Huffel, X.; Imberechts, H.; Dierick, K.; et al. Antimicrobial Resistance in the Food Chain: A Review. *Int. J. Environ. Res. Public Health* **2013**, *10*, 2643–2669. [CrossRef]
5. Brown, K.; Uwiera, R.R.E.; Kalmokoff, M.L.; Brooks, S.P.J.; Inglis, G.D. Antimicrobial growth promoter use in livestock: A requirement to understand their modes of action to develop effective alternatives. *Int. J. Antimicrob. Agents* **2017**, *49*, 12–24. [CrossRef]
6. Tian, M.; He, X.M.; Feng, Y.Z.; Wang, W.T.; Chen, H.S.; Gong, M.; Liu, D.; Clarke, J.L.; van Eerde, A. Pollution by Antibiotics and Antimicrobial Resistance in LiveStock and Poultry Manure in China, and Countermeasures. *Antibiotics* **2021**, *10*, 539. [CrossRef] [PubMed]
7. Taniguchi, A.; Onishi, H.; Eguchi, M. Quantitative PCR assay for the detection of the parasitic ciliate Cryptocaryon irritans. *Fish. Sci.* **2011**, *77*, 607–613. [CrossRef]
8. Zasloff, M. Antimicrobial peptides of multicellular organisms. *Nature* **2002**, *415*, 389–395. [CrossRef]
9. Shabir, U.; Ali, S.; Magray, A.R.; Ganai, B.A.; Firdous, P.; Hassan, T.; Nazir, R. Fish antimicrobial peptides (AMP'S) as essential and promising molecular therapeutic agents: A review. *Microb. Pathog.* **2018**, *114*, 50–56. [CrossRef]
10. Batoni, G.; Maisetta, G.; Esin, S. Antimicrobial peptides and their interaction with biofilms of medically relevant bacteria. *Biochim. Biophys. Acta* **2016**, *1858*, 1044–1060. [CrossRef]
11. Lu, S.; Walters, G.; Parg, R.; Dutcher, J.R. Nanomechanical response of bacterial cells to cationic antimicrobial peptides. *Soft Matter* **2014**, *10*, 1806–1815. [CrossRef]
12. Hanson, M.A.; Dostalova, A.; Ceroni, C.; Poidevin, M.; Kondo, S.; Lemaitre, B. Synergy and remarkable specificity of antimicrobial peptides in vivo using a systematic knockout approach. *Elife* **2019**, *8*, e44341. [CrossRef] [PubMed]
13. Li, H.X.; Lu, X.J.; Li, C.H.; Chen, J. Molecular characterization of the liver-expressed antimicrobial peptide 2 (LEAP-2) in a teleost fish, *Plecoglossus altivelis*: Antimicrobial activity and molecular mechanism. *Mol. Immunol.* **2015**, *65*, 406–415. [CrossRef] [PubMed]
14. Pan, C.Y.; Wu, J.L.; Hui, C.F.; Lin, C.H.; Chen, J.Y. Insights into the antibacterial and immunomodulatory functions of the antimicrobial peptide, epinecidin-1, against Vibrio vulnificus infection in zebrafish. *Fish. Shellfish Immunol.* **2011**, *31*, 1019–1025. [CrossRef] [PubMed]
15. Li, H.X.; Lu, X.J.; Li, C.H.; Chen, J. Molecular characterization and functional analysis of two distinct liver-expressed antimicrobial peptide 2 (LEAP-2) genes in large yellow croaker (*Larimichthys crocea*). *Fish. Shellfish Immunol.* **2014**, *38*, 330–339. [CrossRef]
16. Lin, F.Y.; Gao, Y.; Wang, H.; Zhang, Q.X.; Zeng, C.L.; Liu, H.P. Identification of an anti-lipopolysacchride factor possessing both antiviral and antibacterial activity from the red claw crayfish *Cherax quadricarinatus*. *Fish. Shellfish Immunol.* **2016**, *57*, 213–221. [CrossRef]

17. Shan, Z.; Zhu, K.; Peng, H.; Chen, B.; Liu, J.; Chen, F.; Ma, X.; Wang, S.; Qiao, K.; Wang, K. The New Antimicrobial Peptide SpHyastatin from the Mud Crab Scylla paramamosain with Multiple Antimicrobial Mechanisms and High Effect on Bacterial Infection. *Front. Microbiol.* **2016**, *7*, 1140. [CrossRef] [PubMed]
18. Long, S.; Chen, F.Y.; Wang, K.J. Characterization of a new homologous anti-lipopolysaccharide factor SpALF7 in mud crab *Scylla paramamosain*. *Aquaculture* **2021**, *534*, 736333. [CrossRef]
19. Yang, Y.; Chen, F.; Chen, H.Y.; Peng, H.; Hao, H.; Wang, K.J. A Novel Antimicrobial Peptide Scyreprocin From Mud Crab *Scylla paramamosain* Showing Potent Antifungal and Anti-biofilm Activity. *Front. Microbiol.* **2020**, *11*, 1589. [CrossRef] [PubMed]
20. Pan, C.Y.; Tsai, T.Y.; Su, B.C.; Hui, C.F.; Chen, J.Y. Study of the Antimicrobial Activity of Tilapia Piscidin 3 (TP3) and TP4 and Their Effects on Immune Functions in Hybrid Tilapia (*Oreochromis* spp.). *PLoS ONE* **2017**, *12*, e0169678. [CrossRef]
21. Chen, S.W.; Liu, C.H.; Hu, S.Y. Dietary administration of probiotic Paenibacillus ehimensis NPUST1 with bacteriocin-like activity improves growth performance and immunity against *Aeromonas hydrophila* and *Streptococcus iniae* in Nile tilapia (*Oreochromis niloticus*). *Fish. Shellfish Immunol.* **2019**, *84*, 695–703. [CrossRef]
22. Schittek, B.; Hipfel, R.; Sauer, B.; Bauer, J.; Kalbacher, H.; Stevanovic, S.; Schirle, M.; Schroeder, K.; Blin, N.; Meier, F.; et al. Dermcidin: A novel human antibiotic peptide secreted by sweat glands. *Nat. Immunol.* **2001**, *2*, 1133–1137. [CrossRef] [PubMed]
23. Destoumieux-Garzon, D.; Saulnier, D.; Garnier, J.; Jouffrey, C.; Bulet, P.; Bachere, E. Crustacean immunity—Antifungal peptides are generated from the C terminus of shrimp hemocyanin in response to microbial challenge. *J. Biol. Chem.* **2001**, *276*, 47070–47077. [CrossRef] [PubMed]
24. Wang, K.J.; Huang, W.S.; Yang, M.; Chen, H.Y.; Bo, J.; Li, S.J.; Wang, G.Z. A male-specific expression gene, encodes a novel anionic antimicrobial peptide, scygonadin, in *Scylla serrata*. *Mol. Immunol.* **2007**, *44*, 1961–1968. [CrossRef] [PubMed]
25. Qiao, K.; Xu, W.F.; Chen, H.Y.; Peng, H.; Zhang, Y.Q.; Huang, W.S.; Wang, S.P.; An, Z.; Shan, Z.G.; Chen, F.Y.; et al. A new antimicrobial peptide SCY2 identified in *Scylla paramamosain* exerting a potential role of reproductive immunity. *Fish Shellfish Immunol.* **2016**, *51*, 251–262. [CrossRef]
26. Samakovlis, C.; Kylsten, P.; Kimbrell, D.A.; Engstrom, A.; Hultmark, A. The andropin gene and its product, a male-specific antibacterial peptide in Drosophila melanogaster. *EMBO J.* **1991**, *10*, 163–169. [CrossRef]
27. Felgenhauer, B.E. Internal anatomy of the Decapoda: An overview. *Microsc. Anat. Invertebr.* **1992**, *10*, 45–75.
28. Braga, A.; Nakayama, C.L.; Poersch, L.; Wasielesky, W. Unistellate spermatozoa of decapods: Comparative evaluation and evolution of the morphology. *Zoomorphology* **2013**, *132*, 261–284. [CrossRef]
29. Sun, C.; Xu, W.T.; Zhang, H.W.; Dong, L.P.; Zhang, T.; Zhao, X.F.; Wang, J.X. An anti-lipopolysaccharide factor from red swamp crayfish, *Procambarus clarkii*, exhibited antimicrobial activities in vitro and in vivo. *Fish Shellfish Immunol.* **2011**, *30*, 295–303. [CrossRef]
30. Liu, N.; Lan, J.F.; Sun, J.J.; Jia, W.M.; Zhao, X.F.; Wang, J.X. A novel crustin from *Marsupenaeus japonicus* promotes hemocyte phagocytosis. *Dev. Comp. Immunol.* **2015**, *49*, 313–322. [CrossRef]
31. Li, M.; Ma, C.X.; Zhu, P.; Yang, Y.H.; Lei, A.Y.G.; Chen, X.H.; Liang, W.W.; Chen, M.; Xiong, J.H.; Li, C.Z. A new crustin is involved in the innate immune response of shrimp *Litopenaeus vannamei*. *Fish Shellfish Immunol.* **2019**, *94*, 398–406. [CrossRef] [PubMed]
32. Li, J.; Koh, J.J.; Liu, S.; Lakshminarayanan, R.; Verma, C.S.; Beuerman, R.W. Membrane Active Antimicrobial Peptides: Translating Mechanistic Insights to Design. *Front. Neurosci.* **2017**, *11*, 73. [CrossRef]
33. Shan, Z.G.; Zhu, K.X.; Chen, F.Y.; Liu, J.; Chen, B.; Qiao, K.; Peng, H.; Wang, K.J. In vivo activity and the transcriptional regulatory mechanism of the antimicrobial peptide SpHyastatin in *Scylla paramamosain*. *Fish Shellfish Immunol.* **2016**, *59*, 155–165. [CrossRef]
34. Pushpanathan, M.; Gunasekaran, P.; Rajendhran, J. Antimicrobial peptides: Versatile biological properties. *Int. J. Pept.* **2013**, *2013*, 675391. [CrossRef] [PubMed]
35. Lin, M.C.; Lin, S.B.; Lee, S.C.; Lin, C.C.; Hui, C.F.; Chen, J.Y. Antimicrobial peptide of an anti-lipopolysaccharide factor modulates of the inflammatory response in RAW264.7 cells. *Peptides* **2010**, *31*, 1262–1272. [CrossRef] [PubMed]
36. Pan, C.Y.; Chao, T.T.; Chen, J.C.; Chen, J.Y.; Liu, W.C.; Lin, C.H.; Kuo, C.M. Shrimp (*Penaeus monodon*) anti-lipopolysaccharide factor reduces the lethality of *Pseudomonas aeruginosa* sepsis in mice. *Int. Immunopharmacol.* **2007**, *7*, 687–700. [CrossRef] [PubMed]
37. Vallespi, M.G.; Alvarez-Obregon, J.C.; Rodriguez-Alonso, I.; Montero, T.; Garay, H.; Reyes, O.; Arana, M.J. A Limulus anti-LPS factor-derived peptide modulates cytokine gene expression and promotes resolution of bacterial acute infection in mice. *Int. Immunopharmacol.* **2003**, *3*, 247–256. [CrossRef]
38. Li, W.X. Canonical and non-canonical JAK-STAT signaling. *Trends Cell Biol.* **2008**, *18*, 545–551. [CrossRef]
39. Chu, S.H.; Liu, L.; Abbas, M.N.; Li, Y.Y.; Kausar, S.; Qian, X.Y.; Ye, Z.Z.; Yu, X.M.; Li, X.K.; Liu, M.; et al. Peroxiredoxin 6 modulates Toll signaling pathway and protects DNA damage against oxidative stress in red swamp crayfish (*Procambarus clarkii*). *Fish Shellfish Immunol.* **2019**, *89*, 170–178. [CrossRef] [PubMed]
40. Ruan, Z.C.; Wan, Z.C.; Yang, L.; Li, W.W.; Wang, Q. JAK/STAT signalling regulates antimicrobial activities in *Eriocheir sinensis*. *Fish Shellfish Immunol.* **2019**, *84*, 491–501. [CrossRef]
41. Dharmaraja, A.T. Role of Reactive Oxygen Species (ROS) in Therapeutics and Drug Resistance in Cancer and Bacteria. *J. Med. Chem.* **2017**, *60*, 3221–3240. [CrossRef] [PubMed]
42. Kanzaki, H.; Wada, S.; Narimiya, T.; Yamaguchi, Y.; Katsumata, Y.; Itohiya, K.; Fukaya, S.; Miyamoto, Y.; Nakamura, Y. Pathways that Regulate ROS Scavenging Enzymes, and Their Role in Defense Against Tissue Destruction in Periodontitis. *Front. Physiol.* **2017**, *8*, 351. [CrossRef] [PubMed]

43. Jiang, H.S.; Zhang, Q.; Zhao, Y.R.; Jia, W.M.; Zhao, X.F.; Wang, J.X. A new group of anti-lipopolysaccharide factors from Marsupenaeus japonicus functions in antibacterial response. *Dev. Comp. Immunol.* **2015**, *48*, 33–42. [CrossRef]
44. Liu, N.; Zhang, R.R.; Fan, Z.X.; Zhao, X.F.; Wang, X.W.; Wang, J.X. Characterization of a type-I crustin with broad-spectrum antimicrobial activity from red swamp crayfish *Procambarus clarkii*. *Dev. Comp. Immunol.* **2016**, *61*, 145–153. [CrossRef]
45. Guo, Z.L.; Qiao, X.; Cheng, R.M.; Shi, N.N.; Wang, A.L.; Feng, T.T.; Chen, Y.; Zhang, F.; Yu, H.; Wang, Y.P. As-CATH4 and 5, two vertebrate-derived natural host defense peptides, enhance the immuno-resistance efficiency against bacterial infections in Chinese mitten crab, *Eriocheir sinensis*. *Fish Shellfish Immunol.* **2017**, *71*, 202–209. [CrossRef]
46. Xu, W.F.; Qiao, K.; Huang, S.P.; Peng, H.; Huang, W.S.; Chen, F.Y.; Zhang, N.; Wang, G.Z.; Wang, K.J. The expression pattern of scygonadin during the ontogenesis of *Scylla paramamosain* predicting its potential role in reproductive immunity. *Dev. Comp. Immunol.* **2011**, *35*, 1076–1088. [CrossRef]
47. Chen, F.Y.; Liu, H.P.; Bo, J.; Ren, H.L.; Wang, K.J. Identification of genes differentially expressed in hemocytes of *Scylla paramamosain* in response to lipopolysaccharide. *Fish Shellfish Immunol.* **2010**, *28*, 167–177. [CrossRef]
48. Livak, K.J.; Schmittgen, T.D. Analysis of relative gene expression data using real-time quantitative PCR and the 2(-Delta Delta C(T)) Method. *Methods* **2001**, *25*, 402–408. [CrossRef]
49. Liu, S.S.; Chen, G.X.; Xu, H.D.; Zou, W.B.; Yan, W.R.; Wang, Q.Q.; Deng, H.W.; Zhang, H.Q.; Yu, G.J.; He, J.G.; et al. Transcriptome analysis of mud crab (*Scylla paramamosain*) gills in response to Mud crab reovirus (MCRV). *Fish Shellfish Immunol.* **2017**, *60*, 545–553. [CrossRef]
50. Wei, L.; Yang, J.; He, X.; Mo, G.; Hong, J.; Yan, X.; Lin, D.; Lai, R. Structure and function of a potent lipopolysaccharide-binding antimicrobial and anti-inflammatory peptide. *J. Med. Chem.* **2013**, *56*, 3546–3556. [CrossRef] [PubMed]
51. Deepika, A.; Makesh, M.; Rajendran, K.V. Development of primary cell cultures from mud crab, *Scylla serrata*, and their potential as an in vitro model for the replication of white spot syndrome virus. *In Vitro Cell Dev. Biol.-Anim.* **2014**, *50*, 406–416. [CrossRef] [PubMed]
52. Qiu, W.; Chen, F.; Chen, R.; Li, S.; Zhu, X.; Xiong, M.; Wang, K.J. A New C-Type Lectin Homolog SpCTL6 Exerting Immunoprotective Effect and Regulatory Role in Mud Crab *Scylla paramamosain*. *Front. Immunol.* **2021**, *12*, 661823. [CrossRef] [PubMed]

International Journal of
Molecular Sciences

MDPI

Article

Two Male-Specific Antimicrobial Peptides SCY2 and Scyreprocin as Crucial Molecules Participated in the Sperm Acrosome Reaction of Mud Crab *Scylla paramamosain*

Ying Yang [1], Fangyi Chen [1,2], Kun Qiao [1], Hua Zhang [1], Hui-Yun Chen [1,2] and Ke-Jian Wang [1,2,*]

[1] State Key Laboratory of Marine Environmental Science, College of Ocean and Earth Sciences, Xiamen University, Xiamen 361102, China; yvonneyang0803@gmail.com (Y.Y.); chenfangyi@xmu.edu.cn (F.C.); qiaokun@xmu.edu.cn (K.Q.); zhanghua0209@stu.xmu.edu.cn (H.Z.); hychen@xmu.edu.cn (H.-Y.C.)

[2] State-Province Joint Engineering Laboratory of Marine Bioproducts and Technology, College of Ocean and Earth Sciences, Xiamen University, Xiamen 361102, China

* Correspondence: wkjian@xmu.edu.cn

Abstract: Antimicrobial peptides (AMPs) identified in the reproductive system of animals have been widely studied for their antimicrobial activity, but only a few studies have focused on their physiological roles. Our previous studies have revealed the in vitro antimicrobial activity of two male gonadal AMPs, SCY2 and scyreprocin, from mud crab Scylla paramamosain. Their physiological functions, however, remain a mystery. In this study, the two AMPs were found co-localized on the sperm apical cap. Meanwhile, progesterone was confirmed to induce acrosome reaction (AR) of mud crab sperm in vitro, which intrigued us to explore the roles of the AMPs and progesterone in AR. Results showed that the specific antibody blockade of scyreprocin inhibited the progesterone-induced AR without affecting intracellular Ca^{2+} homeostasis, while the blockade of SCY2 hindered the influx of Ca^{2+}. We further showed that SCY2 could directly bind to Ca^{2+}. Moreover, progesterone failed to induce AR when either scyreprocin or SCY2 function was deprived. Taken together, scyreprocin and SCY2 played a dual role in reproductive immunity and sperm AR. To our knowledge, this is the first report on the direct involvement of AMPs in sperm AR, which would expand the current understanding of the roles of AMPs in reproduction.

Keywords: invertebrate; antimicrobial peptide (AMP); fertilization; sperm; acrosome reaction; progesterone; SCY2; scyreprocin

Citation: Yang, Y.; Chen, F.; Qiao, K.; Zhang, H.; Chen, H.-Y.; Wang, K.-J. Two Male-Specific Antimicrobial Peptides SCY2 and Scyreprocin as Crucial Molecules Participated in the Sperm Acrosome Reaction of Mud Crab *Scylla paramamosain*. *Int. J. Mol. Sci.* **2022**, *23*, 3373. https://doi.org/10.3390/ijms23063373

Academic Editor: Helena Felgueiras

Received: 27 February 2022
Accepted: 17 March 2022
Published: 21 March 2022

1. Introduction

Reproduction is a precisely regulated serial process in all animals, and the step that guarantees sperm–egg fusion is called acrosome reaction (AR) [1]. The sperm AR was first described in sea urchin by Dan [2]; afterwards, this profound structural change of sperm has been identified in many species. The acrosome, a specialized organelle located at the tip of the head of sperm, has been described in a diverse array of species, including Arthropoda (crabs, shrimps, etc.), Mollusca, Annelida, Echinoderma, Cephalochordata, Chordata, and some Vertebrata. In response to certain stimuli (hormones, alkaline environment, or physical contact with the egg envelope), the acrosome undergoes AR [2]. During AR, sperm experiences the protruding of the acrosome, exocytosis of the acrosome vesicle (AV) which releases factors that facilitate penetration of the vitelline coat, thus completing sperm–egg fusion. However, some taxa such as teleost fish have no sperm acrosome [3], whereas some species such as insects possess sperm acrosome but do not undergo AR to penetrate the egg coat [4].

The AR mechanism varies among different species due to their diverse gamete structures and sites of fertilization [5]. Sea urchin, a marine invertebrate executing external fertilization, has made a great contribution to our understanding of AR [6–8]. It is now clear that the AR of sea urchin is triggered by the binding of fucose homopolymers in egg jelly to its receptor (REJ-1) on sperm [9]. The AR-inducing substances (ARIS) differ among animal species, and progesterone (PG) is one of the common ARIS in different species. In situ study of mammalian sperm, AR is generally not feasible, and mouse sperm are often used as the model of choice. Cumulative data showed that the AR in mammalian sperm could be triggered by the alkaline environment in the female reproductive tract, zona pellucida, and directly activated by low molecular weight compounds such as PG [10–12]. In vitro investigations on the AR of human sperm also indicate that PG and neurotransmitters are necessary for AR [13,14]. It is widely accepted that AR requires Ca^{2+} influx [15] and the intracellular Ca^{2+} concentration ($\{Ca^{2+}\}_i$) is the most important factor regulating sperm activity and changes throughout all steps of sperm activity [16,17]. The sperm-specific ion channel, CatSper, was reported to be involved in PG sensation and Ca^{2+} influx during mammalian sperm AR [18,19]. The CatSper also contributes to the chemotaxis of sea urchin sperm [20] and is therefore considered to be a universal channel associated with sperm function. However, although a number of AR-associated molecules have been found in different species, most of them have not been clearly elucidated yet [21–23].

Mud crab, *Scylla paramamosain*, is a typical marine arthropod and an important economic aquatic species with high commercial value in southeast China and Asian countries. Mud crabs molt over 20 times in their lifetime. The last molt (reproductive molt) of the female crabs initiates the mating process and stimulates ovarian development including oogenesis. After mating, sperm are transferred into the female spermathecae where they stay for one or several months until eggs maturity and then released at ovulation to complete the sperm–egg fusion [24]. Mud crabs undergo internal fertilization and produce alflagellate sperm [25]. To our knowledge, some key AR-associated molecules such as CatSper have not been reported in mud crab and we also failed to identify it even after a sincere analysis of the mud crab genome. Thus, mud crab may have a different AR molecular basis due to the lack of certain key AR-associated components that have been identified in other species.

To date, a number of antimicrobial peptides (AMPs) have been identified in the male reproductive system in different species. These reproduction-associated AMPs are proved to participate in not only reproductive tract host defense but also other biological events such as sperm maturation [26,27] and sperm motility [28,29]. Although the AMPs identified in the reproductive system of marine animals have been widely studied for their antimicrobial activities, less is known about their potential functions in the reproductive process. SCY2 is a novel AMP identified from *S. paramamosain* in our previous study [30]. It is male specific and dominantly expressed in the ejaculatory duct (ED). During mating, SCY2 showed cross-gender transmission and was thought to exert reproductive immune functions [30]. Interestingly, the expression level of SCY2 is found significantly induced by PG, but not by lipopolysaccharides (LPS) [30]. Those previous results led us to presume whether SCY2 may not only exert antimicrobial activity but also have multiple functions in reproductive processes, especially in hormone-modulated post-mating events. Meanwhile, a novel SCY2-interacting protein, scyreprocin (MH488960), was revealed and proved to exert potent, broad-spectrum antibacterial, antifungal, and antibiofilm activities in vitro by multiple action modes [31]. Unexpectedly, recombinant products of SCY2 and scyreprocin showed no synergistic antimicrobial activity in vitro [31]. Considering both AMPs were dominantly expressed in the male reproductive system, whether their synergistic functions were reflected in other aspects of the reproduction processes as reported in other animals attracted us to explore their potential physiological roles in the present study.

In this work, the in vivo expression profiles of scyreprocin and SCY2 were investigated to confirm their roles in the reproductive immunity of mud crab. Interestingly, we found that both scyreprocin and SCY2 were also expressed in sperm, and their localizations were dynamically changed during the AR. To better understand sperm AR of mud crab, we used flow cytometry and Ca^{2+} fluorescent probes to investigate whether PG was one of the ARIS of crab sperm and to assess the change in $\{Ca^{2+}\}_i$ during AR. The potential functions of scyreprocin and SCY2 in AR were further explored by antibody blockade assays. In addition, the binding properties of scyreprocin and SCY2 to PG and Ca^{2+} were evaluated via functional experiments to further verify their roles in PG-induced AR.

2. Results

2.1. Expression Pattern of Scyreprocin and SCY2 In Vivo

Under natural conditions, the scyreprocin transcript was predominantly expressed in male gonads, with the highest expression level in testes, followed by anterior vas deferens, while relatively low expression was observed in female crabs, with the highest expression in ovaries (Figure 1A). High levels of scyreprocin protein expression were detected in gonads of adult male crabs, while no scyreprocin expression was detected in adult female crabs. (Figure 1B). In juvenile male crabs, scyreprocin was mainly expressed in spermatophores isolated from testes and seminal plasma isolated from ED (Figure 1C). In adult males, scyreprocin was detected in the spermatophore, and seminal plasma was collected from anterior vas deferens, seminal vesicle, ED, and posterior ejaculatory duct (Figure 1C). Detection of in situ expression indicated that scyreprocin was mainly expressed in spermatophores and epithelial cells of the testis, while SCY2 was expressed in interspaces between spermatophores in the testes of adult mud crabs (Figure 1D). Only weak signals of both proteins were detected in testicular sections of juvenile males (Figure 1D). Scyreprocin and SCY2 were not detected in spermathecae of pre-mating females. In post-mating females, scyreprocin and SCY2 signals were detected in the contents of spermathecae, moreover, strong SCY2 fluorescent signals were observed in epithelial cells (Figures 1E and S1).

2.2. Scyreprocin and SCY2 Responded to Bacterial Infection In Vivo

A primary testicular cell culture method was established in this study (Figure S2). Microbial growth occurred during the first two days in several samples of cultured testicular cells. The endogenous microbes were isolated and identified as *Pseudomonas putida* (Figure S3), which was an aquatic pathogen. The isolated endogenous bacteria *P. putida* isolate X1 was susceptible to recombinant SCY2 (rSCY2) and recombinant Scyreprocin (rScyreprocin) treatments (Table 1). Scanning electron microscopy (SEM) observation revealed significant morphological changes in the bacterial membrane induced by rSCY2 and rScyreprocin treatments (Figure 2A). After being challenged with the *P. putida* isolate X1, in vitro cultured spermatophores showed a significant increase in scyreprocin and SCY2 expression (Figure 2B). Expression levels of SCY2 and scyreprocin were induced in testes and EDs after in vivo challenge with *P. putida* isolate X1 (Figure 2C,D). These results showed that scyreprocin and SCY2 could effectively inhibit and kill the pathogenic bacteria of mud crab and had a positive in vivo response to pathogen infection, indicating their roles in reproductive immunity.

Table 1. Antimicrobial Activity of rScyreprocin, rSCY2 and rScyreprocin/rSCY2.

Microorganisms	rScyreprocin		rSCY2		rScyreprocin/rSCY2	
	MIC [a] (μM)	MBC [a] (μM)	MIC (μM)	MBC (μM)	MIC (μM)	MBC (μM)
Pseudomonas putida isolate X1	<0.5	2–4	6.25–12.5	>50	0.5–1	2–4

[a] MIC and MBC were presented as an interval [A]–[B]: [A] was the highest concentration tested with visible microbial growth, while [B] was determined as the lowest concentration without visible microbial growth (n = 3).

2.3. Subcellular Localization of Scyreprocin and SCY2 in Mud Crab Sperm

Spermatids at various spermiogenesis stages were observed in cultured testicular cells (Figure 3A). In the early proacrosomal granule phase, SCY2 and scyreprocin were co-localized in the cytoplasm. In the preacrosomal vesicle phase, the nucleus shape started to change and preacrosomal granules (PGs) aggregated to form a proacrosomal vesicle (PV). SCY2 and scyreprocin signals were detected on PGs and PV, but rarely co-localized. In the preacrosomal phase, the nucleus developed into a cup-like shape and enwrapped the PV. SCY2 was expressed on the outer edge of the PV, while scyreprocin was located in unaggregated PGs (Figure 3A). The two later spermiogenesis stages (acrosome phase and mature phase) were not observed in the in vitro cultured testicular cells in the present study.

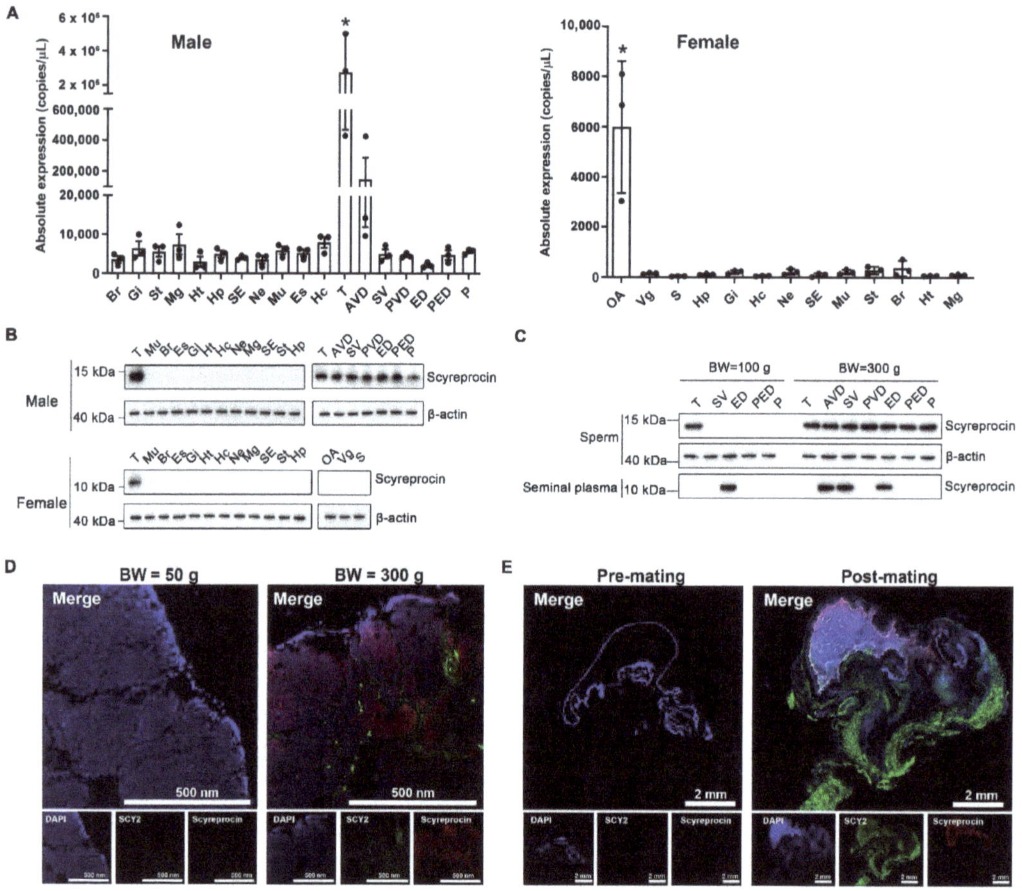

Figure 1. Scyreprocin and SCY2 expressed in reproductive system of adult male mud crabs and transferred to female spermathecae via mating. (**A**) Scyreprocin transcriptional expression level in adult male ($n = 3$) and female ($n = 3$) *Scylla paramamosain* under natural conditions. Data are presented as the mean ± standard deviation (SD). * $p < 0.05$, one-way analysis of variance (ANOVA) and Tukey post-test. (**B**) Scyreprocin expression profiles in different tissues of adult male and female crabs ($n = 3$). (**C**) Scyreprocin expression profiles in semen (sperm and seminal plasma) collected from adult and juvenile males ($n = 3$). BW, body weight. (**D**) In situ expression of SCY2 (green) and scyreprocin (red) in testes of juvenile and adult males. (**E**) In situ expression of SCY2 (green) and scyreprocin (red) in spermathecae of pre- and post-mating females. In panels (**D**,**E**), nucleus is shown in blue color. Abbreviations: Br, brain; Gi, gill; St, stomach; Mg, midgut; Ht, heart; Hp, hepatopancreas; SE, subcuticular epidermis; Ne, thoracic ganglion mass; Mu, muscle; Es, eyestalk; Hc, hemolymph cell; T, testis; AVD, anterior vas deferens; SV, seminal vesicle; PVD, posterior vas deferens; ED, ejaculatory duct; PED, posterior ejaculatory duct; P, penis; S, spermatheca; OA, ovary; Vg, vagina.

In mature sperm, organelle staining assays revealed that scyreprocin and SCY2 were co-localized in the endoplasmic reticulum (ER), Golgi apparatus, and mitochondria (Figure 3B). Transmission electron microscopy (TEM) observations yielded a refined image of scyreprocin and SCY2 localization in single sperm, where they showed co-localization in mitochondria, central tube, and apical cap (AC) (Figure 3C).

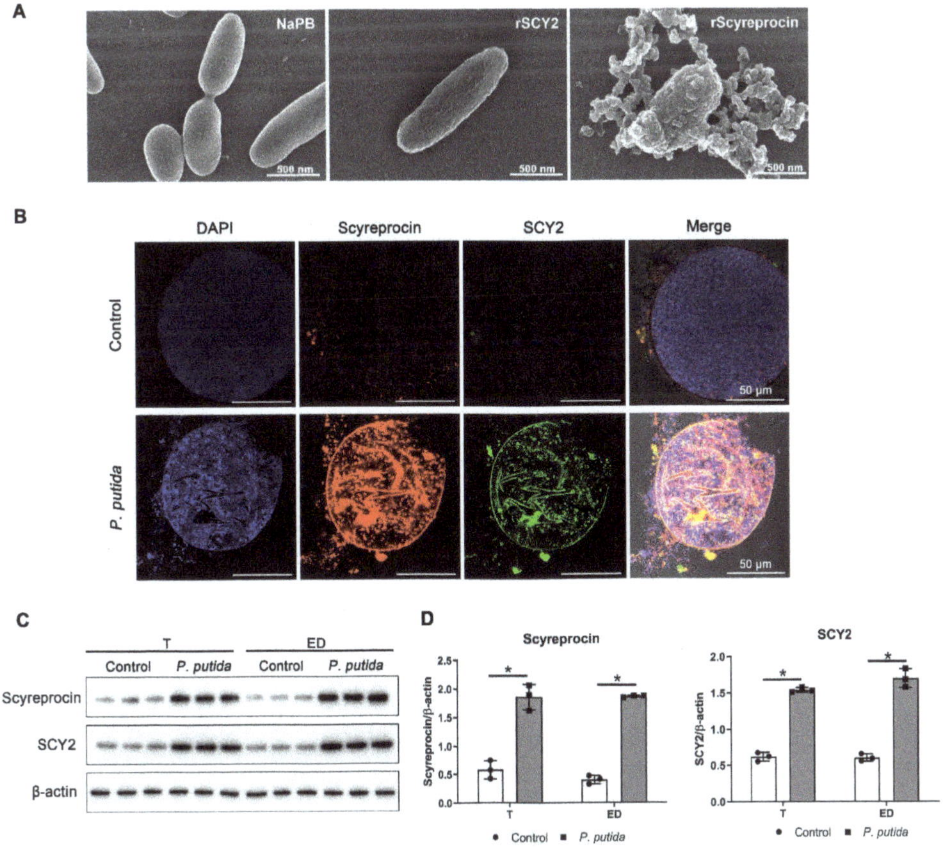

Figure 2. Scyreprocin and SCY2 responded to bacterial infections. (**A**) Morphological changes induced by recombinant scyreprocin (rScyreprocin) and SCY2 (rSCY2) in *Pseudomonas putida* isolate X1 (n = 3). *P. putida* isolate X1 (5 × 10^5 cfu mL^{-1}) was incubated with rScyreprocin (2 μM) or rSCY2 (4 μM) for 30 min and observed by a scanning electron microscopy. (**B**) Induction of SCY2 and scyreprocin expression levels in in vitro cultured spermatophores after *P. putida* isolate X1 challenge (n = 3). The in vitro cultured spermatophore were incubated with *P. putida* isolate X1 (100 cfu $well^{-1}$) for 24 h before subjected to immunofluorescence assay. (**C**) Induction of SCY2 and scyreprocin expression levels in testis (T) and ejaculatory duct (ED) by in vivo *P. putida* isolate X1 challenge (n = 3). Adult male crabs were challenged with *P. putida* isolate X1 (3 × 10^3 cfu $crab^{-1}$). After 24 h, T and ED were sampled and subjected to Western blot analysis. (**D**) Quantification of the blots in (**C**) by ImageJ. Data are presented as the mean ± standard deviation (SD). * $p < 0.05$, two-way analysis of variance (ANOVA) and Bonferroni post-test.

2.4. Progesterone Induced In Vitro Sperm Acrosome Reaction of *S. paramamosain*

To investigate the potential roles of SCY2 and scyreprocin in sperm AR, sperm collected from male gonad and female spermathecae were used for in vitro AR-induction tests (Figure 4A). When treated with artificial seawater containing 0.3% (w/v) Ca^{2+} (ASW), the AR ratio (%AR) increased significantly in sperm collected from spermathecae, whereas those collected from males showed no statistical difference compared to the control group

(Figure 4B,C). These results suggested that some components in spermathecae might be requisite for sperm AR.

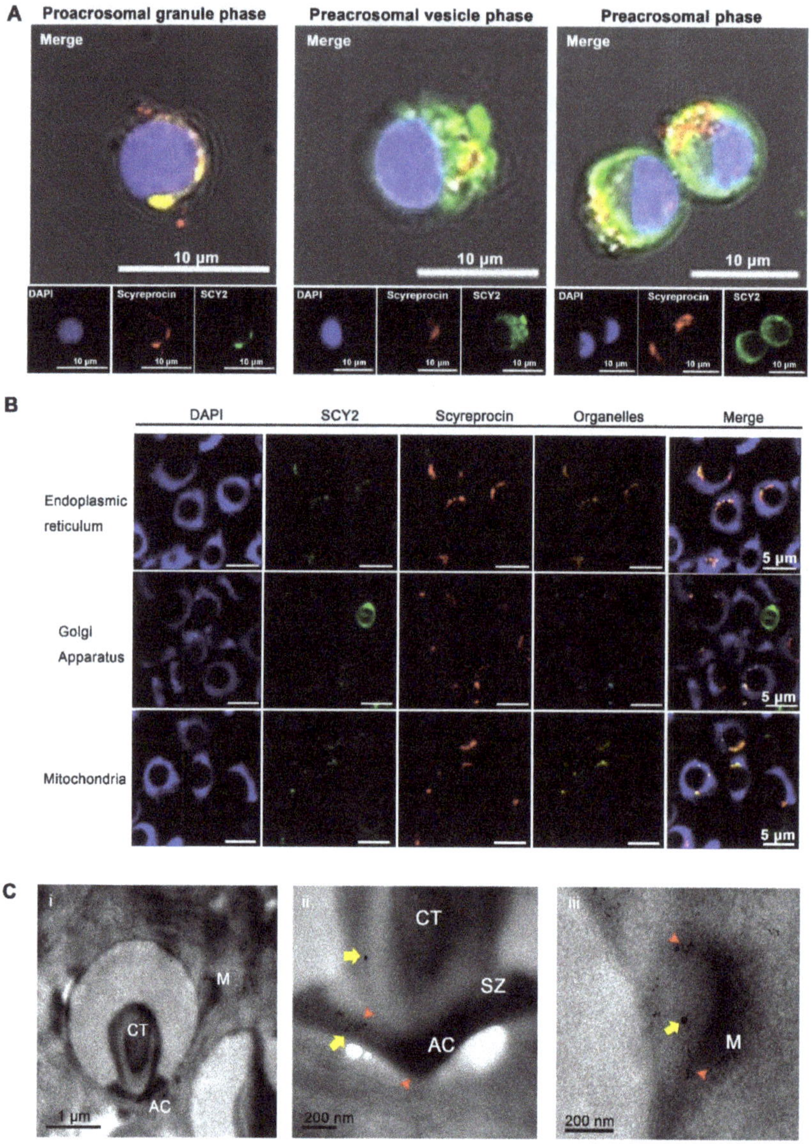

Figure 3. Subcellular location of scyreprocin and SCY2 in male gametes. (**A**) In situ expression of scyreprocin (red) and SCY2 (green) in spermatids at different spermiogenesis stages, nucleus was stained with DAPI (blue). In vitro cultured testicular cells (seeded at 2×10^6 cells well^{-1} for 3 days) were subjected to immunofluorescence assay. (**B**) SCY2 and scyreprocin co-localized with organelles in sperm. Sperm were freshly isolated from seminal vesicles of adult male crabs and subjected to immunofluorescence assay. (**C**) In situ expression of scyreprocin and SCY2 observed by transmission electron microscope (TEM) in mud crab sperm: i, intact sperm; ii, apical cap (AC); iii, mitochondria (M). Red arrows: scyreprocin; yellow arrows, SCY2. Abbreviations: SZ, sub-cap zone; CT, central tube.

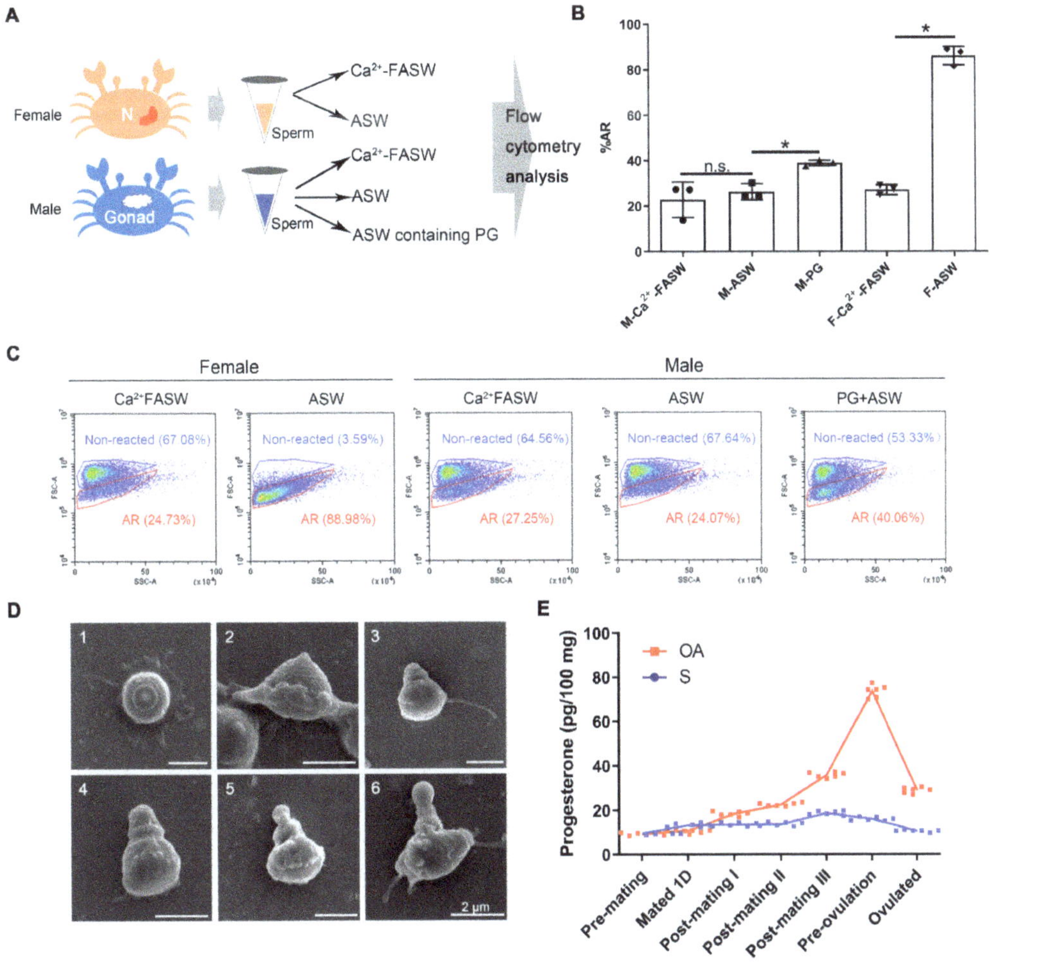

Figure 4. Progesterone (PG) was a crucial acrosome reaction (AR)-induced substance for crab sperm. (**A**) Schematic presentation of the AR ratio (%AR) evaluation on the sperm collected from male and female crabs. N, spermathecae; ASW, artificial seawater; Ca^{2+}-FASW, Ca^{2+}-free ASW. (**B**) Statistical analysis on %AR of sperm collected from female spermathecae and male gonads ($n = 3$). Data are presented as the mean ± standard deviation (SD). * $p < 0.05$, one-way analysis of variance (ANOVA) and Tukey post-test; n.s., not significant. M, male; F, female. (**C**) Flow cytometry assessment on %AR of sperm collected from female spermathecae and male gonads ($n = 3$). Sperm samples were treated with ASW, Ca^{2+}-FASW (male- and female-derived sperm), or ASW containing 20 µg mL^{-1} PG (male-derived sperm) for 24 h before subjected to flow cytometry analysis. (**D**) Ultrastructural changes of crab sperm during AR observed by scanning electron microscope (SEM). Male-derived sperm after PG treatment in (**C**) were subjected for SEM observation: 1–2, unreacted sperm; 3, acrosome protruding stage; 4, acrosomal vesicle valgus stage; 5, central tube extension stage; 6, reacted sperm. (**E**) Changes in PG level in spermatheca (S) and ovary (OA) at pre- and post-mating stages. Spermathecae and ovaries from un-mated females, female crabs at the day after mating, post-mating stage I, II, III, pre-ovulation, and post-ovulation stage, were collected ($n = 6$). The samples (~30 mg) were subjected to PG level analysis. Data are presented as the mean ± SD.

In a year-long investigation on SCY2 expression in male crabs, the highest transcriptional level of SCY2 was observed during mating seasons (May–July, October–December) (Figure S4) and the change in the SCY2 expression level is consistent with that of the hormones [30], indicating the correlation between PG and SCY2 expression levels. In post-mating female crabs, the PG level in the ovary increased during oogenesis, with the highest PG level occurring near ovarian maturation (pre-ovulation) (Figure 4E). Therefore, we further investigated whether PG could induce AR. Compared with the control group (mean $\pm$ SD = 22.76 $\pm$ 7.82%), the %AR of sperm collected from males was significantly induced by ASW containing PG (38.92 $\pm$ 1.22%) (Figure 4B,C), and sperm at different AR stages were observed by SEM (Figure 4D). The in vivo assay showed that sperm $\{Ca^{2+}\}_i$ increased significantly when males were directly injected with PG (Figure S5). These results indicated that PG could induce the AR of mud crab sperm, and $\{Ca^{2+}\}_i$ could be used as an indicator for mud crab sperm AR.

2.5. Localizations of SCY2 and Scyreprocin in Sperm during Sperm Acrosome Reaction

Sperm collected from spermathecae were treated with ASW to induce AR. Subcellular locations of SCY2 and scyreprocin were revealed by cellular immunofluorescence and immuno-colloidal gold technique. At AC protruding stage, SCY2 was detected in the AC, and scyreprocin was found in the cytoplasm. Scyreprocin was detected in the AV at the AV valgus stage and all the subsequent AR stages (Figure 5A). TEM observation showed that scyreprocin could be detected not only in AV but also in the acrosomal vesicle membrane and mitochondria (Figure 5B).

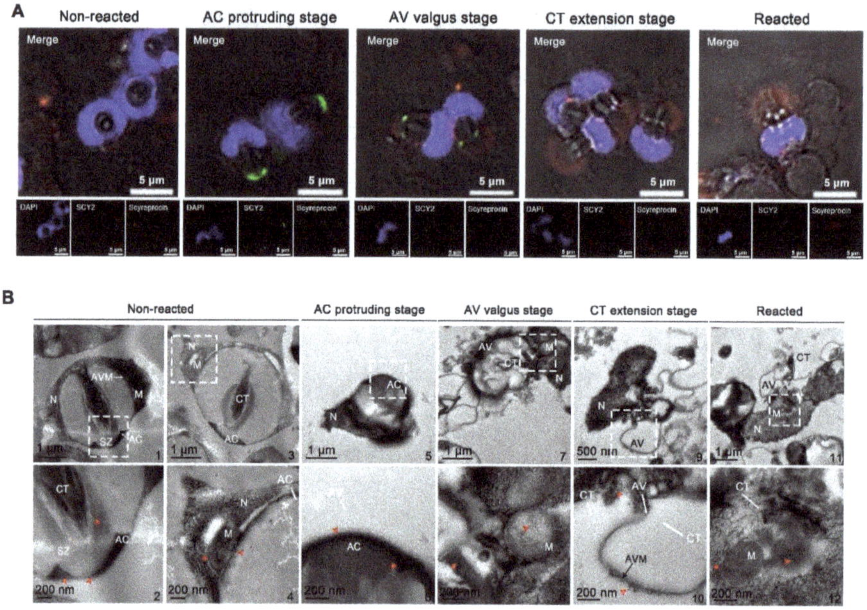

Figure 5. Expression pattern of scyreprocin and SCY2 in sperm during the acrosome reaction (AR). (**A**) Subcellular localization of scyreprocin and SCY2 in sperm at different AR stages (blue, nucleus; red, scyreprocin; green, SCY2). Male-derived sperm were treated with artificial seawater (ASW) containing 20 μg mL^{-1} PG for 24 h before subjected to immunofluorescence assay. (**B**) Subcellular localization of scyreprocin (red arrows) in sperm at different AR stages, from transmission electron microscopy (TEM) observation. Dashed lines indicate the zoom-in regions. Abbreviations: AC, apical cap; CT, central tube; M, mitochondria; SZ, sub-cap zone; AV, acrosomal vesicle; N, nucleus; AVM, acrosomal vesicle membrane.

2.6. SCY2 and Scyreprocin Participated in Progesterone-Induced Acrosome Reaction

To investigate the possible roles of SCY2 and scyreprocin in sperm AR, sperm (collected from males) were incubated with Ca^{2+}-free ASW (Ca^{2+}-FASW) containing SCY2 and/or scyreprocin antibodies and then treated with PG to induce AR. Samples were analyzed for the %AR and $\{Ca^{2+}\}_i$ (Figure 6A).

In the antibody control groups, sperm co-incubated with scyreprocin antibody showed no change in $\{Ca^{2+}\}_i$, while sperm treated with the SCY2 antibody showed a significant decrease in $\{Ca^{2+}\}_i$ (Figure 6B–D). Hence, scyreprocin and SCY2 played different roles in maintaining intracellular Ca^{2+} homeostasis.

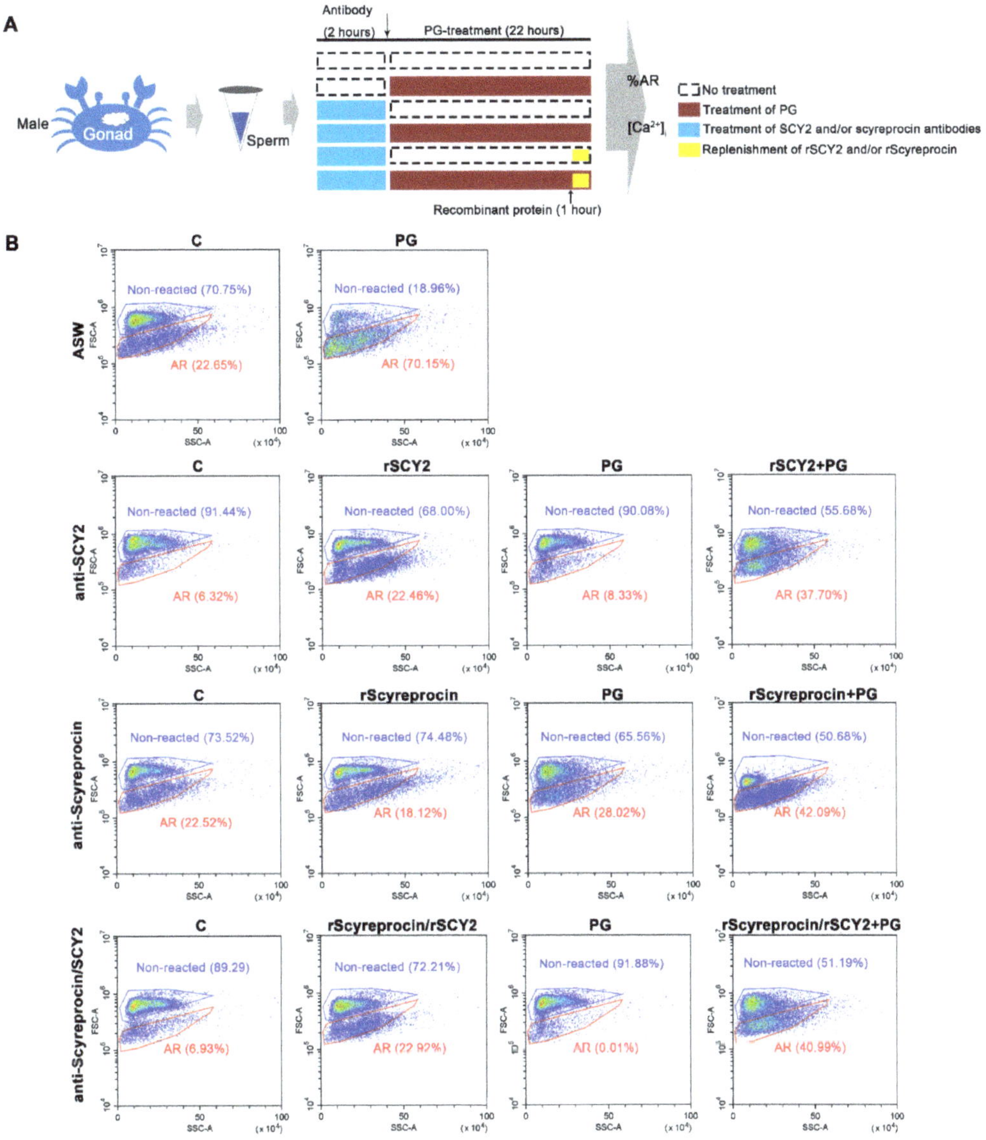

Figure 6. *Cont.*

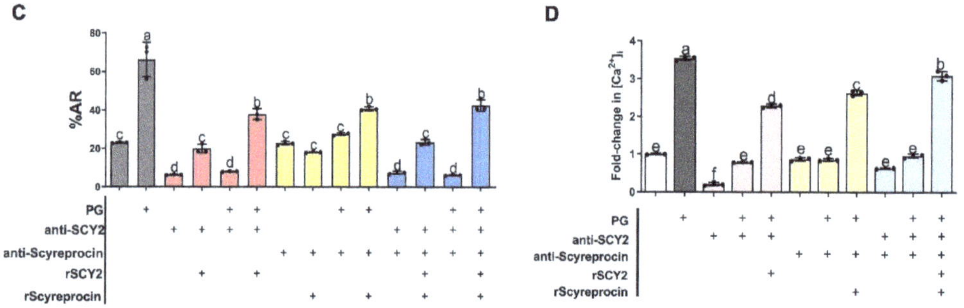

Figure 6. Scyreprocin and SCY2 functioned as critical molecules in progesterone (PG)-induced sperm acrosome reaction (AR). (**A**) Schematic presentation of the AR ratio (%AR) and intracellular Ca^{2+} concentration ($\{Ca^{2+}\}_i$) evaluation of the sperm collected from male and female crabs. (**B**) Flow cytometry analysis of the sperm %AR after different treatments. Male-derived sperm samples (~1×10^6 cells mL^{-1}) were pre-treated with SCY2 antibody (1:500) and/or scyreprocin antibody (1:1000) for 2 h and incubated with PG (50 μg mL^{-1} in artificial seawater) for 22 h. Samples were subjected to flow cytometry analysis. (**C**) Statistical analyses of the flow cytometry data presented in (**B**) (n = 3). Data are presented as the mean ± standard deviation (SD). (**D**) Evaluation of $\{Ca^{2+}\}_i$ in sperm samples in (**B**) (n = 3). In panels (**C**,**D**), "+" represents the addition of the corresponding component, data are presented as the mean ± SD. Letters denote significant differences, one-way analysis of variance (ANOVA), and Tukey post-test.

Progesterone significantly induced sperm AR (66.27 ± 8.88% reacted) after 22 h in comparison with the untreated control (23.00 ± 0.32% reacted) (Figure 6B,C), but it could not induce the AR of the sperm pretreated with either SCY2 antibody (8.13 ± 0.20% reacted) or scyreprocin antibody (27.64 ± 0.75% reacted) (Figure 6B,C). After replenishing recombinant proteins to the corresponding antibody-treated samples, both %AR and $\{Ca^{2+}\}_i$ were restored (Figure 6B–D). Although antibody blockade of scyreprocin did not affect the $\{Ca^{2+}\}_i$ of unreacted sperm, it did hinder PG from inducing sperm AR (Figure 6B–D). These results indicated that scyreprocin might act as an important mediator in initiating PG-induced AR. Similarly, PG could not trigger sperm AR when scyreprocin and SCY2 were inhibited simultaneously (6.34 ± 0.28% reacted). Later replenishment of both rScyreprocin and rSCY2 allowed the increase in %AR (42.66 ± 2.96% reacted) and $\{Ca^{2+}\}_i$ (Figure 6B–D). Besides, SCY1, the SCY2 homologous protein, showed different localization from SCY2 in sperm (Figure S6A) and had no detectable effect on the PG-induced $\{Ca^{2+}\}_i$ increase (Figure S6B).

2.7. Progesterone Binding Capacity of SCY2 and Scyreprocin

Progesterone has been shown to induce SCY2 expression in our previous study [30]. We performed a modified ELISA assay to further determine the interaction of PG with rSCY2 and rScyreprocin, respectively. Scatchard plot analysis showed that the PG-binding affinity of rScyreprocin/rSCY2 mixture (calculated equilibrium dissociation constant, K_D = 72.2 nM) was stronger than that of rScyreprocin (K_D = 258.9 nM) and rSCY2 (K_D = 143.0 nM) alone, thus indicating that the PG-binding affinity was enhanced in the presence of both proteins.

2.8. SCY2 was Involved in Calcium Influx during Acrosome Reaction

Antibody blockade of SCY2 resulted in a significant decrease in sperm $\{Ca^{2+}\}_i$ (Figure 6D). To investigate its possible functions, sperm were treated with the SCY2 antibody or Ni^{2+} (set up as a Ca^{2+} channel inhibition control group). The samples were analyzed for the $\{Ca^{2+}\}_i$ (Figure 7C) and %AR (Figure 7D,E).

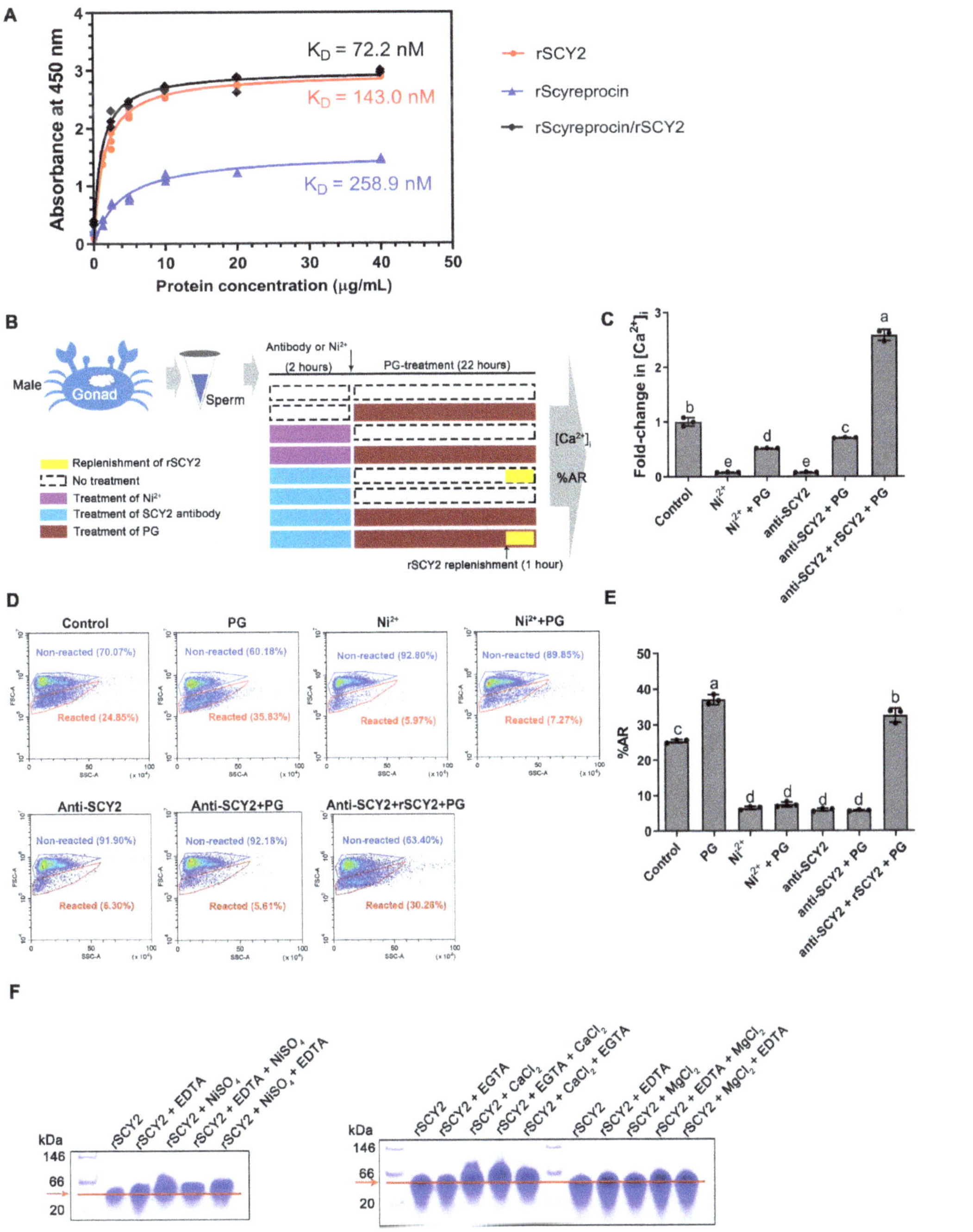

Figure 7. Interplay of scyreprocin, SCY2, progesterone (PG), and Ca^{2+}. (**A**) Comparative examination of PG binding capacity of rScyreprocin, rSCY2 and rScyreprocin/rSCY2 mixture by a modified enzyme-linked immunosorbent assay (ELISA) ($n = 3$). (**B**) Schematic presentation of the intracellular Ca^{2+} concentration ($[Ca^{2+}]_i$) evaluation and acrosome reaction ratio (%AR) analysis. (**C**) Evaluation of $[Ca^{2+}]_i$ in the sperm pretreated with SCY2 antibody or Ni^{2+} ($n = 3$). Sperm (2×10^7 sperm mL^{-1}) were

pre-treated with Ni^{2+} (5 μM) or SCY2 antibody (1:500) for 2 h, and incubated with PG (50 μg mL^{-1} in artificial seawater) for 22 h. Samples were subjected to $\{Ca^{2+}\}_i$ evaluation. (**D**) Flow cytometry analysis of the %AR (n = 3) of the samples in (**C**). (**E**) Statistical analysis of the data presented in (**D**). In panels C and E, data are presented as the mean ± SD. Letters denote significant differences, one-way ANOVA and Tukey post-test. (**F**) Electrophoretic mobility shift assays on the binding properties of rSCY2 with Ca^{2+}, Mg^{2+}, and Ni^{2+}. rSCY2 (2 μg) was incubated in Tris-HCl containing $CaCl_2$, $MgCl_2$, or $NiCl_2$ (0.1 mM) for 3 h and then supplemented with EGTA or EDTA (0.1 mM) for 10 min. Samples were subjected to native gel electrophoresis.

After SCY2 antibody treatment, the sperm $\{Ca^{2+}\}_i$ was markedly reduced to a level similar to that of the positive control (Ni^{2+}-treated group), and the Ca^{2+} influx induced by PG treatment was inhibited, suggesting the association between SCY2 and Ca^{2+} influx (Figure 7C). Similarly, flow cytometry analysis showed that treatments of Ni^{2+} and SCY2 antibody inhibited %AR of the sperm samples (Figure 7D,E). In the Ca^{2+}-dependent gel-shifting assay, an overt band-shift of rSCY2 was observed in the presence of $CaCl_2$, which was more distinct in the presence of both ethylene glycol tetraacetic acid (EGTA) and $CaCl_2$ (Figure 7F). It is worth noting that SCY2 showed no binding affinity to Mg^{2+} (Figure 7F).

3. Discussion

The mating behavior of marine animals provides an opportunity for pathogens in the aquatic environment to infect sperm and enter the female reproductive system. Crab sperm experience long-term storage (weeks to months) in the spermathecae before insemination [32], thus, bioactive molecules such as AMPs in the reproductive system are requisite for sperm health. As AMPs are highly expressed in male gonads, scyreprocin and SCY2 could efficiently inhibit the growth of aquatic pathogens such as the isolated *P. putida* strain X1 (Table 1). Both AMPs could be transferred to female spermathecae during mating and maintained in spermathecae until ovulation (Figure S1), thus it would be inferred that they may provide prolonged protection for the reproduction process of mud crab. Unlike other AMPs identified in mud crabs [31,33,34], rSCY2 only had moderate antimicrobial activity in vitro [30], and unexpectedly, showed no in vitro synergistic antimicrobial activity with rScyreprocin [31]. These findings prompt us to explore whether the interaction between SCY2 and Scyreprocin is reflected in other reproductive processes beyond reproductive immunity.

With numerous reproductive-associated AMPs being successively identified in the past decades, the fact that the male-specific AMPs, such as SCY2 and scyreprocin [30], are often highly expressed in the genital system during breeding seasons seems to raise a contradiction against reproduction-immunity trade-offs [35]. In recent years, AMPs have been shown to function beyond their antimicrobial activity during reproduction. The potential dual roles of β-defensins in the regulation of infection and control of sperm function is compelling [36]. Rat epididymis-specific β-defensin 15 plays a dual role in both sperm maturation and pathogen defense in rat epididymis [29]. Rat Bin1b is proved important for the acquisition of sperm motility and the initiation of sperm maturation [27]. Moreover, human cathelicidin 18 in seminal plasma is processed to generate a 38-amino acid AMP (ALL-38), transferred to the female reproductive tract, and enzymatically activated upon exposure to the vaginal milieu, preventing infection following sexual intercourse [37]. SCY2 shares similar cross-gender transmission patterns with ALL38 and its expression is regulated by PG but not LPS [30]. Therefore, we hypothesized that SCY2 may play an unrevealed role in hormone-regulated post-mating events in addition to its antimicrobial activity. In this study, we found that scyreprocin and SCY2 were presented not only in seminal plasma but also on the sperm apical cap (Figure 3) and were detected in the sperm apical cap (both AMPs) and acrosomal vesicle (scyreprocin) during PG-induced AR (Figure 5). These findings strongly support our prior presumption. We have confirmed that scyreprocin and SCY2 existing in seminal plasma provide anti-infection protection (Figure 2), but what are the potential biological functions of the AMPs located on sperm during AR?

Acrosome reaction, one of the hormone-associated sperm activities, is finely regulated by hormones, ion channels, and preassemble signal pathways [5,20,38,39]. It is now well known that in mammals and sea urchins, the sperm AR requires the collaboration of hormones (e.g., PG) and cationic channels (e.g., CatSper). In most species, egg water containing a variety of reproduction-related hormones is considered the main contributor to sperm activities [40]. PG is considered an important factor to endow sperm fecundity by initiating sperm capacitation (motility), hyperactivation, and AR [41,42]. Crab sperm is non-flagellated and thus lacks motility [25]. Researchers have tried to induce the AR of crab sperm isolated from the male reproductive system by means of ionic carriers and extracted infraspecific egg-water, but results were inconsistent among different crab species [24,43–47]. Therefore, it is still controversial as to what triggers the AR of crab sperm. In the present study, sperm isolated from spermathecae but not the sperm isolated from the male reproductive system could directly undergo AR after ASW treatment (Figure 4B,C), suggesting certain components in spermathecae were requisite for sperm AR. Consistent with previous reports [48], this study showed that the PG level of the female ovary gradually increased after mating and peaked before ovulation (Figure 4E). After PG treatment, sperm collected from males showed a significant increase in %AR (Figure 4B,C), suggesting that PG may be one of the ARIS for mud crab sperm.

PG induces AR through its membrane receptors on human sperm [1]. Screening of PG membrane receptors has been the focus of the study on the PG non-genomic effects. Some PG-binding proteins have been identified on the sperm membrane, among which CatSper and PAQR7 are thought to be the most promising candidates as PG receptors [18,49]. Since the AR-associated molecules (e.g., CatSper) have not been identified in mud crab, the molecular basis of PG-induced AR of mud crab remains unclarified. Although some AMPs have been proven to play vital roles in various sperm activities (e.g., sperm maturation and motility) [27–29], to our knowledge, there are no reports that they are directly involved in sperm AR in any animal species. Based on our findings, questions were then raised: is there a close relationship between SCY2, scyreprocin, PG, and PG-induced AR? Do SCY2 and scyreprocin exert a similar role in crab sperm AR as the AR-associated components in other species?

In this study, we found that antibody blockade of either scyreprocin or SCY2 led to failure in PG-induced AR and $\{Ca^{2+}\}_i$ increase. Notably, antibody blockade of SCY2, rather than scyreprocin, led to a significant decrease in sperm $\{Ca^{2+}\}_i$ before PG treatment at levels similar to those in the Ni^{2+}-treated group (Figure 7C). Later functional studies revealed the Ca^{2+}-binding capacity of rSCY2 (Figure 7F). These findings strongly implied that SCY2 was important for the maintenance of Ca^{2+} homeostasis in mud crab sperm and participated in the Ca^{2+} influx during AR. Based on these results, it could be inferred that SCY2 may be involved in the active Ca^{2+} transportation and is a key component of the Ca^{2+} channel in mud crab sperm. Thus, further genomic screening of scygonadin homologous proteins and structural analysis of SCY2 may shed light on its basis for Ca^{2+} selectivity and its actual role in Ca^{2+} regulation.

Although antibody blockade of scyreprocin had no effect on $\{Ca^{2+}\}_i$ before PG induction, it could not induce AR in the absence of scyreprocin (Figure 6D). It was inferred that scyreprocin may be involved in the process of sperm receiving progesterone signals. Later functional studies confirmed the PG binding capacity of rScyreprocin and rSCY2 (Figure 7A), indicating that PG could bind to scyreprocin on the sperm and subsequently initiate the SCY2-mediated Ca^{2+} influx. Previous research has shown that the calcium channel CatSper is also a non-genomic PG receptor of human sperm [50]. SCY2 and scyreprocin were a pair of interacting proteins. Whether the complexes they formed play a similar role in sperm AR as CatSper is worth further exploration.

Elevation of $\{Ca^{2+}\}_i$ during AR is caused not only by the influx of extracellular Ca^{2+} but also by the following Ca^{2+}-induced Ca^{2+} release (CICR); that is, the Ca^{2+} would further induce the release of Ca^{2+} from intracellular Ca^{2+} stores such as acrosome and mitochondria [17]. In the present study, we did not permeabilize the sperm before antibody treatments; therefore, only scyreprocin and SCY2 on the cell surface were inhibited. Scyreprocin and SCY2 on sperm AC assumed crucial roles in the initial influx of Ca^{2+}. Given that these two AMPs were also co-located with organelles in crab sperm (Figure 2), it remains to be investigated whether they would take part in the following CICR process.

During sperm AR, scyreprocin was seen in the AV (Figure 5A). The acrosomal vesicle is known to contain a variety of enzymes that dissolve the oolemma and assist in successful sperm–egg fusion [51]. Our preliminary experiments indicated that rScyreprocin exerted acid phosphatase and superoxide dismutase activity (54.84 U $gprot^{-1}$ and 118.12 U $mgprot^{-1}$, respectively). More studies are required to verify if scyreprocin in the AV exerts a similar function. During the mating season, male crabs expressed a synchronous increase in SCY2 in parallel with elevated PG levels [30]. Similarly, a significant increase in the SCY2 fluorescent signal was detected in the spermathecal epithelium after mating (Figure 1E). In a prior study on spermatophore transplantation, it was found that spermatophores could be absorbed into the spermathecal epithelium by endocytosis, and thus some spermatophore degradation products could enter the vessel lumen and further modulate female reproductive behavior [52]. It remains to be determined whether SCY2 detected in the spermathecal epithelium was a result of spermatophore degradation absorption or in situ expression. The origin and other possible physiological functions of SCY2 in the spermathecal epithelium thus also need further investigation.

4. Materials and Methods

4.1. Animals

Mud crab (*S. paramamosain*) were obtained from the Xiamen aquatic products market, Fujian, China. Crabs were acclimated in cement tanks containing seawater for 1–2 days before experiments. Before sampling, mud crabs were anesthetized by ice-bathing for 15 min and all efforts were made to minimize suffering. All animal experiments were carried out in strict accordance with the National Institute of Health Guidelines for the Care and Use of Laboratory Animals and were approved by the Animal Welfare and Ethics Committee of Xiamen University.

4.2. Isolation of Spermatophores and Seminal Plasma

Semen was divided into seminal plasma and spermatophores following the prior descriptions [53]. Spermatophores were treated with 0.25% trypsin (prepared in Ca^{2+}-FASW) to obtain single sperm. Seminal plasma was stored at −20 °C and sperm were stored at 4 °C before use.

4.3. Preparation of Recombinant Proteins and Polycolonal Antibodies

Recombinant His-tagged scyreprocin (rScyreprocin) and SCY2 (rSCY2) were generated following prior descriptions [31,54]. Purified proteins were dialyzed, concentrated, and stored in 50 mM phosphate buffer (PB, pH 8.0) at −80 °C. Protein concentration was determined by the Bradford assay [55]. The scyreprocin antibody and SCY2 antibody were prepared as previously described [30,31].

4.4. Quantitative PCR

To investigate the expression profile of scyreprocin transcripts, tissues from three adult males and three adult females (300 ± 20 g in weight) were sampled. Tissues were flash-frozen in liquid nitrogen and stored at −80 °C. Total RNA and protein of each tissue (30 mg) were extracted by the Tripure reagent (Roche, Mannheim, Germany) following the manufacturer's instruction. Real-time quantitative PCR (RT-qPCR) was performed on a Roto-Gene Q platform (QIAGEN, Hilden, Germany) using the SYBR Green assay

(Roche, Mannheim, Germany). The primer sequences are listed in Table S1. Absolute qPCR was carried out to evaluate the expression profile of scyreprocin in different tissues of healthy adult male and female crabs ($n = 3$) as previously described [56]. For relative qPCR, the target gene Scyreprocin (GenBank Accession No. MH488960) was detected, and the Sp-β-actin (GenBank Accession No. GU992421) was chosen as the reference gene. Data were analyzed using the algorithm of the $2^{-\Delta\Delta Ct}$ method [57].

4.5. Antimicrobial Assays

The antimicrobial activity of the rScyreprocin, rSCY2, and rSCY2/rScyreprocin isomolar concentration mixture (e.g., the 1 μM mixture was composed of 1 μM rSCY2 and 1 μM rScyreprocin) against the isolated endogenous bacteria was evaluated. The MIC and MBC values were determined in triplicate on separate occasions following the prior descriptions [54]. After 30 min-treatment with rScyreprocin (2 μM) or rSCY2 (4 μM), the morphological changes of the isolated endogenous bacteria were observed using a Zeiss Supra™ 55 Scanning Electron Microscope (Carl Zeiss Microscopy GmbH, Oberkochen, Germany) as described earlier [31,58]. Experiments were performed three times on different occasions.

4.6. Western Blotting

To study the expression profile of scyreprocin, total proteins extracted from the tissues of adult male and female crabs ($n = 3$) were submitted to the Tricine-SDS-PAGE assay and transferred to a polyvinylidene difluoride (PVDF) membrane (Amersham, Sunnyvale, CA, USA). Immune detection of Sp-β-actin and scyreprocin was carried out using β-actin antibody (Santa Cruz Biotechnology, Santa Cruz, CA, USA) and scyreprocin antibody (dilution factors = 1:1000) following the standard Western blotting procedures. To evaluate expression level of scyreprocin in semen, seminal plasma and spermatophores were isolated from adult (300 ± 10 g) and juvenile male crabs (100 ± 10 g). Total protein extracted from spermatophores and 5 μg seminal plasma protein ($n = 3$) were detected for scyreprocin expression as described above. To investigate the expression profile of scyreprocin and SCY2 after bacterial infection, *P. putida* isolate X1 was injected into adult male crabs (250 ± 10 g) at 3×10^3 cfu crab^{-1}. Crab saline injections were performed as controls ($n = 3$). After 24 h, testes and ED samples ($n = 3$) were subjected for scyreprocin and SCY2 detection, and blots were quantified and analyzed using ImageJ (National Institutes of Health, Bethesda, MD, USA).

4.7. Immunofluorescence Assay

To explore the in situ expression profile of scyreprocin and SCY2, testes of juvenile (50 ± 10 g) and adult males (300 ± 10 g), spermathecae of female crabs on the day after mating, post-mating stage I, post-mating stage II, post-mating stage III, pre-ovulation stage were collected and sectioned (8–10 μm) for immunofluorescence assay. To investigate the in situ expression of scyreprocin and SCY2 in male gametes, in vitro-cultured testicular cells (seeded at 2×10^6 cells well^{-1} for 3 days, Text S1) and sperm isolated from male crabs (250 ± 10 g) were fixed with 4% paraformaldehyde (prepared in crab saline), permeabilized with 0.1% Triton X-100. To study the expression of scyreprocin and SCY2 after bacterial infection, the in vitro cultured spermatophore were incubated with *P. putida* isolate X1 (100 cfu well^{-1}) for 24 h before being subjected to immunofluorescence assay. Immunofluorescence assay was carried out based on a prior description [30]. Briefly, samples were blocked with 5% bovine serum albumin (BSA), incubated with a mixture containing SCY2 and scyreprocin antibodies (1:400) or unimmunized serum (1:100) for 4 h at 37 °C in a humidified chamber. After washing with phosphate-buffered saline (PBS, pH 7.4), samples were incubated with Dylight 488 conjugated goat anti-mouse IgG and Dylight 650 conjugated goat anti-rabbit IgG secondary antibodies (1:1000) (Thermo Fisher Scientific, Waltham, MA, USA) for 1 h. Slides were mounted with coverslips using Vectashield®

antifade mounting medium with DAPI (Vector Labs, Burlingame, CA, USA), and observed by a confocal laser scanning microscope (Zeiss Lsm 780 NLO; Carl Zeiss, Jena, Germany).

4.8. Hormone Level Examination

In every month of the year 2012, EDs from 3 crabs (300 $\pm$ 20 g) were tested for PG, testosterone, and estradiol levels using ELISA kits (Cayman Chemical Company, Ann Arbor, MI, USA). Tissues (~50 mg) were ground in liquid nitrogen and mixed with 1 mL of ELISA buffer (Cayman Chemical Company, Ann Arbor, MI, USA); supernatants were subjected to ELISA following the manufacturer's instructions. Analyses were carried out in duplicate. For evaluation of PG level in pre- and post-mating females, spermathecae and ovaries from un-mated females, female crabs at the day after mating, post-mating stage I, II, III, pre-ovulation, and post-ovulation stage, were collected (n = 6). The samples (~30 mg) were analyzed as described above.

4.9. Enzyme-Linked Immunosorbent Assay

To test if rSCY2, rScyreprocin, and/or rSCY2/rScyreprocin could bind to PG (Sigma-Aldrich, St. Louis, MO, USA), a modified ELISA assay was performed following a prior description [31]. Briefly, a flat bottom 96-well ELISA plate was coated with PG (3 μg), blocked with 5% BSA, and incubated with serial dilutions of rScyreprocin, rSCY2, and rSCY2/rScyreprocin (0–24 μM, 100 μL well^{-1}). After washing with PBS (50 mM, pH 7.4), plates were incubated with 100 μL mixture containing scyreprocin antibody (1:2000) and SCY2 antibody (1:1000) for 2 h before incubating with a mixture of HRP-labeled goat anti-rabbit IgG and HRP-labeled goat anti-mouse IgG (1:5000) for 1 h. After the colorimetric reaction, absorbance at 450 nm was measured using a multifunctional microplate reader (TECAN GENios; Tecan Group Ltd., Männedorf, Switzerland). The assays were carried out in triplicate and the results were analyzed using Scatchard plot analysis.

4.10. Transmission Electron Microscopy (TEM) Observation

Sperm freshly collected from mature male crabs (250 $\pm$ 10 g) were fixed in 4% paraformaldehyde. For TEM observation, samples were subjected to ultrathin sections and negative stained following standard protocols before being observed by a transmission electron microscope (FEI, Tecnai G2 F20, Eindhoven, the Netherlands) [59]. For the immunocolloidal gold assay, ultrathin sections were blocked with 5% BSA (prepared in PBS, pH 7.4) for 30 min and incubated overnight with a mixture of scyreprocin antibody (1:100) and SCY2 antibody (1:50) at 4 °C. The scyreprocin antibody was recognized by the specific secondary antibody coupled with 6 nm of colloidal gold (Electron Microscopy Sciences, Ft. Washington, PA, USA), and the SCY2 antibody was revealed with a 25 nm colloidal gold-coupled secondary antibody (Electron Microscopy Sciences, Ft. Washington, PA, USA). Sections were post-fixed with 4% paraformaldehyde, negative stained, and subjected for TEM observation.

4.11. SCY2-Calcium Binding Property

A modified electrophoretic mobility shift assay (EMSA) was used to investigate the Ca^{2+} binding property of SCY2. rSCY2 (2 μg) and rSCY2 incubated in Tris-HCl (10 mM, pH 7.5) containing EGTA (0.1 mM) at room temperature for 3 h, were set up as blank and experimental controls, respectively. Samples of (1) rSCY2 incubated in Tris-HCl containing $CaCl_2$ (0.1 mM) for 3 h, (2) rSCY2 first incubated with $CaCl_2$ (0.1 mM) for 3 h and then supplemented with EGTA (final concentration = 0.1 mM) for 10 min, and (3) an experimental group designed in reverse order were subjected to native gel electrophoresis. Similar assays using (1) Mg^{2+} and EDTA, and (2) Ni^{2+} and EDTA were carried out as described above.

4.12. Evaluation of Sperm Intracellular Calcium Concentration and Acrosome Reaction Ratio

Methods were developed in the present study to assess the sperm %AR and $\{Ca^{2+}\}_i$. A modified method based on flow cytometry was set up to analyze %AR. Sperm samples were analyzed using a CytoFLEX LX (Beckman Coulter Inc., Brea, CA, USA) and data were acquired with CytExpert software (Version 2.0). Samples were stained with DAPI (Thermo Fisher Scientific) and events with DAPI fluorescence were gated as intact sperm (valid counted events). The number of events was set to 8000 and recorded. The recorded sperm population was divided into two non-overlapping sub-populations representing acrosome-reacted and non-reacted sperm. For $\{Ca^{2+}\}_i$ evaluation, sperm samples were loaded with Fluo-4/AM following the manufacturer's instruction, and fluorescence intensity was measured using a microplate reader (TECAN GENios; Tecan Group Ltd.).

4.13. *In Vitro AR Induction*

Sperm were freshly collected and randomly divided into aliquots. To investigate the difference in %AR between sperm samples (2×10^7 sperm mL^{-1}) collected from male gonads (n = 3) and female spermathecae (n = 3), (1) control groups (male- and female-derived sperm suspended in Ca^{2+}-FASW for 24 h), (2) ASW groups (male- and female-derived sperm suspended in ASW for 24 h), and (3) PG-treatment groups (male-derived sperm suspended in ASW containing 20 μg mL^{-1} PG for 24 h) were analyzed for %AR and $\{Ca^{2+}\}_i$ as described before. Male-derived sperm after PG treatment were subjected for SEM observation following prior description [58].

4.14. *Antibody Blockade Assay*

Sperm were collected from male gonads, washed in Ca^{2+}-FASW, randomly divided into aliquots, and used to study the functions of scyreprocin and SCY2 in the AR process. To explore the possible role of SCY2 in Ca^{2+} influx during PG-induced AR, Ni^{2+} (final concentration = 5 μM) was applied as a Ca^{2+} channel inhibitor. Sperm (from 3 crabs) were adjusted to 2×10^7 sperm mL^{-1} and experimental groups were set up as follows: (1) non-treatment control group (sperm incubated in ASW for 24 h), (2) positive control group (sperm treated with Ni^{2+} for 2 h then incubated in ASW for 22 h), (3) positive PG-treated group (sperm treated with Ni^{2+} for 2 h then incubated in ASW containing 50 μg mL^{-1} PG for 22 h), (4) SCY2-blocked group (sperm treated with SCY2 antibody for 2 h then incubated in ASW containing 50 μg mL^{-1} PG for 22 h), and (5) SCY2-blocked PG-treated group (sperm treated with the SCY2 antibody for 2 h then incubated in ASW containing 50 μg mL^{-1} PG for 22 h). The dilution factor of the SCY2 antibody applied was 1:500 (Text S1). Samples were analyzed for %AR and $\{Ca^{2+}\}_i$ as described previously.

To investigate the involvement of scyreprocin and SCY2 during AR, sperm (~1×10^6 cells mL^{-1} in Ca^{2+}-FASW) were treated with scyreprocin antibody (1:1000), SCY2 antibody (1:500), and scyreprocin (1:1000)/SCY2 (1:500) antibody mixture for 2 h, respectively, before PG treatment (50 μg mL^{-1} in ASW) for 22 h. Optimization of antibody concentration was confirmed by a preliminary study (Figure S7). Samples were subjected to $\{Ca^{2+}\}_i$ and %AR elevation. To confirm the physiological function of SCY2 and scyreprocin, the corresponding protein (4 μM) was replenished at 1 h before %AR and $\{Ca^{2+}\}_i$ evaluation.

4.15. *Statistical Analysis*

Statistical analyses were performed using IBM SPSS statistics (Version 22; IBM Corp., Armonk, NY, USA) and GraphPad Prism software (version 5.01; GraphPad Software Inc., San Diego, CA, USA). One-way analysis of variance (ANOVA) followed by Tukey post-test were used to compare the scyreprocin expression profile in different tissues of *S. paramamosain* and the levels of %AR and $\{Ca^{2+}\}_i$ of sperm samples after different treatments. Two-way ANOVA followed by Bonferroni post-test was performed to analyze the changes in scyreprocin and SCY2 in vivo expression levels before and after bacterial infection. Significant levels were accepted at $p < 0.05$.

5. Conclusions

The present study revealed that two male gonadal AMPs play a dual role in both reproductive immunity and PG-induced AR of mud crab *S. paramamosain* (Figure 8). Adult male crabs expressed SCY2 and scyreprocin in sperm and seminal plasma. The AMPs exerted their antimicrobial activity to provide anti-infection protection during reproduction. In post-mating females, PG level increased, reaching a peak value before ovulation, and inducing sperm AR upon sperm–egg attachment. Scyreprocin and SCY2 expressed on sperm directly participated in PG-induced AR. During the process, PG bound to scyreprocin and then triggered SCY2-mediated Ca^{2+} influx. The increase in $\{Ca^{2+}\}_i$ led to the AR and ultimately sperm–egg fusion. It was worth noting that PG failed to induce AR when either scyreprocin or SCY2 function was absent. Although the detailed functions of scyreprocin and SCY2 in sperm AR remain to be elucidated, the observed dual effect of scyreprocin and SCY2 attest to the importance of the reproduction-associated AMPs in *S. paramamosain*. Thus, a particular protein may exert distinct functions alone and/or with the assistance of its interacting partners under different physiological stages and at different action sites. This reproductive strategy of mud crabs may have evolved over millions of years to cope with their complex habitat. At present, there is a very limited understanding of the mechanism for crab sperm action, and the results of this study indicate that it may differ from that in well-studied mammals, sea urchins, and amphibians (Figure 9). Due to technical obstacles, we are currently unable to perform direct functional verification by constructing scyreprocin- or SCY2-deficient crabs. However, the suggestion that AMPs, beyond their antimicrobial activity, may participate in post-mating sperm activation may shed new light on the intricate interplay between immunity and reproduction. Moreover, given that AMP expression is under endocrine regulation and controls the breeding process in mammals, birds, and invertebrates [60,61], the results of the present study will be relevant for future studies on how reproductive hormones control the tradeoffs between reproduction and immunity.

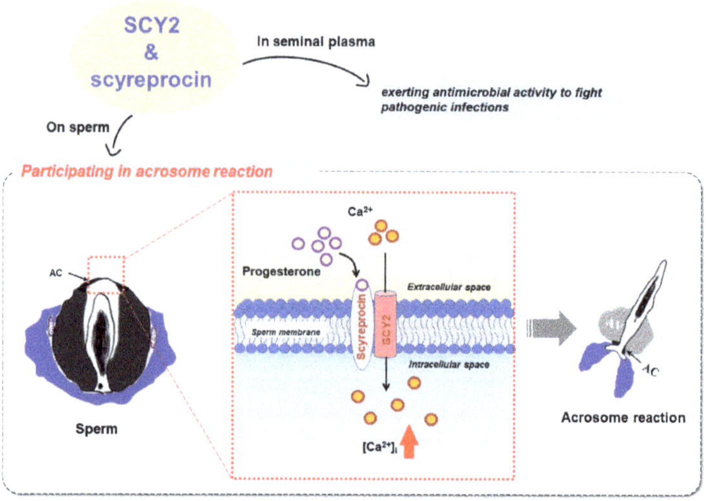

Figure 8. Roles of scyreprocin and SCY2 in the sperm acrosome reaction (AR) of *Scylla paramamosain*. Adult male crabs expressed scyreprocin and SCY2 in semen, which were then transferred to female spermatheca via mating. Scyreprocin and SCY2 in seminal plasma were proved to maintain gamete health by exerting antimicrobial activity. In sperm, scyreprocin and SCY2 showed co-localization on the apical cap and mitochondria, and are proven to participate in the initiation of progesterone-induced AR. In un-reacted sperm, SCY2 was responsible for maintaining intracellular Ca^{2+} homeostasis. Upon sperm–egg attachment, scyreprocin bound to progesterone, with SCY2 cooperatively strengthening the binding affinity. SCY2 bound to extracellular Ca^{2+} and transported it into the sperm. The increase in $\{Ca^{2+}\}_i$ ultimately initiated AR and allowed completion of sperm–egg fusion. Abbreviations: AC, apical cap; AV, acrosomal vesicle; $\{Ca^{2+}\}_i$, intracellular Ca^{2+} concentration.

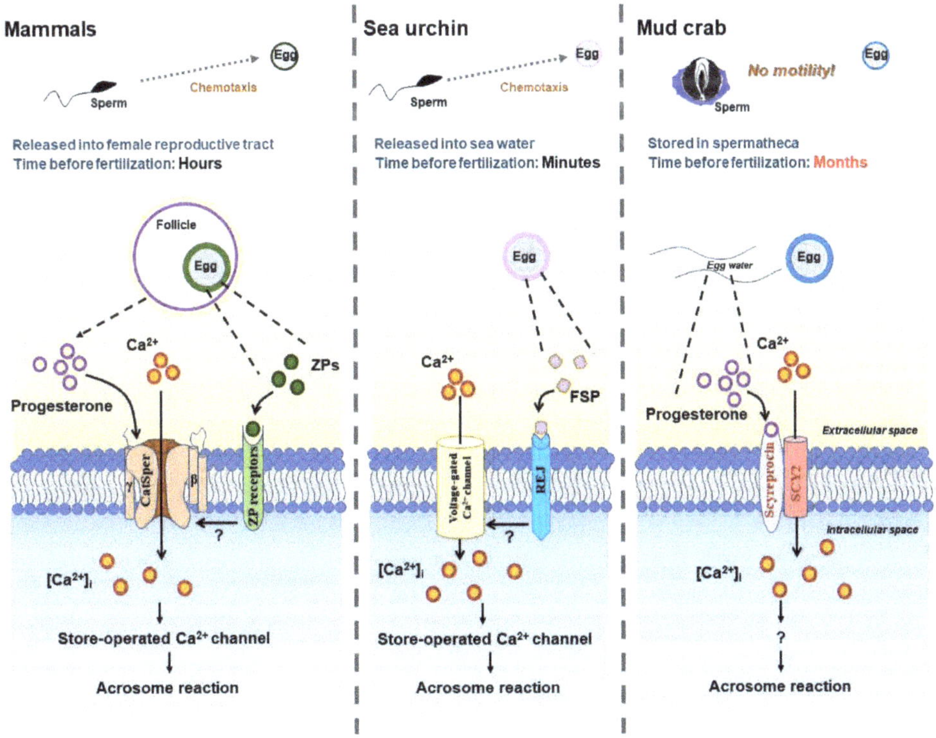

Figure 9. Brief comparison of sperm acrosome reaction (AR) mechanism in mammals, sea urchin, and mud crab. In mammals, progesterone and egg zona pellucida proteins (ZPs) interact with their corresponding receptors (i.e., CatSper, ZP receptors) on the sperm membrane, activate CatSper, and induce Ca^{2+} influx. Increase in intracellular Ca^{2+} concentration ($\{Ca^{2+}\}_i$) then leads to the release of Ca^{2+} from intracellular Ca^{2+} store, and thus completes sperm AR. In sea urchins, sperm AR is induced by the interaction of fucose sulfated glycoconjugate from egg-coat (FSG) and its specific receptor (REJ) on the sperm membrane, which opens a Ca^{2+}-selective channel and a store-operated Ca^{2+} channel and leads to vesicular fusion. In mud crab, progesterone interacts with scyreprocin on the sperm surface, thus inducing Ca^{2+} influx mediated by SCY2 and initiating sperm AR. The AR molecular basis of mud crab *Scylla paramamosain* revealed in the present study is different from that of other species.

Supplementary Materials: The following supporting information can be downloaded at: https://www.mdpi.com/article/10.3390/ijms23063373/s1. (References [30,54,56] are cited in the supplementary materials).

Author Contributions: Conceptualization, K.-J.W. and Y.Y.; methodology, Y.Y.; software, Y.Y. and H.-Y.C.; validation, Y.Y., K.Q., H.-Y.C. and F.C.; formal analysis, Y.Y. and K.Q.; investigation, Y.Y. and H.Z.; writing—original draft preparation, Y.Y.; writing—review and editing, K.-J.W. and F.C.; supervision, project administration and funding acquisition, K.-J.W. All authors have read and agreed to the published version of the manuscript.

Funding: This research was funded by the National Natural Science Foundation of China (grant number 41676158), the Fundamental Research Funds from Central Universities (grant number 20720190109), Fujian Marine Economic Development Subsidy Fund Project from the Fujian Ocean and Fisheries Department (grant number FJHJF-L-2019-1) and the Xiamen Science and Technology Planning Project (grant number 3502Z20203012).

Institutional Review Board Statement: All animal experiments were carried out in strict accordance with the National Institute of Health Guidelines for the Care and Use of Laboratory Animals and were approved by the Animal Welfare and Ethics Committee of Xiamen University.

Informed Consent Statement: Not applicable.

Data Availability Statement: Not applicable.

Acknowledgments: We thank Hua Hao, Hui Peng and Zhi-yong Lin for their help in the preparation of recombinant proteins, and V. Monica Bricelj, for her help in editing of the manuscript.

Conflicts of Interest: The authors declare no conflict of interest.

References

1. Stival, C.; Puga Molina, L.D.C.; Paudel, B.; Buffone, M.; Visconti, P.; Krapf, D. Sperm capacitation and acrosome reaction in mammalian sperm. *Sperm Acrosome Biog. Funct. Dur. Fertil.* **2016**, *220*, 93–106.
2. Dan, J.C. Studies on the acrosome. I. Reaction to egg-water and other stimuli. *Biol. Bull.* **1952**, *103*, 54–66. [CrossRef]
3. Ryuzo, Y.; Gary, C.; Takahiro, M.; Tadashi, A.; Tatsuo, H.; Carol, V.; Murali, P.; Frederick, G.; Hajime, M.; Tina, W. Sperm attractant in the micropyle region of fish and insect eggs. *Biol. Reprod.* **2013**, *88*, 47. [CrossRef]
4. Wilson, K.L.; Fitch, K.R.; Bafus, B.T.; Wakimoto, B.T. Sperm plasma membrane breakdown during Drosophila fertilization requires sneaky, an acrosomal membrane protein. *Development* **2006**, *133*, 4871–4879. [CrossRef]
5. Hirohashi, N.; Yanagimachi, R. Sperm acrosome reaction: Its site and role in fertilization. *Biol. Reprod.* **2018**, *99*, 127–133. [CrossRef]
6. Schackmann, R.W.; Christen, R.; Shapiro, B.M. Membrane potential depolarization and increased intracellular pH accompany the acrosome reaction of sea urchin sperm. *Proc. Natl. Acad. Sci. USA* **1981**, *78*, 6066–6070. [CrossRef]
7. Chang, M.C.; Berkery, D.; Schuel, R.; Laychock, S.G.; Zimmerman, A.M.; Zimmerman, S.; Schuel, H. Evidence for a cannabinoid receptor in sea urchin sperm and its role in blockade of the acrosome reaction. *Mol. Reprod. Dev.* **1993**, *36*, 507–516. [CrossRef]
8. Vacquier, V.D.; Swanson, W.J.; Hellberg, M.E. What have we learned about sea urchin sperm bindin? *Dev. Growth Differ.* **2003**, *37*, 1–10. [CrossRef]
9. Vacquier, V.D.; Moy, G.W. The fucose sulfate polymer of egg jelly binds to sperm REJ and is the inducer of the sea urchin sperm acrosome reaction. *Dev. Biol.* **1997**, *192*, 125–135. [CrossRef]
10. Bleil, J.D.; Wassarman, P.M. Mammalian sperm-egg interaction: Identification of a glycoprotein in mouse egg zonae pellucidae possessing receptor activity for sperm. *Cell* **1980**, *20*, 873–882. [CrossRef]
11. Murphy, S.J.; Yanagimachi, R. The pH dependence of motility and the acrosome reaction of guinea pig spermatozoa. *Mol. Reprod. Dev.* **1984**, *10*, 1–8. [CrossRef]
12. Primakoff, P.; Myles, D.G. Penetration, adhesion, and fusion in mammalian sperm-egg interaction. *Science* **2002**, *296*, 2183–2185. [CrossRef] [PubMed]
13. Meizel, S.; Turner, K.O. Progesterone acts at the plasma membrane of human sperm. *Mol. Cell. Endocrinol.* **1991**, *77*, R1–R5. [CrossRef]
14. Meizel, S. The sperm, a neuron with a tail: 'neuronal' receptors in mammalian sperm. *Biol. Rev.* **2004**, *79*, 713–732. [CrossRef]
15. Dan, J.C. Studies on the Acrosome. III. Effect of Calcium Deficiency. *Biol. Bull* **1954**, *107*, 335–349. [CrossRef]
16. Correia, J.; Michelangeli, F.; Publicover, S. Regulation and roles of Ca^{2+} stores in human sperm. *Reproduction* **2015**, *150*, R65–R76. [CrossRef]
17. Costello, S.; Michelangeli, F.; Nash, K.; Lefievre, L.; Morris, J.; Machado-Oliveira, G.; Barratt, C.; Kirkman-Brown, J.; Publicover, S. Ca^{2+}-stores in sperm: Their identities and functions. *Reproduction* **2009**, *138*, 425–437. [CrossRef]
18. Miller, M.R.; Mannowetz, N.; Iavarone, A.T.; Safavi, R.; Gracheva, E.O.; Smith, J.F.; Hill, R.Z.; Bautista, D.M.; Kirichok, Y.; Lishko, P.V. Unconventional endocannabinoid signaling governs sperm activation via the sex hormone progesterone. *Science* **2016**, *352*, 555–559. [CrossRef]
19. Strunker, T.; Goodwin, N.; Brenker, C.; Kashikar, N.D.; Weyand, I.; Seifert, R.; Kaupp, U.B. The CatSper channel mediates progesterone-induced Ca^{2+} influx in human sperm. *Nature* **2011**, *471*, 382–386. [CrossRef]
20. Seifert, R.; Flick, M.; Bonigk, W.; Alvarez, L.; Trotschel, C.; Poetsch, A.; Muller, A.; Goodwin, N.; Pelzer, P.; Kashikar, N.D.; et al. The CatSper channel controls chemosensation in sea urchin sperm. *EMBO J.* **2015**, *34*, 379–392. [CrossRef]
21. Mcleskey, S.B.; Dowds, C.; Carballada, R.; White, R.R.; Saling, P.M. Molecules involved in mammalian sperm-egg interaction. *Int. Rev. Cytol. A Surv. Cell Biol.* **1997**, *177*, 57–113. [CrossRef]
22. Hirohashi, N.; Kamei, N.; Kubo, H.; Sawada, H.; Matsumoto, M.; Hoshi, M. Egg and sperm recognition systems during fertilization. *Dev. Growth Differ.* **2008**, *50*, S221–S238. [CrossRef]
23. Töpfer-Petersen, E. Molecules on the sperm's route to fertilization. *J. Exp. Zool. Part A Ecol. Genet. Physiol.* **2015**, *285*, 259–266. [CrossRef]
24. Li, S.J.; Wang, G.Z. Studies on reproductive biology and artificial culture of mud crab, Scylla Serrata. *J. Xiamen Univ.* **2001**, *40*, 552–565.
25. Shang-guan, B.; Li, S. Study on ultrastrcture of the sperm of Scylla serrata (Crustacea, Decapoda, Brachyura). *Curr. Zool.* **1994**, *1*, 7–11.
26. Li, P.; Chan, H.C.; He, B.; So, S.C.; Chung, Y.W.; Shang, Q.; Zhang, Y.D.; Zhang, Y.L. An antimicrobial peptide gene found in the male reproductive system of rats. *Science* **2001**, *291*, 1783–1785. [CrossRef]
27. Zhou, C.X.; Zhang, Y.L.; Xiao, L.Q.; Zheng, M.; Leung, K.M.; Chan, M.Y.; Lo, P.S.; Tsang, L.L.; Wong, H.Y.; Ho, L.S. An epididymis-specific β-defensin is important for the initiation of sperm maturation. *Nat. Cell Biol.* **2004**, *6*, 458–464. [CrossRef]

28. Tollner, T.L.; Venners, S.A.; Hollox, E.J.; Yudin, A.I.; Liu, X.; Tang, G.; Xing, H.; Kays, R.J.; Lau, T.; Overstreet, J.W. A Common Mutation in the Defensin DEFB126 Causes Impaired Sperm Function and Subfertility. *Sci. Transl. Med.* **2011**, *3*, 92ra65. [CrossRef]
29. Zhao, Y.; Diao, H.; Ni, Z.; Hu, S.G.; Yu, H.G.; Zhang, Y.L. The epididymis-specific antimicrobial peptide β-defensin 15 is required for sperm motility and male fertility in the rat (*Rattus norvegicus*). *Cell. Mol. Life Sci. Cmls* **2010**, *68*, 697–708. [CrossRef]
30. Qiao, K.; Xu, W.F.; Chen, H.Y.; Peng, H.; Zhang, Y.Q.; Huang, W.S.; Wang, S.P.; An, Z.; Shan, Z.G.; Chen, F.Y.; et al. A new antimicrobial peptide SCY2 identified in Scylla paramamosain exerting a potential role of reproductive immunity. *Fish Shellfish Immun.* **2016**, *51*, 251–262. [CrossRef]
31. Yang, Y.; Chen, F.Y.; Chen, H.Y.; Peng, H.; Hao, H.; Wang, K.J. A novel antimicrobial peptide scyreprocin from mud crab Scylla paramamosain showing potent antifungal and anti-biofilm activity. *Front. Microbiol.* **2020**, *11*, 1589. [CrossRef] [PubMed]
32. Cheng, Y.; Li, S.J.; Wang, G.Z. Ultrastructure of the female spermatheca and its storage spermatozoa after spawning of mud crab Scylla serrata. *J. Shanghai Fish. Univ.* **2000**, *9*, 69–71.
33. Ma, X.W.; Hou, L.; Chen, B.; Fan, D.Q.; Chen, Y.C.; Yang, Y.; Wang, K.J. A truncated Sph12–38 with potent antimicrobial activity showing resistance against bacterial challenge in Oryzias melastigma. *Fish Shellfish Immun.* **2017**, *67*, 561–570. [CrossRef] [PubMed]
34. Shan, Z.; Zhu, K.; Peng, H.; Chen, B.; Liu, J.; Chen, F.; Ma, X.; Wang, S.; Qiao, K.; Wang, K. The new antimicrobial peptide SpHyastatin from the mud crab Scylla paramamosain with multiple antimicrobial mechanisms and high effect on bacterial infection. *Front. Microbiol.* **2016**, *7*, 1140. [CrossRef] [PubMed]
35. Brokordt, K.; Defranchi, Y.; Espósito, I.; Cárcamo, C.; Schmitt, P.; Mercado, L.; Erwin, F.O.; Rivera-Ingraham, G.A. Reproduction immunity trade-off in a mollusk: Hemocyte energy metabolism underlies cellular and molecular immune responses. *Front. Physiol.* **2019**, *10*, 77. [CrossRef] [PubMed]
36. Dorin, J.R.; Barratt, C.L.R. Importance of β-defensins in sperm function. *Mol. Hum. Reprod.* **2014**, *20*, 821–826. [CrossRef]
37. Sørensen, O.E.; Gram, L.; Johnsen, A.H.; Andersson, E.; Bangsbøll, S.; Tjabringa, G.S.; Hiemstra, P.S.; Malm, J.; Egesten, A.; Borregaard, N. Processing of seminal plasma hCAP-18 to ALL-38 by gastricsin: A novel mechanism of generating antimicrobial peptides in vagina. *J. Biol. Chem.* **2003**, *278*, 28540–28546. [CrossRef]
38. Eisenbach, M.; Giojalas, L.C. Sperm guidance in mammals-an unpaved road to the egg. *Nat. Rev. Mol. Cell Biol.* **2006**, *7*, 276–285. [CrossRef]
39. Kaupp, U.B.; Kashikar, N.D.; Weyand, I. Mechanisms of sperm chemotaxis. *Annu. Rev. Physiol.* **2008**, *70*, 93–117. [CrossRef]
40. Kekalainen, J.; Evans, J.P. Female-induced remote regulation of sperm physiology may provide opportunities for gamete-level mate choice. *Evolution* **2017**, *71*, 238–248. [CrossRef]
41. Teves, M.E.; Guidobaldi, H.A.; Unates, D.R.; Sanchez, R.; Miska, W.; Publicover, S.J.; Garcia, A.A.M.; Giojalas, L.C. Molecular mechanism for human sperm chemotaxis mediated by progesterone. *PLoS ONE* **2009**, *4*, e8211. [CrossRef]
42. Foresta, C.; Rossato, M.; Mioni, R.; Zorzi, M. Progesterone induces capacitation in human spermatozoa. *Andrologia* **1992**, *24*, 33–35. [CrossRef]
43. Talbot, P.; Summers, R.G.; Hylander, B.L.; Keough, E.M.; Franklin, L.E. The role of calcium in the acrosome reaction: An analysis using ionophore A23187. *J. Exp. Zool.* **1976**, *198*, 383–392. [CrossRef] [PubMed]
44. Du, N.H.; Lai, W.; Xue, L.H. Acrosome reaction of the sperm in the Chinese mitten-handed crab, Eriocheir sinensis (Crustacea, Decapoda). *Acta Zool. Sin.* **1987**, *33*, 9–13. [CrossRef]
45. Clark, W.H.; Griffin, F.J. The morphology and physiology of the acrosome reaction in the sperm of the Decapod, Sicyonia ingentis. *Dev. Growth Differ.* **1988**, *30*, 451–462. [CrossRef]
46. Medina, A.; Rodriguez, A. Structural-changes in sperm from the fiddler crab, Uca tangeri (Crustacea, Brachyura), during the acrosome reaction. *Mol. Reprod. Dev.* **1992**, *33*, 195–201. [CrossRef]
47. Du, N.S.; Lai, W.; An, Y.; Jiang, H.W. Studies on the cytology of fertilization in the Chinese mitten-handed crab, Eriocheir sinensis (Crustacea, Decapoda). *Sci. China Ser. B* **1993**, *36*, 288–296.
48. Ye, H.H.; Song, P.; Ma, J.; Huang, H.Y.; Wang, G.Z. Changes in progesterone levels and distribution of progesterone receptor during vitellogenesis in the female mud crab (*Scylla paramamosain*). *Mar. Freshw. Behav. Physiol.* **2010**, *43*, 25–35. [CrossRef]
49. Lishko, P.V.; Botchkina, I.L.; Kirichok, Y. Progesterone activates the principal Ca^{2+} channel of human sperm. *Nature* **2011**, *471*, 387–391. [CrossRef]
50. Smith, J.F.; Kirichok, Y.; Lishko, P.V. Calcium channel CatSper is a non-genomic progesterone receptor of human sperm. *Biophys. J.* **2012**, *102*, 338a. [CrossRef]
51. Ralt, D.; Goldenberg, M.; Fetterolf, P.; Thompson, D.; Dor, J.; Mashiach, S.; Garbers, D.L.; Eisenbach, M. Sperm attraction to a follicular factor(s) correlates with human egg fertilizability. *Proc. Natl. Acad. Sci. USA* **1991**, *88*, 2840–2844. [CrossRef] [PubMed]
52. Adams, E.M.; Wolfner, M.F. Seminal proteins but not sperm induce morphological changes in the Drosophila melanogaster female reproductive tract during sperm storage. *J. Insect Physiol.* **2007**, *53*, 319–331. [CrossRef]
53. Senarai, T.; Vanichviriyakit, R.; Miyata, S.; Sato, C.; Sretarugsa, P.; Weerachatyanukul, W.; Kitajima, K. Alpha-2 macroglobulin as a region-specific secretory protein in male reproductive tract, and its dynamics during sperm transit towards the female spermatheca in the blue crab. *Mol. Reprod. Dev.* **2017**, *84*, 585–595. [CrossRef] [PubMed]
54. Peng, H.; Liu, H.P.; Chen, B.; Hao, H.; Wang, K.J. Optimized production of scygonadin in Pichia pastoris and analysis of its antimicrobial and antiviral activities. *Protein Expr. Purif.* **2012**, *82*, 37–44. [CrossRef]
55. Kruger, N.J. The Bradford method for protein quantitation. In *Basic Protein and Peptide Protocols. Methods in Molecular Biology*; Walker, J.M., Ed.; Humana Press: Totowa, NJ, USA, 1994; Volume 32, pp. 9–15.

56. Xu, W.F.; Qiao, K.; Huang, S.P.; Peng, H.; Huang, W.S.; Chen, B.; Chen, F.Y.; Bo, J.; Wang, K.J. Quantitative gene expression and in situ localization of scygonadin potentially associated with reproductive immunity in tissues of male and female mud crabs, Scylla paramamosain. *Fish Shellfish. Immun.* **2011**, *31*, 243–251. [CrossRef] [PubMed]
57. Arocho, A.; Chen, B.Y.; Ladanyi, M.; Pan, Q.L. Validation of the 2-DDCt calculation as an alternate method of data analysis for quantitative PCR of BCR-ABL P210 transcripts. *Diagn. Mol. Pathol.* **2006**, *15*, 56–61. [CrossRef]
58. Lin, W.; Yang, J.; He, X.; Mo, G.; Jing, H.; Yan, X.; Lin, D.; Ren, L. Structure and function of a potent lipopolysaccharide-binding antimicrobial and anti-inflammatory peptide. *J. Med. Chem.* **2013**, *9*, 3546–3556. [CrossRef]
59. Chen, H.M.; Chan, S.C.; Lee, J.C.; Chang, C.C.; Jack, R.W. Transmission electron microscopic observations of membrane effects of antibiotic Cecropin B on Escherichia coli. *Microsc. Res. Tech.* **2003**, *62*, 423–430. [CrossRef]
60. Lawniczak, M.K.N.; Barnes, A.I.; Linklater, J.R.; Boone, J.M.; Wigby, S.; Chapman, T. Mating and immunity in invertebrates. *Trends Ecol. Evol.* **2007**, *22*, 48–55. [CrossRef]
61. Harshman, L.G.; Zera, A.J. The cost of reproduction: The devil in the details. *Trends Ecol. Evol.* **2007**, *22*, 80–86. [CrossRef]

International Journal of *Molecular Sciences*

Article

Optimized Silica-Binding Peptide-Mediated Delivery of Bactericidal Lysin Efficiently Prevents *Staphylococcus aureus* from Adhering to Device Surfaces

Wan Yang [1], Vijay Singh Gondil [2], Dehua Luo [1], Jin He [1], Hongping Wei [2,3] and Hang Yang [2,3,*]

1 State Key Laboratory of Agricultural Microbiology, College of Life Science and Technology, Huazhong Agricultural University, Wuhan 430070, China; yw13618649009@hotmail.com (W.Y.); luode_hua@webmail.hzau.edu.cn (D.L.); hejin@mail.hzau.edu.cn (J.H.)
2 CAS Key Laboratory of Special Pathogens and Biosafety, Center for Biosafety Mega-Science, Wuhan Institute of Virology, Chinese Academy of Sciences, Wuhan 430071, China; vjgondal@gmail.com (V.S.G.); hpwei@wh.iov.cn (H.W.)
3 University of Chinese Academy of Sciences, Beijing 100049, China
* Correspondence: yangh@wh.iov.cn; Tel.: +86-27-51861078

Abstract: Staphylococcal-associated device-related infections (DRIs) represent a significant clinical challenge causing major medical and economic sequelae. Bacterial colonization, proliferation, and biofilm formation after adherence to surfaces of the indwelling device are probably the primary cause of DRIs. To address this issue, we incorporated constructs of silica-binding peptide (SiBP) with ClyF, an anti-staphylococcal lysin, into functionalized coatings to impart bactericidal activity against planktonic and sessile *Staphylococcus aureus*. An optimized construct, SiBP1-ClyF, exhibited improved thermostability and staphylolytic activity compared to its parental lysin ClyF. SiBP1-ClyF-functionalized coatings were efficient in killing MRSA strain N315 (>99.999% within 1 h) and preventing the growth of static and dynamic *S. aureus* biofilms on various surfaces, including siliconized glass, silicone-coated latex catheter, and silicone catheter. Additionally, SiBP1-ClyF-immobilized surfaces supported normal attachment and growth of mammalian cells. Although the recycling potential and long-term stability of lysin-immobilized surfaces are still affected by the fragility of biological protein molecules, the present study provides a generic strategy for efficient delivery of bactericidal lysin to solid surfaces, which serves as a new approach to prevent the growth of antibiotic-resistant microorganisms on surfaces in hospital settings and could be adapted for other target pathogens as well.

Keywords: lysin; *Staphylococcus aureus*; silica-binding peptide; antimicrobial agents immobilization; surface functionalization; antimicrobial agents; biofilm

Citation: Yang, W.; Gondil, V.S.; Luo, D.; He, J.; Wei, H.; Yang, H. Optimized Silica-Binding Peptide-Mediated Delivery of Bactericidal Lysin Efficiently Prevents *Staphylococcus aureus* from Adhering to Device Surfaces. *Int. J. Mol. Sci.* **2021**, *22*, 12544. https://doi.org/10.3390/ijms222212544

Academic Editor: Helena Felgueiras

Received: 18 October 2021
Accepted: 16 November 2021
Published: 21 November 2021

1. Introduction

Medical devices play a pivotal role in the management of healthcare-associated patients in modern medicine. Indwelling urinary and central venous catheters are the most frequently employed invasive devices, which have revolutionized medical treatment, especially post-operative care [1]. These catheters remain continuously interacting with body fluids for a long duration, which is critical for the success of these implants [2]. However, long-term catheterization also favors microbial colonization and dissemination, leading to the failure of implant and further increasing the treatment cost and the severity of ailment [3]. For instance, a 3–6% per day increased risk of bacterial colonization has been estimated in urinary catheterization and 7–10 days of catheterization may result in catheter-associated infections in 50% of the hospitalized patients [4,5]. Bacterial colonization on surface of central venous catheters presents more serious complications as compared to urinary catheters, as relatively small number of colonized bacteria can successfully establish the central line associated blood stream infections [6], which commonly links to higher life-threatening risk and cost [7].

In general, different types of implantable biomedical device-related infections (DRIs) have linked to varied bacterial species. For example, cardiovascular implantable devices and joint prosthesis are often colonized by Staphylococci, Streptococci, Enterococci, and *Candida* spp. [8]. However, Staphylococci are one of the major causes of medical DRIs due to strong capacity to form device-related biofilms, and the most pathogenic and aggressive one is methicillin-resistant *S. aureus* (MRSA) [9]. Various strategies have been employed to reduce bacterial colonization on surfaces of devices, such as increased hygiene, optimized dwelling measures, and biocidal agent-based surface modifications [10]. However, the antimicrobial resistance and biofilm-forming ability of *S. aureus* brought the efficacy of these strategies into question [11]. Therefore, designing novel antibacterial and antibiofouling coating is needed to counter the mounting menace of drug-resistant *S. aureus*-mediated DRIs.

It has been demonstrated in the past two decades that the bacteriophage-encoded peptidoglycan hydrolase, i.e., endolysin or lysin, is a promising candidate to overcome antimicrobial resistance [12,13]. The primary function of lysin is to release the virion progeny from the host cytoplasm by digesting its peptidoglycan, but in recent years, lysin is immensely exploited as an antibacterial agent due to its unique mechanisms of action. A good example is the chimeric lysin ClyF that possesses high activity against planktonic and biofilm *S. aureus* both in vitro and in vivo models [14]. ClyF composes the catalytic domain (CD) from Ply187 lysin (GenBank: CAA69022.1, UniProtKB: O56785, the N-terminal 157 aa) with a putative CHAP (cysteine, histidine-dependent amidohydrolase/peptidase) catalytic activity and the cell wall binding domain (CBD) from PlySs2 lysin (NCBI No.: WP_170238997.1, UniProtKB: A0A0Z8Y0I3, the C-terminal 99 aa) that possesses high affinity for *S. aureus*. Because of rapid activity, high specificity, proteinaceous nature, and not yet reported case of resistance [15], lysin could be presented as a potent alternative agent for immobilization on surface of devices to prevent DRIs.

Lysins have been well investigated in various in vitro and in vivo infection models against a range of potent Gram-positive and Gram-negative pathogens over the decades [16–21]. Continuous work has well established that the second generation of lysin could be engineered to possess improved bactericidal activity and/or broad spectrum of function [22,23]. Whilst the third generation of lysin could be continuously engineered and developed to gain improved pharmacological properties [24]. Few studies demonstrated the activity of phage-derived lysins stored in complexes with block-copolymers of poly-L-glutamic acid and polyethylene glycol [25], or after fusing with matrix-binding protein, such as cellulose binding domain [26]; however, there is a knowledge void in the activity as well as the possibility of immobilized lysins on solid surfaces. The current study was designed to fill the existing knowledge void and investigated the potential of bactericidal lysins immobilization on biomedical surfaces as a means to combat medical DRIs.

Short solid binding peptides are popular molecular linkers for the fabrication of bioactive proteins onto solid surfaces via multiple weak noncovalent interactions [27]. These peptides increase the affinity of bioactive proteins for their targeted solid matrix and confers orientation, flexibility, and directionality to proteins without impeding their activity [28,29]. Therefore, in the present study, ClyF was used as a model lysin to be modified with three different silica-binding peptides (SiBPs) [14] to convene the conception of bactericidal lysin-functionalized surfaces as a new approach to block device-related bacterial colonization (Figure 1). Specifically, three peptides reported to have high affinity for silica surfaces were selected fusing to the C-terminal of ClyF, and SiBP-fused ClyF variants were then immobilized on various silicone-containing surfaces and evaluated for their antibacterial and antibiofilm activities under static and dynamic conditions.

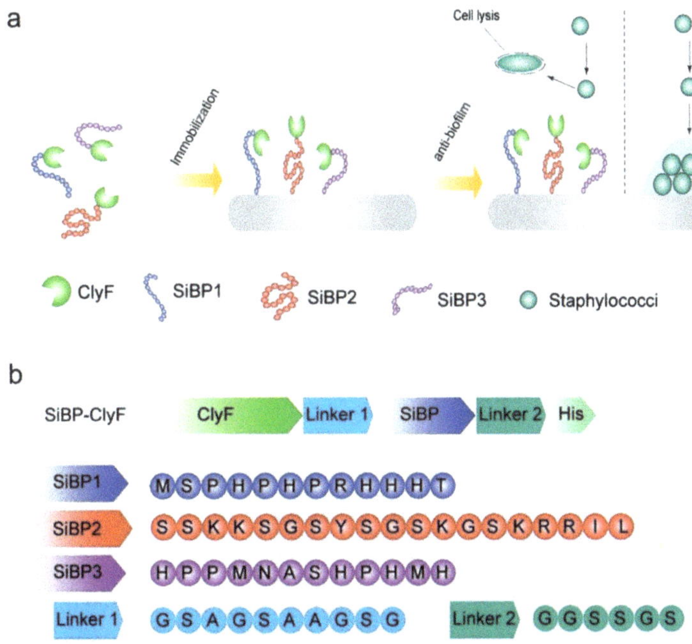

Figure 1. Schematic diagram of experimental design. (**a**) Silica-binding peptide-mediated fixation of ClyF imparts antistaphylococcal propriety to solid surfaces. (**b**) Construction and composition of SiBP-fused ClyF variants. The amino acid sequences of SiBP1, SiBP2, SiBP3, linker between ClyF and SiBP (Linker 1), and linker between SiBP and His tag (Linker 2) are shown.

2. Results

2.1. Construction and Biochemical Characterization of ClyF Variants

Previously, we demonstrated that the chimeric lysin ClyF is highly active against various staphylococcal strains [14], highlighting its potential as an alternative antistaphylococcal agent. Considering the epidemiology and threats of staphylococci-primed device-related infections (DRIs) in model healthcare settings, we further explored the antistaphylococcal capacity of surface-immobilized ClyF by using solid surface directed silica-binding peptide (SiBP). To this end, three peptides varying in charge and length, i.e., a 12-residue peptide SiBP1 (MSPHPHPRHHHT; Z = +1) [30], a 19-residue peptide SiBP2 (SSKKSGSYSGSKGSKRRIL; Z = +6) [31], and another 12-residue peptide SiBP3 (HPPMNASHPHMH; Z = 0) [32], were selected fusing to the C-terminal of ClyF lysin (Figure 1). To adjust the compatibility of ClyF lysin and silica-binding peptide, a separate flexible linker was incorporated before and after each peptide sequence, and a C-terminal 6×his-tag was attached for affinity purification of each construct (Figure 1). All ClyF constructs were expressed in *E. coli* BL21(DE3) cells as soluble proteins and purified using Ni-NTA affinity chromatography (Figure S1).

Because the bactericidal activity of ClyF depends on the proper folding of its two functional domains, we thus assessed the effects of SiBP on the structural conformation of ClyF variants by circular dichroism. Results showed that the spectra of ClyF, SiBP2-ClyF and SiBP3-ClyF almost resemble each other and that the spectra of SiBP1-ClyF showed minor differences due to difference in the molar ellipticity intensities (Figure 2a). However, all four proteins had UV peaks at 215 nm, suggesting similar folding in all four. Additional analysis revealed that the composition of the secondary structural components for all four enzymes is nearly identical (Table S1), indicating that SiBP-fusing only introduces a minor influence on the folding profile of ClyF domains. We further used RoseTTAFold to perform structural predictions for ClyF and its variants. Each prediction showed a similar structure with a hydrophobic cleft in the catalytic domain and an Ig-like structure in the CBD (Figure S2). However, the predicted surface shape of SiBP2-ClyF is a bit different from that of the other variants, showing a L-like shape, while the others displayed a V-like shape (Figure S2).

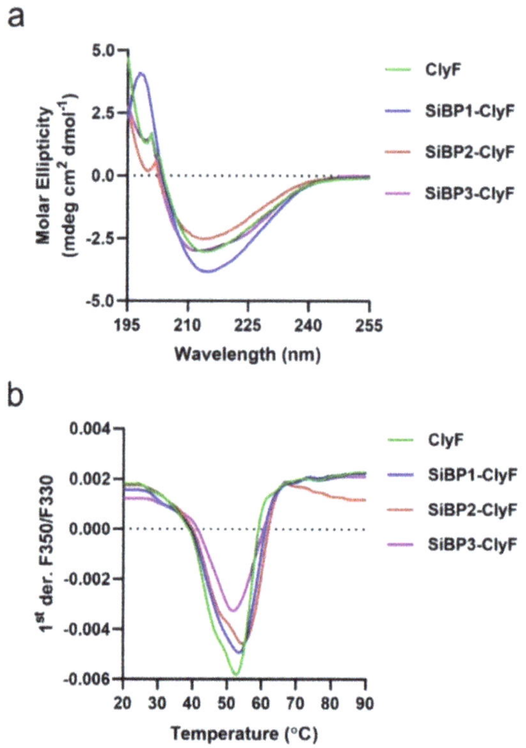

Figure 2. Biochemical properties of ClyF and its variants. (**a**) Circular dichroism spectra of ClyF and its variants. The UV spectra of ClyF and its variants were scanned from 190–260 nm (0.1 cm path length) at room temperature. (**b**) Thermal unfolding profiles for ClyF and its variants. The profiles of all proteins were determined by nanoDSF from 25–90 °C. The *Y*-axis represents the first derivative of the ratio of fluorescence at 350 nm and 330 nm.

Next, we evaluated the influence of these peptides on the thermostability of ClyF using nano-differential scanning fluorimetry. Results showed that the thermal transition temperature increases from 52.1 °C for ClyF to 54.3 °C for SiBP2-ClyF, the variant with the highest positively charged peptide, while the other two ClyF variants, SiBP1-ClyF and SiBP2-ClyF, exhibit similar thermal transition temperatures with their parental ClyF lysin (Figure 2b and Table S2). The single peaks noted for ClyF and its three SiBP-fused variants indicate that the two constitutive domains of ClyF unfold together in all four (Figure 2b).

2.2. Bactericidal Activities of Free ClyF Variants

Initially, we tested the bacteriolytic of ClyF and its variants against eight representative *S. aureus* strains with different genetic profiles (Table S3), results showed that SiBP1-ClyF and SiBP2-ClyF exhibit improved lytic activities in all strains tested compared to the native ClyF (Figure S3). In contrast, an impaired activity was observed in SiBP3-ClyF, which could be associated to its slightly different circular dichroism curve (Figure 2a) and 3D modeling structure (Figure S2). We then evaluated the bactericidal activities of ClyF and its variants against three staphylococcal strains, WHS11032, WHS11103, and N315, under equal molar concentrations. In consistent with the bacteriolytic assays, the variant SiBP3-ClyF maintained impaired bactericidal activity compared to that of the parental ClyF lysin, effecting a 1- to 3-log10 decrement in bacterial viability in 60 min, depending on the strain (Figure 3). In contrast, SiBP1-ClyF and SiBP2-ClyF exhibited significantly ($p < 0.001$) elevated bactericidal activity, effecting a 1.36- and 0.87-log10 increase in killing activity for *S. aureus* N315, respectively, compared to the activity of their parental ClyF (Figure 3). As both SiBP1 (Z = +1) and SiBP2 (Z = +6) are positively charged, presumably, the neutrally charged SiBP3 (Z = 0) prevents the direction of the cell-wall binding domain (CBD) in SiBP3-ClyF to its bacterial cell wall substrates.

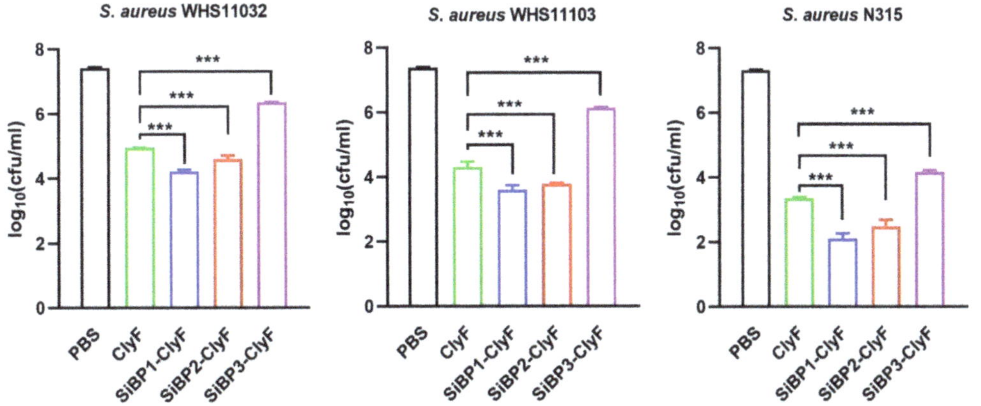

Figure 3. Bactericidal activities of ClyF and its SiBP-fused variants. *S. aureus* strains WHS11032, WHS11103, and N315 were treated with equal molar concentration (0.7 μM) of each protein for 1 h at 37 °C, residual number of viable bacteria was determined by plating serial dilutions on LB agar. Data are shown as means ± standard deviations and *** represents $p < 0.001$.

2.3. Bactericidal Capacities of Immobilized ClyF Variants against Planktonic S. aureus

Next, we compared the bacteriostatic activities of immobilized ClyF and its variants against the growth of planktonic *S. aureus*, under an equal molar concentration. As shown in Figure 4a, immobilized SiBP1-ClyF and SiBP2-ClyF showed significantly improved bacteriostatic activities, with rare notable bacterial growth even after 20 h of co-incubation at 37 °C, as compared to the native ClyF. In contrast, the variant SiBP3-ClyF showed attenuated bacteriostatic ability, priming a 2-h-earlier visible growth of *S. aureus* N315, compared to the parental ClyF (Figure 4a). Notably, compared to the PBS-treated group, minor bacteriostatic activity was observed in ClyF-immobilized wells, implying a non-specific binding of ClyF to supporting surfaces. In addition, we determined the viable bacterial number in lysin-immobilized wells after co-cultured for 1 h to further confirm their bacteriostatic activities. Results showed that, the variants SiBP1-ClyF and SiBP2-ClyF exhibit improved bactericidal activities, leading to a killing of 3.37- and 2.99-log10 (Figure 4b), corresponding to a reduction of 53.36% and 47.39% in log10 (Figure 4c), respectively, compared to the killing of 2.24-log10 and reduction of 35.52% in log10 in the parental ClyF. As expected, SiBP3-ClyF maintained impaired bactericidal activity in comparison to the wild type ClyF (Figure 4b,c), which is relatively consistent with the attenuated bacteriostatic activity in immobilized SiBP3-ClyF.

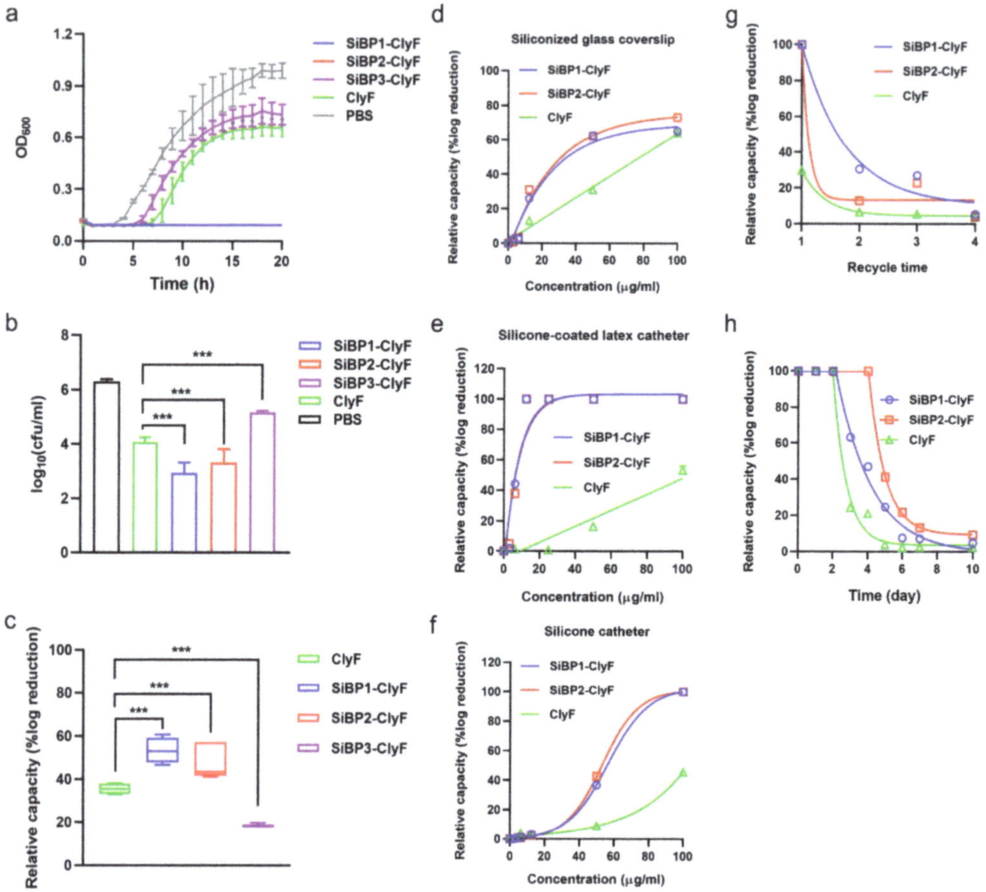

Figure 4. Bactericidal activities of immobilized ClyF and its variants against planktonic *S. aureus* on different surfaces. (**a**) Bacteriostatic activities of ClyF and its variants immobilized on siliconized glass surface against *S. aureus* N315. (**b**,**c**) Bactericidal capacities of ClyF and its variants immobilized on siliconized glass surface against *S. aureus* N315. ClyF and its SiBP-fused variants were immobilized on siliconized glass surfaces and cocultured with *S. aureus* N315 for 1 h at 37 °C, residual number of viable bacteria was determined by plating serial dilutions on LB agar (**b**), and the relative capacity of each protein was presented as the percentage of log reduction in lysin-immobilized groups in comparison to the mock-immobilized PBS-treated controls (**c**). (**d**–**f**) Bactericidal capacities of ClyF and its variants on different immobilized surfaces. Different concentrations of ClyF, SiBP1-ClyF, and SiBP2-ClyF were immobilized on surfaces of siliconized glass coverslip (**d**), silicone-coated latex catheter (**e**), and silicone catheter (**f**) for 2 h at room temperature, the bactericidal capacity of each surface after co-culture with *S. aureus* N315 for 1 h was then determined by plating assay. (**g**) Recycle capacity of ClyF, SiBP1-ClyF, and SiBP2-ClyF immobilized glass 96-well plates. (**h**) Bactericidal activities of ClyF, SiBP1-ClyF, and SiBP2-ClyF immobilized glass 96-well plates after stored different times at 4 °C. Data are shown as means ± standard deviations and *** represents $p < 0.001$.

As the above observations collectively showed that immobilized SiBP1-ClyF and SiBP2-ClyF possess a higher relative capacity on the solid surface than SiBP3-ClyF and ClyF (Figure 4c), we further characterized their performance in multiple clinically relevant surfaces, including siliconized glass, silicone-coated latex catheter, and silicone catheter. Results showed that immobilized SiBP1-ClyF and SiBP2-ClyF exhibit similar dose-dependent anti-staphylococcal responses and significantly elevated capacities in all three surfaces tested, compared to the parental ClyF (Figure 4d–f). Comparable capacities were observed in siliconized glass coverslip under higher immobilization concentration (up to 100 μg/mL) for all three lysins (Figure 4d), indicating strong non-specific binding of positively charged ClyF CBD to glass surfaces. On the surface of silicone-coated catheter, SiBP1-ClyF and SiBP2-ClyF showed high bactericidal activities under low concentrations, almost achieving their maximal bactericidal capacity at 12.5 μg/mL for both proteins, causing a reduction of 5.52-log10 in viable bacterial number (>99.999% removing efficacy), compared to the activity of ClyF (Figure 4e). Likewise, high anti-staphylococcal activities were also observed in SiBP1-ClyF- and SiBP2-ClyF-coated surfaces of silicone catheter (Figure 4f).

In addition, a recycle evaluation assay showed that the relative capacity of lysin-functionalized surfaces decreased along with the recycle times, and rare bactericidal activity was observed after 4 recycles (Figure 4g). Nonetheless, the bactericidal activity of SiBP1-ClyF-immobilized wells after three recycles was still comparable to that of the ClyF-immobilized wells in its first cycle (Figure 4g). Like other protein-functionalized surfaces, immobilized lysins lose bactericidal activity in a time-dependent manner and were almost inactivated after 7 days of storage at 4 °C (Figure 4h), although SiBP1-ClyF- and SiBP2-ClyF-immobilized wells showed improved tolerance than that of ClyF-coated wells. Taken together, immobilization of ClyF on silicone-containing surfaces via SiBP1 and SiBP2 could bring high antimicrobial activity and stability against planktonic *S. aureus*.

2.4. *Antibiofilm Capacity of Immobilized SiBP1-ClyF against Static S. aureus Biofilms*

As *S. aureus* biofilm is the most common cause of surgical site infections and medical DRIs initiated by bacterial adherence to surfaces [33], we thus ascertained the antibiofilm activity of immobilized ClyF, harboring the conception that immobilized ClyF could kill surface Staphylococci and thus prevent biofilm formation. Because immobilized SiBP1-ClyF shows the highest bactericidal capacity against *S. aureus* (Figure 4c), the antibiofouling capacity of ClyF-functionalized surface was carried out by using SiBP1-ClyF in our subsequent studies. In this regard, SiBP1-ClyF was immobilized on surface of siliconized glass coverslips and cocultured with *S. aureus* N315 in the biofilm formation medium. Resulted staphylococcal biofilms of different ages (2, 6, 10, and 24 h), corresponding to different developing stages of *S. aureus* biofilms [34], were analyzed by SEM. As shown in Figure 5a, mock-immobilized groups evidenced the development of *S. aureus* biofilms from initial attachment, multiplication, and exodus to mature biofilms. In contrast, SiBP1-ClyF immobilized group showed a significantly retard development of *S. aureus* biofilms, with fewer *S. aureus* attached to lysin-functionalized surfaces, visible cell deformation, and dead ghost cells caused by the lysis of SiBP1-ClyF (Figure 5a). Notably, the ClyF-coated group showed reduced *S. aureus* attachment and visible signs of cell lysis, probably due to the non-specific bound of ClyF to glass surface, but rare inhibitory effects on the maturation of *S. aureus* biofilms were observed (Figure 5a). To more accurately reflect the antibiofilm capacity of SiBP1-ClyF-immobilized surfaces, we stained *S. aureus* biofilms aged 10 h by Live/Dead bacterial viability kit and imaged using confocal fluorescence microscopy. Results showed that a lawn of confluent bright green stained cells, indicating viable *S. aureus*, was observed in the mock-immobilized PBS-treated control group (Figure 5b), which could be correlated with the high bacterial load and the successful establishment of bacterial biofilms. In contrast, rare green fluorescent signal was detected in SiBP1-ClyF immobilized group, but multiple scattered red fluorescent spots were observed, representing dead *S. aureus* cells (Figure 5b). These observations collectively showed that the SiBP1-ClyF-immobilized surface has a potent antibiofouling capacity against static *S. aureus* biofilms.

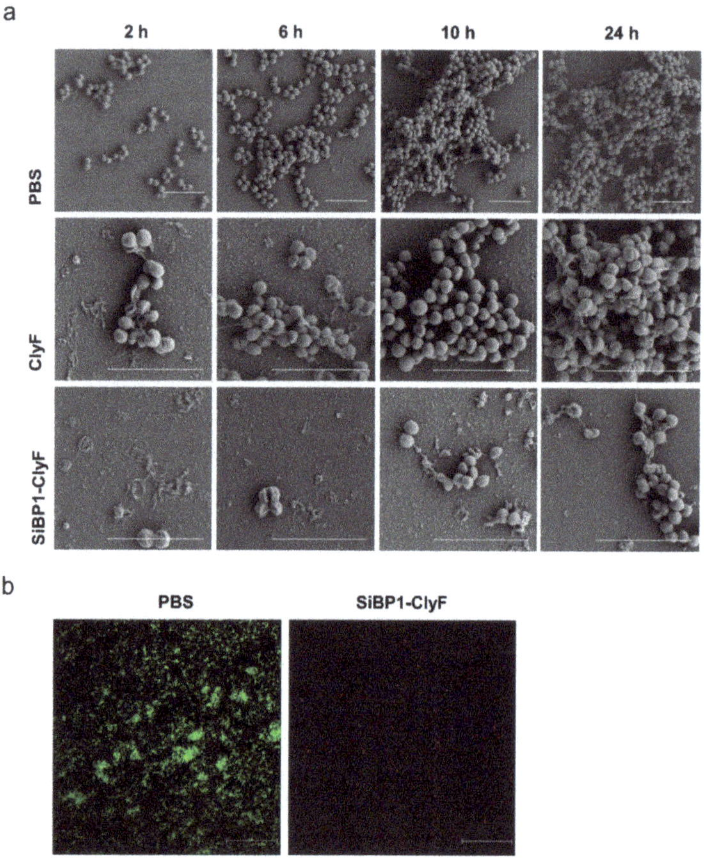

Figure 5. Antibiofouling activity of SiBP1-ClyF-immobilized surfaces against static *S. aureus* biofilms. (**a**,**b**) Analysis of antibiofilm activity of SiBP1-ClyF-immobilized surfaces. Siliconized glass coverslips were coated with 100 μg/mL of SiBP1-ClyF for 2 h at room temperature, and then incubated with *S. aureus* N315 in TBSG at 37 °C. Biofilms developed at 2, 6, 10, and 24 h were analyzed by a JSM-6390 scanning electron microscope (**a**). Biofilms developed at 10 h were further stained with Live/Dead bacterial viability kit and visualized by confocal fluorescence microscope (**b**). Bar scalar: 5 μm.

2.5. Antibiofilm Capacity of Immobilized SiBP1-ClyF against Dynamic S. aureus Biofilms

To mimic the in vivo antibiofilm capacity of immobilized SiBP1-ClyF on clinically relevant surfaces, we established a dynamic biofilm model using silicone catheter and evaluated the performance of SiBP1-ClyF. To this end, 100 μg/mL SiBP1-ClyF was immobilized on the surface of silicone catheter for 2 h at room temperature, inoculated with ~10^6 CFU/mL of *S. aureus* N315 for 3 h at room temperature, and then fabricated into a flowing peripherally inserted central catheter with a fluid speed of 0.6 mL/min (Figure 6a). Staphylococcal biofilms formed on the surface of silicone catheter after 24 h of media flow was determined by plating assay. Results showed that a significant drop ($p < 0.001$) in bacterial burden in the SiBP1-ClyF immobilized silicone catheters, indicating an average bacterial load of 2.2-log10 cfu/cm^2, compared to that of the mock-immobilized PBS-treated control catheters (5.8-log10 cfu/cm^2; Figure 6b). The decreased bacterial load can be correlated with the high staphylolytic activity of SiBP1-ClyF on surfaces of silicone catheters in the continuous flow model.

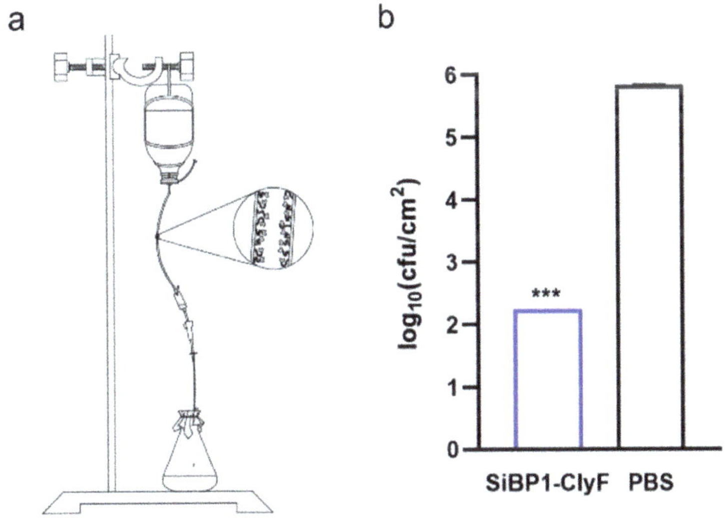

Figure 6. Antibiofouling activity of SiBP1-ClyF-immobilized surfaces against dynamic *S. aureus* biofilms. (**a**) Schematic diagram of fabricated dynamic *S. aureus* biofilm model. Silicone catheter (~5 cm length) was coated with 100 μg/mL of SiBP1-ClyF for 2 h at room temperature, and then incubated with ~10^6 CFU/mL of *S. aureus* N315 for 3 h at room temperature. Afterwards, the silicone catheter was inserted into a peripherally inserted central catheter and flowed with LB at a fluid speed of 0.6 mL/min for 24 h to allow biofilm development. Finally, silicone catheters were removed and underwent an ultrasound bath for 10 min to disturb established biofilms. Resulted viable bacterial number was analyzed by plating serial dilutions on LB agar. PBS-treated mock-coated silicone catheter was used as control. (**b**) Antibiofilm capacity of immobilized SiBP1-ClyF on surface of silicone catheter. Data are shown as means ± standard deviations and *** represents $p < 0.001$.

2.6. SiBP1-ClyF Immobilized Surface Supports Normal Growth of Mammalian Cells

To understand the potency of SiBP1-ClyF-functionalized surface in clinic applications, we evaluated the cytotoxicity of those surfaces by CCK-8 assay. To this end, BHK-21 cells were inoculated in wells immobilized with various concentrations of SiBP1-ClyF for 24 h, the cell viability was then determined. Results showed that rare differences in cell viability were observed from SiBP1-ClyF-immobilized wells and PBS-treated control wells (Figure 7a), suggesting that SiBP1-ClyF-functionalized surface could support the normal growth of mammalian cells. Note that similar biocompatibility was also observed in ClyF-immobilized wells (Figure 7a), indicating the safety profile of native ClyF, which is also consistent with our previous in vivo observations [14]. As expected, SiBP1-ClyF and ClyF immobilized wells supported a normal cell proliferation, with similar confluence to that of the mock-immobilized control wells (Figure 7b).

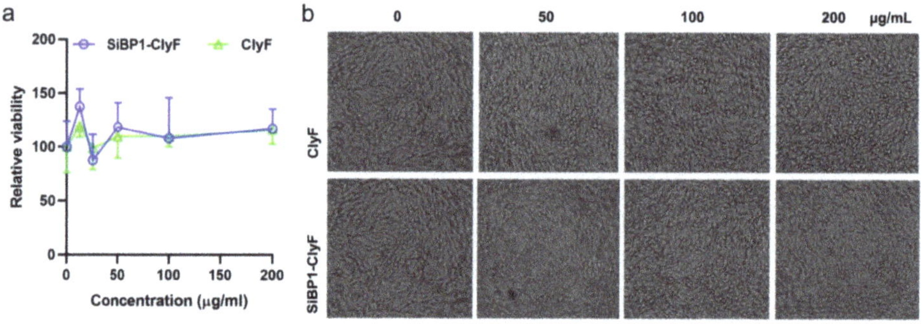

Figure 7. SiBP1-ClyF-immobilized surfaces support normal growth of mammalian cells. Wells were immobilized with various concentrations (0, 12.5, 25, 50, 100, and 200 μg/mL) of SiBP1-ClyF or ClyF overnight at 4 °C and inoculated with 104 cells/well of BHK-21 cells for 24 h, the cell viability of each treatment was then determined by CCK-8 assay (**a**) and the cell confluence of each treatment was captured by microscopy (**b**). Representative images under 10× objective lens from wells immobilized with 0, 50, 100, and 200 μg/mL SiBP1-ClyF or ClyF were shown.

3. Discussion

In recent decades, antibiotic resistance has emerged as a mounting menace for global healthcare [35]. Potential pathogens have established themselves as multidrug-resistant superbugs, which are refractory to conventional antibiotics. With scarce treatment options, many of the untreatable bacterial infections are now primarily cause of mortality globally. The current pipeline for new antibiotics is drying, which is even more vexatious for healthcare professionals. Currently, clinicians and researchers are forced to look for alternative agents to antibiotics, including bacteriophages and their lysins, antibacterial metal nanoparticles, phytochemicals, antimicrobial peptides, nitric oxide, and other secondary metabolites [36–41]. Lysins have gained much popularity because of their high bactericidal properties, rapid killing activity, low risk of resistance, and modular proteinaceous structure. However, the performance of lysins on solid surfaces as a means to address DRIs is still largely unknown. In this study, we evaluated the bactericidal and antibiofilm activity of the chimeric staphylolytic lysin ClyF on various clinic relevant surfaces by genetically engineering with SiBPs and found that lysin-functionalized surfaces gain improved resistant to bacterial adhesion and biofilm formation.

Immobilization of enzymes may reduce their catalytic activities because of the steric restriction and limited access to the substrate to enzymatic site in particular conformation [42]. Therefore, in the present study, ClyF was designed to modulate with different peptides to optimize a suitable one that can help ClyF to conquer steric restriction and conformational hindrance for immobilized bacteriolytic activity. By adopting flexible linkers, peptides could thus take any orientation, including a folding back on the lysin structure. The linker can contribute to an increased autonomy of each moiety, i.e., ClyF for killing and peptide for silica binding. In this regard, two ClyF variants, especially SiBP1-ClyF, exhibited satisfactory properties for immobilization applications, as evidenced by their high antibacterial and antibiofilm capacities against *S. aureus* planktonic cells and biofilms on different surfaces.

Notably, one SiBP-construct, i.e., SiBP3-ClyF showed impaired bactericidal activity. Increase of activity of lysins acting against Gram-positive bacteria by positively charged peptides has been documented previously [43,44]; therefore, the positive charges present in SiBP1 (Z = +1) and SiBP2 (Z = +6) may explain their enhanced activities against planktonic strains. It may thus be the lack of a positive charge and the additional steric hindrance of the fused peptide SiBP3 (Z = 0) that lowers the activity of SiBP3-ClyF, although the detailed mechanisms behind still need further study. However, for the immobilized enzymes, the SiBP is involved in binding the silica-based surfaces, thus would then not be further available to interact with the negatively charged bacterial cell wall. Nonetheless, the influence of the charge of silica-based materials on the observed activity of SiBP-fusions still needs to be established.

A potential shortcoming of the current approach is the limitations of the recycling potential and long-term stability of ClyF-immobilized surfaces. This may be due to the fragility of biological protein molecules which tend to lose their activity when in contact with a support surface [45]. According to the current progress in immobilizing functional enzymes on solid supports, several approaches could be adopted to solve such problem, for instance, optimizing the storing buffer of coated surfaces [26], favoring the molecular orientation of immobilized enzymes through rational design [46], fabricating ClyF to bioactive films by conjugating with nanoparticles [47], self-assembling spider silk protein [48], or programable biofilm-integrated nanofiber [49].

Biofilms are complex 3D structure of bacterial communities, which provides enhanced bacterial colonization on solid surfaces and extravagant the management of infections [50]. Biofilms provide protection to bacteria from host immunity and block the access of antibiotics by producing thick extracellular polymeric substances [51,52]. Medical DRIs are biologically initiated from microorganisms' adherence on surface of interaction. Therefore, preventing bacterial attachment and growth via bactericidal lysin-mediated surface immobilization is a fundamental and efficient strategy to prevent DRIs. Taking *S. aureus* as an example, the present study showed that immobilization staphylolytic lysin ClyF via silica-targeting peptide SiBP1, i.e., SiBP1-ClyF, on surfaces can not only lead to scarce bacterial colonization and growth due to lysis of attached bacteria, but also resulted in significantly reduced mature biofilms developed under both static and dynamic conditions. However, the influence of lysed bacterial debris on the ecosystem in the long run still needs further study.

Because of the nature of phage, lysins are usually specific to their target bacterium, commonly in genus level, which makes them different from broad-spectrum antibiotics. As a proof-of-concept study, we take staphylococci-targeted lysin, ClyF, as an example to show the feasibility of using lysin-functionalized surfaces as a new approach to prevent DRIs. Our current model, in principle, will only be active against bacterial species that are susceptible to the killing of ClyF, but not other strains that lie outside of the lysis spectrum of ClyF. Other bacteria could also form biofilms; our current strategy, however, could be transplanted to another bacterium by using an ideal lysin targeting that bacterium, considering the continuous progress in lysin discovery and engineering. Therefore, the present strategy provides a roadmap for endolysin immobilization to counter device-related drug-resistant infections, which are cumbersome to conventional antibiotic therapy.

4. Materials and Methods

4.1. Construction of SiBP-ClyF Fusions

The ClyF-coding gene was amplified with three different SiBPs by overlap polymerase chain reaction assays with specific primers (Table S4). The amplified SiBP-ClyF gene products were cloned into *Nco*I and *Xho*I sites of pET28b(+) vector and further transformed into *E. coli* BL21(DE3) competent cells. Clones harboring the appropriate sequence were confirmed by sequencing (Table S4) and then processed for further experiments.

4.2. Protein Expression and Purification

A single positive colony for ClyF and its SiBP-ClyF constructs was cultured separately in 5 mL of lysogeny broth (LB) supplemented with 50 μg/mL kanamycin. The tubes were incubated at 220 rpm at 37 °C overnight. The next day, 1 mL of the culture was transferred to 100 mL of fresh LB medium with 50 μg/mL kanamycin and incubated with shaking at 37 °C for 2–3 h. Protein expression was induced with 0.25 mM isopropyl-β-D-thiogalactoside when the optical density (600 nm) of inoculated media reached 0.6–0.8. The flasks were incubated for 16–20 h at 16 °C with 120 rpm of shaking. Cells were harvested by centrifugation at 12,000 rpm at 4 °C for 20 min and cell pellet was washed thrice with Tris-HCl buffer (50 mM sodium phosphate, 500 mM NaCl, pH 8) to remove media components. The cells were lysed using pressure facture and purified by Ni-NTA affinity chromatography with gradient of imidazole solutions. Purified enzyme was dialyzed against 0.1 mM $CaCl_2$ containing phosphate-buffered saline (PBS, pH 7.4) to remove imidazole and confirmed by SDS-PAGE analysis [53]. The dialyzed protein was then filter sterilized using 0.22 μm syringe filters and stored at 4 °C for subsequent experiments.

4.3. Structure Prediction of ClyF and Its Variants

The 3D structure of ClyF and its variants were predicated by RoseTTAFold online service [53] and further analyzed by PyMOL.

4.4. Nano Differential Scanning Fluorimetry

The thermal stability of ClyF and its variants were analysed by a nano differential scanning fluorimetry method using a Prometheus NT.48 instrument (NanoTemper Technologies, San Francisco, CA, USA). The intrinsic emission fluorescence of each protein (200 μg/mL) at 350 and 330 nm was monitored over a temperature range of 25 to 90 °C (increasing step of 1 °C/min), using dialysis buffer as controls. The first derivative of the fluorescence ratio at 350 nm and 330 nm (1st derivative of F350/F330) was calculated automatically by the PR-ThermControl software supplied with the instrumentation. Samples were measured in triplicates. The thermal unfolding transition temperature (Tm) corresponds to peaks of the 1st derivative of F350/F330.

4.5. Circular Dichroism

The circular dichroism spectra of ClyF and its variants (200 μg/mL) were collected with an Applied Photophysics Chirascan Plus circular dichroism spectrometer (Leatherhead, UK) from 190–260 nm (0.1 cm path length) at room temperature. The spectra of air and buffer were recorded as background and baseline, respectively. The secondary structure was analyzed by the CDNN V2.1 software, supplied by the instrument manufacturer.

4.6. Bactericidal Activity of Free ClyF and Its SiBP-Fused Variants

Antibacterial activity of ClyF and its SiBP-fused variants were evaluated by log killing assay as described previously [14]. Briefly, *S. aureus* strains (Table S3) were inoculated in 5 mL of LB broth at 37 °C. Next day, 50 μL of overnight grown culture was inoculated to 5 mL of fresh LB media for 3–4 h at 37 °C with shaking. Cells were then harvested, washed, and resuspended in PBS to an optical density of OD_{600} = 0.6. Bacterial suspension was treated with an equal molar concentration (final concentration of 0.7 μM, corresponding to ClyF concentration of 20 μg/mL) of ClyF and its SiBP-fused variants for 1 h at 37 °C. The turbidity of each treatment was monitored by a Synergy H1 microplate reader and viable bacterial quantification was determined by plating serial 10-fold PBS-diluted dilutions on LB agar. Parallel suspensions that treated with an equal volume of PBS were used as controls.

4.7. Antibacterial Activity of Lysin-Functionalized Surfaces

To evaluate the bactericidal activity of lysin-functionalized silicon glass, ClyF and its SiBP-fused variants were immobilized in glass 96-well plates at an equal molar concentration of 1.75 μM (corresponding to ClyF concentration of 50 μg/mL) for 2 h at room temperature. Wells were then washed twice with PBS, inoculated with ~10^6 CFU/well of *S. aureus* N315 in LB medium, and incubated at 37 °C. The growth of bacteria was determined by monitoring the OD_{600} in each well using a microplate reader for 20 h at intervals of 15 min. Additionally, the viable bacterial number in each well after incubation for 1 h was further confirmed by plating serial dilutions on LB agar. The capacity of immobilized lysin in each treatment was expressed as the percentage of the reduction in bacterial cell count compared to that of the PBS-treated groups (%log reduction).

To evaluate the performance of ClyF variants on different surfaces, siliconized glass coverslip, silicone-coated latex catheter (φ = 6.7 mm, ~1 cm length; 20Fr, STAR, Zhanjiang,

China), and silicone catheter (φ = 6.7 mm, ~1 cm length; 20Fr, STAR, Zhanjiang, China) were coated with different concentrations (0, 20, 40, 60, 80, and 100 μg/mL) of ClyF, SiBP1-ClyF, or SiBP2-ClyF for 2 h at room temperature in 48-well plates. These surfaces were washed twice with PBS and then inoculated with ~10^6 CFU/well of PBS-suspended *S. aureus* N315 for 1 h at 37 °C. Viable bacterial number was quantified by plating serial dilutions on LB agar. Each experiment was carried out in biological triplicates.

4.8. Recycle Capacity and Stability of Lysin-Functionalized Surface

To evaluate the recycle capacity of lysin-functionalized silicon glass, ClyF and its SiBP-fused variants were immobilized in glass 96-well plates at an equal molar concentration of 3.5 μM (corresponding to ClyF concentration of 100 μg/mL) for 2 h at room temperature. Wells were then washed twice with PBS, inoculated repeatedly with ~106 CFU/well of *S. aureus* N315 and incubated at 37 °C for 10 min for 5 cycles. Viable bacterial number from each cycle was further confirmed by plating serial dilutions on LB agar. The relative capacity of each enzyme was compared to the capacity of SiBP1-ClyF (%log reduction) in the first cycle.

To ascertain the stability of lysin-functionalized surface during storage, glass 96-well plates coated with an equal molar concentration of 1.75 μM (corresponding to ClyF concentration of 50 μg/mL) ClyF and its SiBP-fused variants were stored for different times at 4 °C. The relative capacity of lysin-functionalized wells was determined as described above at 0, 1, 2, 3, 4, 5, 6, 7, and 10 days post-immobilization, and normalized to the bactericidal activity of corresponding wells before storage. All experiments were carried out in biological triplicates.

4.9. Prevention of Biofilm Formation on Lysin-Functionalized Surfaces

Siliconized glass coverslips were coated with 100 μg/mL of SiBP1-ClyF for 2 h at room temperature in 6-well plates, washed twice with PBS, and then incubated with ~106 CFU/well of *S. aureus* N315 in 2 mL TBSG (1.5% tryptone, 0.5% soytone, 0.5% NaCl, and 1% glucose) at 37 °C. Biofilms developed at 2, 6, 10, and 24 h were analyzed by a JSM-6390 scanning electron microscope (JEOL, Tendo, Japan) as described previously [54]. Groups coated with ClyF and PBS were used as controls. Additionally, biofilms established for 10 h were further stained with Live/Dead Baclight bacterial viability kit (L13152, Thermo, Shanghai, China) and visualized by an UltraVIEW VoX confocal fluorescence microscope (PerkinElmer, Waltham, MA, USA) as described previously [55]. PBS-treated mock-coated groups were used as controls.

To test the capacity of lysin-coated surface against flow biofilms, silicone catheter (φ = 4 mm, ~4 cm length; 20Fr, STAR, Zhanjiang, China) was coated with 100 μg/mL of SiBP1-ClyF for 2 h at room temperature. The coated catheters were washed twice with PBS and then incubated with ~10^6 CFU/mL of *S. aureus* N315 for 3 h at room temperature to allow bacterial attachment on the catheter surface. Afterwards, the *S. aureus*-containing silicone catheter was inserted into a peripherally inserted central catheter and flowed with LB at a fluid speed of 0.6 mL/min for 24 h to allow the biofilm establishment. Finally, silicone catheters were removed and underwent an ultrasound bath for 10 min to disrupt established biofilms. Resulted viable bacterial number was analyzed by plating serial dilutions on LB agar. PBS-treated mock-coated silicone catheter was used as control.

4.10. Cytotoxicity of Lysin-Functionalized Surface

Various concentrations of ClyF and SiBP1-ClyF (0, 12.5, 25, 50, 100, and 200 μg/mL) were immobilized in 96-well plates overnight at 4 °C. Wells were then washed twice with PBS and inoculated with 10^4 cells/well of BHK-21 cells in Dulbecco's modified Eagle's medium (DMEM; Sigma-Aldrich, Shanghai, China) supplemented with 10% fetal bovine serum, 1% penicillin, and 1% streptomycin in a humidified atmosphere of 5% CO_2 at 37 °C for 24 h. Afterwards, the cell viability of each treatment was determined by CCK-8 assay and the cell confluence was captured by microscopy. For CCK-8 assay, the contents of the plates were replaced with fresh medium containing 10% CCK-8 solution and incubated at 37 °C for 1 h. The final optical density at OD_{450} was noted by a Synergy H1 microplate reader (BioTek, Winooski, VT, USA). The results were expressed as relative cell viability, expressed as a percentage of the growth of cells in control wells immobilized with PBS only. For confluence detection, wells were imaged by an IX51 inverted microscope under 10× objective lens (Olympus, Center Valley, PA, USA). All experiments were carried out in biological triplicates.

4.11. Statistic Analysis

Data analyses were performed by one-way analysis of variance (ANOVA) and layout by GraphPad Prism 8.0.

5. Conclusions

The present study demonstrates the antibacterial and antibiofilm potential of immobilized ClyF on multiple solid surfaces via silica-binding peptides. One such variant, SiBP1-ClyF, showed not only feasible immobilization stability on solid support surfaces, but also retains high antibacterial and antibiofilm abilities. This study supports a promising approach to design innovative antimicrobial surfaces by using bactericidal lysins, which can be highly selective for their target bacteria. The generic approach reported here could also be easily extended to other pathogen-targeted lysins to prevent multiple medical device-related drug-resistant infections.

Supplementary Materials: The following are available online at https://www.mdpi.com/article/10.3390/ijms222212544/s1.

Author Contributions: Conceptualization, H.Y.; Methodology, H.Y. and W.Y.; Investigation, H.Y., D.L. and W.Y.; Formal analysis, H.Y., W.Y. and V.S.G.; Data Curation, H.Y., D.L. and W.Y.; Writing—Original Draft, W.Y., V.S.G. and H.Y.; Writing—Review and Editing, H.Y.; Supervision, H.Y., J.H. and H.W.; Resource, J.H. and H.W.; Funding Acquisition, H.Y. All authors have read and agreed to the published version of the manuscript.

Funding: This research was funded by the National Natural Science Foundation of China (No. 32070187 and No. 31770192), the Youth Innovation Promotion Association CAS, and the Open Research Fund Program of CAS Key Laboratory of Special Pathogens and Biosafety, Wuhan Institute of Virology (2021SPCAS001).

Institutional Review Board Statement: Not applicable.

Informed Consent Statement: Not applicable.

Data Availability Statement: The data presented in this study are available from the corresponding author upon request.

Acknowledgments: We thank Bichao Xu from the Core Facility and Technical Support of Wuhan Institute of Virology for assistance in microscopy studies.

Conflicts of Interest: The authors declare no conflict of interest.

References

1. Saint, S.; Savel, R.H.; Matthay, M.A. Enhancing the safety of critically ill patients by reducing urinary and central venous catheter-related infections. *Am. J. Respir Crit. Care Med.* **2002**, *165*, 1475–1479. [CrossRef] [PubMed]
2. Brisbois, E.J.; Davis, R.P.; Jones, A.M.; Major, T.C.; Bartlett, R.H.; Meyerhoff, M.E.; Handa, H. Reduction in Thrombosis and Bacterial Adhesion with 7 Day Implantation of S-Nitroso-N-acetylpenicillamine (SNAP)-Doped Elast-eon E2As Catheters in Sheep. *J. Mater. Chem. B* **2015**, *3*, 1639–1645. [CrossRef]
3. Parienti, J.J.; Mongardon, N.; Megarbane, B.; Mira, J.P.; Kalfon, P.; Gros, A.; Marque, S.; Thuong, M.; Pottier, V.; Ramakers, M.; et al. Intravascular Complications of Central Venous Catheterization by Insertion Site. *N. Engl. J. Med.* **2015**, *373*, 1220–1229. [CrossRef] [PubMed]
4. Schumm, K.; Lam, T.B. Types of urethral catheters for management of short-term voiding problems in hospitalised adults. *Cochrane Database Syst. Rev.* **2008**, *16*, 2:CD004013.

5. Andersen, M.J.; Flores-Mireles, A.L. Urinary Catheter Coating Modifications: The Race against Catheter-Associated Infections. *Coatings* **2020**, *10*, 23. [CrossRef]
6. Haddadin, Y.; Annamaraju, P.; Regunath, H. *Central Line Associated Blood Stream Infections*; StatPearls: Treasure Island, FL, USA, 2020.
7. Neoh, K.G.; Li, M.; Kang, E.T.; Chiong, E.; Tambyah, P.A. Surface modification strategies for combating catheter-related complications: Recent advances and challenges. *J. Mater. Chem. B* **2017**, *5*, 2045–2067. [CrossRef]
8. Xu, Y.; Larsen, L.H.; Lorenzen, J.; Hall-Stoodley, L.; Kikhney, J.; Moter, A.; Thomsen, T.R. Microbiological diagnosis of device-related biofilm infections. *APMIS* **2017**, *125*, 289–303. [CrossRef]
9. Zheng, Y.; He, L.; Asiamah, T.K.; Otto, M. Colonization of medical devices by staphylococci. *Environ. Microbiol.* **2018**, *20*, 3141–3153. [CrossRef]
10. Durant, D.J. Nurse-driven protocols and the prevention of catheter-associated urinary tract infections: A systematic review. *Am. J. Infect. Control* **2017**, *45*, 1331–1341. [CrossRef]
11. Singh, S.; Singh, S.K.; Chowdhury, I.; Singh, R. Understanding the Mechanism of Bacterial Biofilms Resistance to Antimicrobial Agents. *Open Microbiol. J.* **2017**, *11*, 53–62. [CrossRef]
12. Schmelcher, M.; Loessner, M.J. Bacteriophage endolysins—Extending their application to tissues and the bloodstream. *Curr. Opin. Biotechnol.* **2021**, *68*, 51–59. [CrossRef] [PubMed]
13. Linden, S.B.; Alreja, A.B.; Nelson, D.C. Application of bacteriophage-derived endolysins to combat streptococcal disease: Current state and perspectives. *Curr. Opin. Biotechnol.* **2021**, *68*, 213–220. [CrossRef] [PubMed]
14. Yang, H.; Zhang, H.; Wang, J.; Yu, J.; Wei, H. A novel chimeric lysin with robust antibacterial activity against planktonic and biofilm methicillin-resistant Staphylococcus aureus. *Sci. Rep.* **2017**, *7*, 40182. [CrossRef] [PubMed]
15. Gondil, V.S.; Harjai, K.; Chhibber, S. Endolysins as emerging alternative therapeutic agents to counter drug-resistant infections. *Int. J. Antimicrob. Agents* **2020**, *55*, 105844. [CrossRef] [PubMed]
16. Yang, H.; Linden, S.B.; Wang, J.; Yu, J.; Nelson, D.C.; Wei, H. A chimeolysin with extended-spectrum streptococcal host range found by an induced lysis-based rapid screening method. *Sci. Rep.* **2015**, *5*, 17257. [CrossRef]
17. Huang, L.; Luo, D.; Gondil, V.S.; Gong, Y.; Jia, M.; Yan, D.; He, J.; Hu, S.; Yang, H.; Wei, H. Construction and characterization of a chimeric lysin ClyV with improved bactericidal activity against Streptococcus agalactiae in vitro and in vivo. *Appl. Microbiol. Biotechnol.* **2020**, *104*, 1609–1619. [CrossRef]
18. Loeffler, J.M.; Djurkovic, S.; Fischetti, V.A. Phage lytic enzyme Cpl-1 as a novel antimicrobial for pneumococcal bacteremia. *Infect. Immun.* **2003**, *71*, 6199–6204. [CrossRef]
19. Gondil, V.S.; Dube, T.; Panda, J.J.; Yennamalli, R.M.; Harjai, K.; Chhibber, S. Comprehensive evaluation of chitosan nanoparticle based phage lysin delivery system; a novel approach to counter, S. pneumoniae infections. *Int. J. Pharm.* **2020**, *573*, 118850. [CrossRef]
20. Guo, M.; Feng, C.; Ren, J.; Zhuang, X.; Zhang, Y.; Zhu, Y.; Dong, K.; He, P.; Guo, X.; Qin, J. A Novel Antimicrobial Endolysin, LysPA26, against Pseudomonas aeruginosa. *Front. Microbiol.* **2017**, *8*, 293. [CrossRef]
21. Ghose, C.; Euler, C.W. Gram-Negative Bacterial Lysins. *Antibiotics* **2020**, *9*, 74. [CrossRef]
22. Gerstmans, H.; Criel, B.; Briers, Y. Synthetic biology of modular endolysins. *Biotechnol. Adv.* **2018**, *36*, 624–640. [CrossRef] [PubMed]
23. Sao-Jose, C. Engineering of Phage-Derived Lytic Enzymes: Improving Their Potential as Antimicrobials. *Antibiotics* **2018**, *7*, 29. [CrossRef] [PubMed]
24. De Maesschalck, V.; Gutierrez, D.; Paeshuyse, J.; Lavigne, R.; Briers, Y. Advanced engineering of third-generation lysins and formulation strategies for clinical applications. *Crit. Rev. Microbiol.* **2020**, *46*, 548–564. [CrossRef]
25. Filatova, L.Y.; Donovan, D.M.; Ishnazarova, N.T.; Foster-Frey, J.A.; Becker, S.C.; Pugachev, V.G.; Balabushevich, N.G.; Dmitrieva, N.F.; Klyachko, N.L. A Chimeric LysK-Lysostaphin Fusion Enzyme Lysing Staphylococcus aureus Cells: A Study of Both Kinetics of Inactivation and Specifics of Interaction with Anionic Polymers. *Appl. Biochem. Biotechnol.* **2016**, *180*, 544–557. [CrossRef] [PubMed]
26. Abouhmad, A.; Mamo, G.; Dishisha, T.; Amin, M.A.; Hatti-Kaul, R. T4 lysozyme fused with cellulose-binding module for antimicrobial cellulosic wound dressing materials. *J. Appl. Microbiol.* **2016**, *121*, 115–125. [CrossRef]
27. Johnson, A.K.; Zawadzka, A.M.; Deobald, L.A.; Crawford, R.L.; Paszczynski, A.J. Novel method for immobilization of enzymes to magnetic nanoparticles. *J. Nanopart. Res.* **2008**, *10*, 1009–1025. [CrossRef]
28. Care, A.; Bergquist, P.L.; Sunna, A. Solid-binding peptides: Smart tools for nanobiotechnology. *Trends Biotechnol.* **2015**, *33*, 259–268. [CrossRef]
29. Cetinel, S.; Caliskan, H.B.; Yucesoy, D.T.; Donatan, A.S.; Yuca, E.; Urgen, M.; Karaguler, N.G.; Tamerler, C. Addressable self-immobilization of lactate dehydrogenase across multiple length scales. *Biotechnol. J.* **2013**, *8*, 262–272. [CrossRef]
30. Naik, R.R.; Brott, L.L.; Clarson, S.J.; Stone, M.O. Silica-precipitating peptides isolated from a combinatorial phage display peptide library. *J. Nanosci. Nanotechnol.* **2002**, *2*, 95–100. [CrossRef] [PubMed]
31. Kroger, N.; Deutzmann, R.; Sumper, M. Polycationic peptides from diatom biosilica that direct silica nanosphere formation. *Science* **1999**, *286*, 1129–1132. [CrossRef]
32. Eteshola, E.; Brillson, L.J.; Lee, S.C. Selection and characteristics of peptides that bind thermally grown silicon dioxide films. *Biomol. Eng.* **2005**, *22*, 201–204. [CrossRef] [PubMed]

33. Arciola, C.R.; Campoccia, D.; Montanaro, L. Implant infections: Adhesion, biofilm formation and immune evasion. *Nat. Rev. Microbiol.* **2018**, *16*, 397–409. [CrossRef] [PubMed]
34. Moormeier, D.E.; Bayles, K.W. Staphylococcus aureus biofilm: A complex developmental organism. *Mol. Microbiol.* **2017**, *104*, 365–376. [CrossRef] [PubMed]
35. Talebi Bezmin Abadi, A.; Rizvanov, A.A.; Haertlé, T.; Blatt, N.L. World Health Organization Report: Current Crisis of Antibiotic Resistance. *BioNanoScience* **2019**, *9*, 778–788. [CrossRef]
36. Romero-Calle, D.; Guimarães Benevides, R.; Góes-Neto, A.; Billington, C. Bacteriophages as Alternatives to Antibiotics in Clinical Care. *Antibiotics* **2019**, *8*, 138. [CrossRef]
37. Gondil, V.S.; Kalaiyarasan, T.; Bharti, V.K.; Chhibber, S. Antibiofilm potential of Seabuckthorn silver nanoparticles (SBT@AgNPs) against Pseudomonas aeruginosa. *3 Biotech* **2019**, *9*, 402. [CrossRef]
38. Simoes, M.; Bennett, R.N.; Rosa, E.A. Understanding antimicrobial activities of phytochemicals against multidrug resistant bacteria and biofilms. *Nat. Prod. Rep.* **2009**, *26*, 746–757. [CrossRef]
39. Gondil, V.S.; Asif, M.; Bhalla, T.C. Optimization of physicochemical parameters influencing the production of prodigiosin from Serratia nematodiphila RL2 and exploring its antibacterial activity. *3 Biotech* **2017**, *7*, 338. [CrossRef]
40. Mahlapuu, M.; Håkansson, J.; Ringstad, L.; Björn, C. Antimicrobial Peptides: An Emerging Category of Therapeutic Agents. *Front. Cell. Infect. Microbiol.* **2016**, *6*, 194. [CrossRef]
41. Douglass, M.; Hopkins, S.; Pandey, R.; Singha, P.; Norman, M.; Handa, H. S-Nitrosoglutathione-Based Nitric Oxide-Releasing Nanofibers Exhibit Dual Antimicrobial and Antithrombotic Activity for Biomedical Applications. *Macromol. Biosci.* **2021**, *21*, e2000248. [CrossRef]
42. Brena, B.; Gonzalez-Pombo, P.; Batista-Viera, F. Immobilization of enzymes: A literature survey. *Methods Mol. Biol.* **2013**, *1051*, 15–31.
43. Rodriguez-Rubio, L.; Chang, W.L.; Gutierrez, D.; Lavigne, R.; Martinez, B.; Rodriguez, A.; Govers, S.K.; Aertsen, A.; Hirl, C.; Biebl, M.; et al. 'Artilysation' of endolysin lambdaSa2lys strongly improves its enzymatic and antibacterial activity against streptococci. *Sci. Rep.* **2016**, *6*, 35382. [CrossRef]
44. Diez-Martinez, R.; de Paz, H.D.; Bustamante, N.; Garcia, E.; Menendez, M.; Garcia, P. Improving the lethal effect of cpl-7, a pneumococcal phage lysozyme with broad bactericidal activity, by inverting the net charge of its cell wall-binding module. *Antimicrob. Agents Chemother.* **2013**, *57*, 5355–5365. [CrossRef]
45. Talbert, J.N.; Goddard, J.M. Enzymes on material surfaces. *Colloids Surf. B Biointerfaces* **2012**, *93*, 8–19. [CrossRef] [PubMed]
46. Liu, Y.; Ogorzalek, T.L.; Yang, P.; Schroeder, M.M.; Marsh, E.N.; Chen, Z. Molecular orientation of enzymes attached to surfaces through defined chemical linkages at the solid-liquid interface. *J. Am. Chem. Soc.* **2013**, *135*, 12660–12669. [CrossRef] [PubMed]
47. Pangule, R.C.; Brooks, S.J.; Dinu, C.Z.; Bale, S.S.; Salmon, S.L.; Zhu, G.; Metzger, D.W.; Kane, R.S.; Dordick, J.S. Antistaphylococcal nanocomposite films based on enzyme-nanotube conjugates. *ACS Nano* **2010**, *4*, 3993–4000. [CrossRef] [PubMed]
48. Nileback, L.; Widhe, M.; Seijsing, J.; Bysell, H.; Sharma, P.K.; Hedhammar, M. Bioactive Silk Coatings Reduce the Adhesion of Staphylococcus aureus while Supporting Growth of Osteoblast-like Cells. *ACS Appl. Mater. Interfaces* **2019**, *11*, 24999–25007. [CrossRef]
49. Nguyen, P.Q.; Botyanszki, Z.; Tay, P.K.; Joshi, N.S. Programmable biofilm-based materials from engineered curli nanofibres. *Nat. Commun.* **2014**, *5*, 4945. [CrossRef]
50. Trautner, B.W.; Darouiche, R.O. Role of biofilm in catheter-associated urinary tract infection. *Am. J. Infect. Control* **2004**, *32*, 177–183. [CrossRef]
51. Costerton, J.W.; Stewart, P.S.; Greenberg, E.P. Bacterial biofilms: A common cause of persistent infections. *Science* **1999**, *284*, 1318–1322. [CrossRef]
52. Stewart, P.S.; Costerton, J.W. Antibiotic resistance of bacteria in biofilms. *Lancet* **2001**, *358*, 135–138. [CrossRef]
53. Baek, M.; DiMaio, F.; Anishchenko, I.; Dauparas, J.; Ovchinnikov, S.; Lee, G.R.; Wang, J.; Cong, Q.; Kinch, L.N.; Schaeffer, R.D.; et al. Accurate prediction of protein structures and interactions using a three-track neural network. *Science* **2021**, *373*, 871–876. [CrossRef] [PubMed]
54. Yang, H.; Zhang, Y.; Huang, Y.; Yu, J.; Wei, H. Degradation of methicillin-resistant Staphylococcus aureus biofilms using a chimeric lysin. *Biofouling* **2014**, *30*, 667–674. [CrossRef] [PubMed]
55. Yang, H.; Bi, Y.; Shang, X.; Wang, M.; Linden, S.B.; Li, Y.; Li, Y.; Nelson, D.C.; Wei, H. Antibiofilm Activities of a Novel Chimeolysin against Streptococcus mutans under Physiological and Cariogenic Conditions. *Antimicrob. Agents Chemother.* **2016**, *60*, 7436–7443. [CrossRef] [PubMed]

International Journal of *Molecular Sciences*

MDPI

Article

Injectable Platelet-Rich Fibrin as a Drug Carrier Increases the Antibacterial Susceptibility of Antibiotic—Clindamycin Phosphate

Karina Egle [1,2], Ingus Skadins [2,3], Andra Grava [1,2], Lana Micko [2,4,5], Viktors Dubniks [1,2], Ilze Salma [2,4,5] and Arita Dubnika [1,2,*]

1 Rudolfs Cimdins Riga Biomaterials Innovations and Development Centre, Institute of General Chemical Engineering, Faculty of Materials Science and Applied Chemistry, Riga Technical University, LV-1007 Riga, Latvia; karina.egle@rtu.lv (K.E.); andra.grava@rtu.lv (A.G.); viktors.dubniks@rtu.lv (V.D.)

2 Baltic Biomaterials Centre of Excellence, Headquarters at Riga Technical University, LV-1048 Riga, Latvia; ingus.skadins@rsu.lv (I.S.); lana.micko@gmail.com (L.M.); ilze.salma@rsu.lv (I.S.)

3 Department of Biology and Microbiology, Riga Stradins University, LV-1007 Riga, Latvia

4 Institute of Stomatology, Riga Stradins University, LV-1007 Riga, Latvia

5 Department of Oral and Maxillofacial Surgery, Riga Stradins University, LV-1007 Riga, Latvia

* Correspondence: arita.dubnika@rtu.lv; Tel.: +371-67089605

Abstract: The aim of this study was to investigate the change in clindamycin phosphate antibacterial properties against Gram-positive bacteria using the platelet-rich fibrin as a carrier matrix, and evaluate the changes in the antibiotic within the matrix. The antibacterial properties of CLP and its combination with PRF were tested in a microdilution test against reference cultures and clinical isolates of *Staphylococcus aureus* (*S. aureus*) or *Staphylococcus epidermidis* (*S. epidermidis*). Fourier-transform infrared spectroscopy (FTIR) and scanning electron microscope (SEM) analysis was done to evaluate the changes in the PRF_CLP matrix. Release kinetics of CLP was defined with ultra-performance liquid chromatography (UPLC). According to FTIR data, the use of PRF as a carrier for CLP ensured the structural changes in the CLP toward a more active form of clindamycin. A significant decrease in minimal bactericidal concentration values (from 1000 µg/mL to 62 µg/mL) against reference cultures and clinical isolates of *S. aureus* and *S. epidermidis* was observed for the CLP and PRF samples if compared to pure CLP solution. In vitro cell viability tests showed that PRF and PRF with CLP have higher cell viability than 70% after 24 h and 48 h time points. This article indicates that CLP in combination with PRF showed higher antibacterial activity against *S. aureus* and *S. epidermidis* compared to pure CLP solution. This modified PRF could be used as a novel method to increase drug delivery and efficacy, and to reduce the risk of postoperative infection.

Keywords: platelet-rich fibrin; antibacterial properties; antibiotic resistance; drug release; CLP

Citation: Egle, K.; Skadins, I.; Grava, A.; Micko, L.; Dubniks, V.; Salma, I.; Dubnika, A. Injectable Platelet-Rich Fibrin as a Drug Carrier Increases the Antibacterial Susceptibility of Antibiotic—Clindamycin Phosphate. *Int. J. Mol. Sci.* **2022**, *23*, 7407. https://doi.org/10.3390/ijms23137407

Academic Editor: Helena Felgueiras

Received: 7 June 2022
Accepted: 29 June 2022
Published: 3 July 2022

1. Introduction

Platelet-rich fibrin (PRF) is an autogenous material derived from human blood and is widely used to promote wound healing and tissue regeneration [1]. The leukocytes in the PRF promote wound healing and PRF contains growth factors that are released over time [2]. In several applications, such as oral and maxillofacial surgery, plastic surgery, cardiac surgery and dentistry, there is a great interest in PRF antimicrobial activity. Until now, most clinical studies have been conducted in dentistry and oral and maxillofacial surgery. Platelet concentrates are used in maxillary sinus floor augmentation, as the filling of teeth extraction sockets, in dental implant surgery, in regenerative endodontic treatment, in peri-implantitis and periodontitis treatment.

During the last decade, the antimicrobial properties of PRF have been described in various studies and different testing methods and bacteria have been used. Not only is injectable platelet-rich fibrin (I-PRF) anti-microbial, but anti-biofilm activity against human oral abscess pathogens has also been described. It was found that I-PRF decreases biofilm production at the minimal inhibitory concentration (MIC) and no biofilm production at the minimal bactericidal concentration (MBC) [3]. Using the disk diffusion method, I-PRF showed notable zones of inhibition, which varied depending on different bacterial species [4]. I-PRF also shows the superiority of antimicrobials against bacteria from the supragingival plate over PRF and PRP [4].

Infections are one of the most common postoperative risks caused by pathogenic and opportunistic bacteria [5,6]. *S. aureus* and *S. epidermidis* are Gram-positive opportunistic bacteria, which are present in the normal human microbiome. With the ability to produce biofilms, these bacteria can evade the host immune system and can cause various local and systemic infections, such as bacteremia, skin and soft tissue infections, osteomyelitis, and implant and device-related infections [7–9]. A lot of these infections can be prevented with antibiotics, especially those where the portals of entry for the bacteria are wounds due to surgery in the hospital environment. For treatment of community-acquired, methicillin-resistant and methicillin-susceptible *S. aureus* infections, clindamycin has been recommended for many years, and it also can increase the susceptibility of methicillin-resistant *S. aureus* clinical isolates [10,11]. The virulence of clinical isolates and their virulence factors, such as surface proteins, determine their ability to cause disease and the severity of the disease [12]. Nowadays, the demand for clindamycin as a medicine is increasing in oral and maxillofacial surgery (including for the prevention and treatment of osteonecrosis of the jaw [13]). It is widely considered as an alternative for patients with an allergic reaction to penicillin [14].

Clindamycin phosphate (CLP) is a prodrug of clindamycin that has no antibacterial activity [15]. As mentioned in the literature, prodrugs can offer many advantages over the parent drug (in our case clindamycin). These benefits include increased solubility, improved stability, reduced side effects, improved bioavailability and better selectivity [16]. CLP can be converted to clindamycin by in vitro hydrolysis of phosphatase esters [15,17]. Rapid in vivo hydrolysis also converts the CLP compound to the antibacterial clindamycin. Hydrolysis of the phosphatase ester is a relatively difficult mechanism (Figure 1). It has been reported that after hydrolysis using alkaline phosphatase, clindamycin phosphate is determined as clindamycin. Following topical, as well as upon intravaginal administration, clindamycin phosphate is slowly hydrolyzed to clindamycin due to limited hydrolysis of the prodrug by the phosphatase enzymes on the surface and within the skin. This prevents the incidence of antibiotic-induced GI side effects [18].

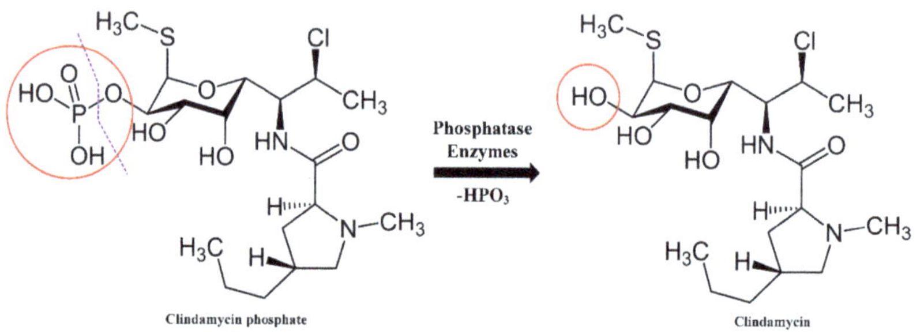

Figure 1. Clindamycin phosphate hydrolysis mechanism.

Clindamycin is known to be obtained by the chemical modification of lincomycin, so the potential impurities are analogs of lincomycin [19]. It is reported that the conversion of clindamycin phosphate to clindamycin in the blood is significantly lower than with oral administration of clindamycin hydrochloride [20,21]. CLP is absorbed as an inactive ester for parenteral use and is rapidly hydrolyzed to the active base in the blood.

CLP has not been widely studied in terms of antibacterial properties. Until now there are only a few studies on CLP's individual antibacterial properties, which show that the

MIC of CLP (w/v %) on *Staphylococcus aureus* is 0.02 ± 0.005% [22]. Nevertheless, it has a broad range of applications in biomaterials: for example, it is used in eye implants [23], periodontal films [24], and particles [25].

The aim of this study was to investigate the change in CLP antibacterial properties against reference culture and clinical isolates of *S. aureus* and *S. epidermidis* using platelet-rich fibrin as a carrier matrix, and evaluate the CLP structural changes, release kinetics and in vitro cytotoxicity within the PRF matrix.

2. Results

2.1. Structural Changes in PRF and PRF_CLP Samples at 37 °C

The FTIR spectrum of PRF and PRF_CLP is shown in Figure 2. The FTIR spectra of the samples in Figure 2A,B show the absorption peaks indicating the fibrin phase: peak at 1641 cm^{-1}—amide I (C=O), maximum at 1535 cm^{-1}—amide II (N-H) and amide III (C-N) (decreases at 1310 cm^{-1} and increases at 1236 cm^{-1}) (Figure 2B). Characteristic changes in the FTIR spectra are due to rearrangements in the secondary structure of the protein. According to other studies [26,27], the absorption of different proteins at higher wavelengths (1633–1645 cm^{-1}, 1531–1539 cm^{-1} and 1240 cm^{-1}) occurs mainly due to α-helical structures, whereas the lower wavenumbers (1651 cm^{-1}, 1539 cm^{-1}) are mostly characteristic of β-structures [28]. Thus, the α-structure is more pronounced in the studied sample. A pronounced absorption maximum at 3281 cm^{-1} indicates the presence of an OH group in the fibrin structure.

CLP and clindamycin have a similar molecular structure, except for the phosphate group. The absorption maximum, specific for both CLP and clindamycin, was observed in PRF_CLP samples incubated for 1, 3, and 7 days at 37 °C. The main structural components of clindamycin molecules are characterized by the vibrations of the pyrrole and saccharide rings, which form skeletal vibrations between 1600 and 600 cm^{-1}. The band group indicated in this region is mainly related to C double bond tensile vibrations. Large changes are observed at about 1047 cm^{-1}, which corresponds to the C-C stretching of the pyrrolidine group. It can be seen that as the incubation time of the PRF_CLP samples increases (from 1 to 7 days), the intensity of the C-C bond also increases. The tensile vibrations of the C-O groups bound to the saccharide ring are observed at 1157 cm^{-1} [23]. The band at 640 cm^{-1} corresponds to the tensile vibrations of the C-Cl groups. In the spectra of the PRF_CLP samples, a wide band with a maximum of 3350 cm^{-1} can also be observed, which corresponds to the vibrations of the O-H groups of aromatic alcohols [29].

It is also observed that the intensity of the phosphate group (PO_4^{3-} at 531 cm^{-1}) from CLP increases in the PRF_CLP sample after 7 days of incubation compared to the PRF_CLP sample after 1 day of incubation (Figure 2B). This may be due to the formation of other CLP degradation products or potential contaminants except clindamycin. Wang et al. [30] state that in addition to clindamycin, two other substances are formed: lincomycin-2-phosphate and clindamycin B-2-phosphate. Brown [19], on the other hand, mentioned the formation of three substances—clindamycin 3-phosphate, clindamycin 4-phosphate and clindamycin 2-phosphate. It can be concluded that the possible degradation products increased the intensity of the PO_4^{3-} absorption peak with increasing degradation time.

It has also been observed that the bands characteristic of clindamycin and CLP at 1673 cm^{-1} (NH-C=O) and at 1568 cm^{-1} (C-C) shift to the right in the presence of PRF. The spectra of the PRF_CLP samples show an increase in the absorption peaks of the above bands, which may have been influenced by the interaction of PRF with CLP. The development of additional intensity at 1080 cm^{-1} C-O cyclic ester galactose sugar elongation [31] was also observed for the PRF_CLP sample after 7 days of incubation. Looking at the CLP and clindamycin spectra, this absorption peak is most indicative of clindamycin. Based on the literature [15,17], CLP induces hydrolysis in the presence of blood and converts to clindamycin. It is possible that this hydrolysis and partial conversion to clindamycin is observed in the spectra of PRF_CLP samples.

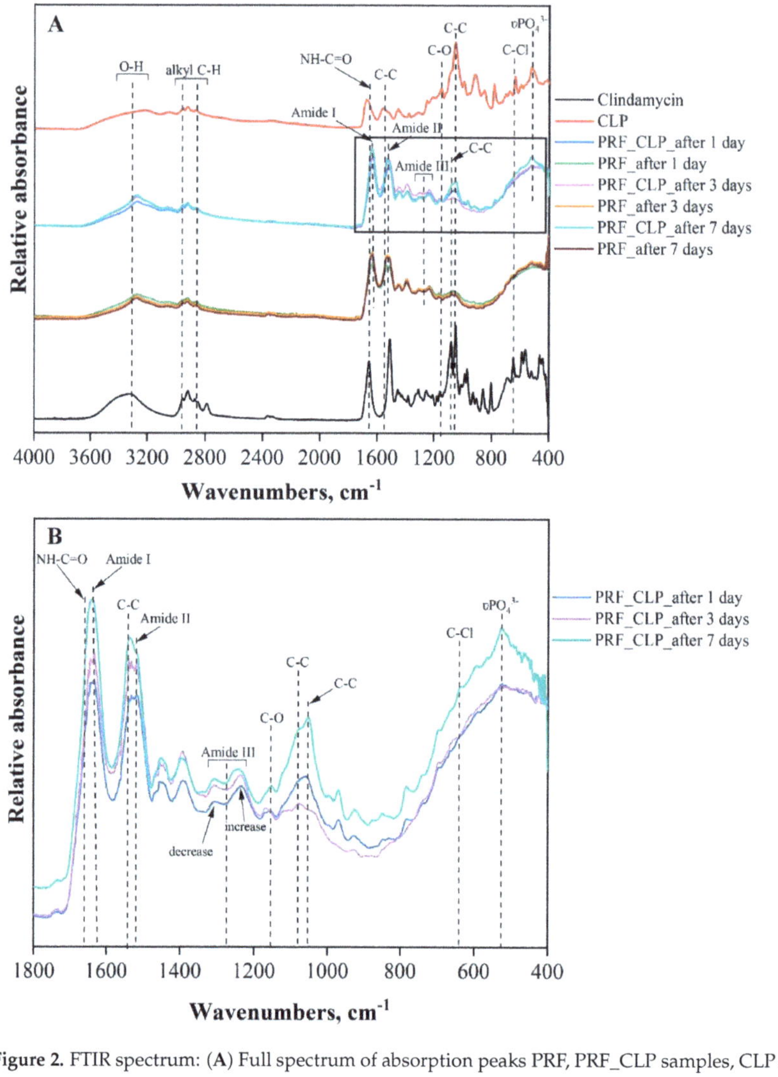

Figure 2. FTIR spectrum: (**A**) Full spectrum of absorption peaks PRF, PRF_CLP samples, CLP and clindamycin; (**B**) FTIR spectrum of PRF_CLP samples at incubation time points.

SEM images of the PRF matrices with and without CLP after incubation and lyophilization are shown in Figure 3. Examining PRF samples with SEM, it can be seen that their surface morphology is irregular with a porous microstructure. There are no visible differences in the structure of the PRF samples depending on the incubation time (1, 3 and 7 days at 37 °C). For PRF_CLP samples after 1-day incubation, crystalline structure formations can be seen on the surface of the sample (marked in the images with a red line), these are also observed after 3 and 7 days.

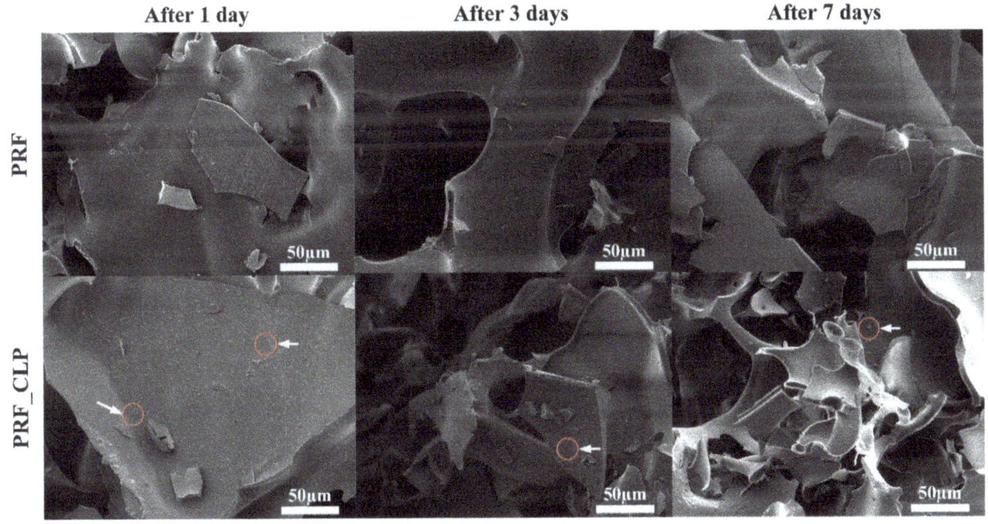

Figure 3. SEM pictures of PRF and PRF_CLP matrix surface; red circles with white arrows indicate the existence of NaCl in the PRF samples.

Comparing the PRF and PRF_CLP samples, it can be seen that the addition of CLP did not significantly affect the structure of the PRF after 1 and 3 days of incubation. In turn, after 7 days of incubation, small network formations are observed on the surface of the PRF_CLP sample. This could be related to the degradation of CLP, thus changing the structure of the PRF.

According to the SEM-EDX data, the crystalline structures present in the PRF_CLP sample contain a large amount of NaCl. PRF contains Na ions and according to Pradid et al., the Cl peaks indicate the presence of clindamycin phosphate [32].

2.2. Drug Release Kinetics

CLP release from PRF matrices was determined by incubating PRF matrices for 0.25, 0.5, 1, 2, 4, 6, 17 and 24 h (Figure 4).

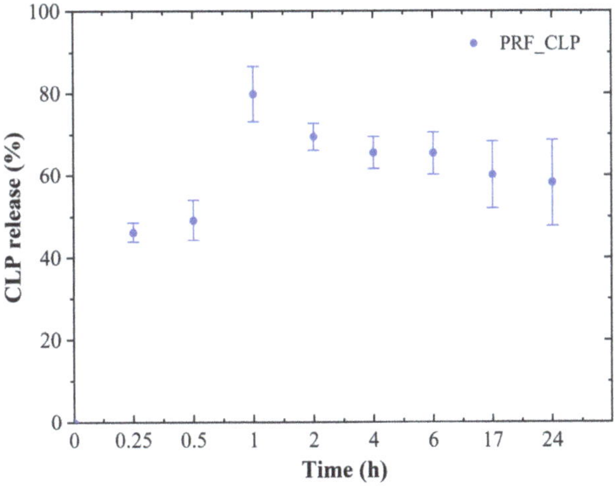

Figure 4. CLP release from PRF matrices in DMEM; average of 3 donor release data.

Burst release of CLP was observed for all PRF_CLP samples in the first incubation hour, when 80% of the encapsulated CLP was released. Based on the obtained data, it is possible to provide local antibacterial activity in a certain place in the first hours, thus reducing the risk of infection during the postoperative period. For long-term treatment, drug delivery systems should be used to prevent burst release during the first hours. ANOVA tests show that at $p < 0.05$, there is no significant difference between drug release from different donor samples.

2.3. Effect of PRF_CLP on Antibacterial Properties

Four Gram-positive bacterial cultures and three donors were used to evaluate and compare the antibacterial properties between CLP, PRF and PRF_CLP samples (Figures 5 and 6).

As shown in Figure 5, the MIC and MBC values for pure CLP solution were first determined to test the ability of the substance to provide an antibacterial effect against selected bacterial cultures. The data showed that against *S. aureus* (ATCC 25923), *S. epidermidis* (ATCC 12228) and *S. epidermidis* (clinical isolate), higher CLP concentrations (1000 μg/mL) were required if compared to *S. aureus* (clinical isolate)—500 μg/mL. In general, high CLP concentrations (1000 μg/mL) are required for maximal effect.

Obtained results showed that negative control (PRF_CLP_broth solution) has an increased level of absorption in the higher concentrations, due to the autologous PRF sample. This is because the PRF has a color that comes from the blood sample. According to the obtained results for each donor's antibacterial properties, MIC and MBC levels for PRF_CLP samples depend on the donor and the bacteria strain. In general, we observed that the incorporation of CLP within the PRF leads to lower MIC and MBC values for all donors and all bacteria strains (Figure 6).

The mean donor MIC values for PRF_CLP samples ranged from 52.1 to 62.5 μg/mL, which are lower than the MIC values for pure CLP samples (ranging from 125 to 250 μg/mL). In turn, the mean MBC values range from 62.5 to 145.8 μg/mL, while for pure CLP samples they are at 500—1000 μg/mL. Differences in MIC and MBC values are affected by the bacteria selected for testing (Figures S1 and S2).

As shown in Figure 6, there is a difference in the MIC value of the donor 1 PRF_CLP samples against *S. aureus* (ATCC 25923). It is lower (31.25 μg/mL) than against three other bacterial cultures (62.5 μg/mL). For donor 2 PRF_CLP samples, lower MIC (31.25 μg/mL) and MBC (62.5 μg/mL) values were observed against *S. epidermidis* (ATCC 12228) than for other donor samples. Finally, for donor 3 PRF_CLP samples, there is a difference in MIC values against *S. epidermidis* (clinical isolate); it is higher (125 μg/mL) than against *S. aureus* (ATCC 25923), *S. aureus* (clinical isolate), *S. epidermidis* (ATCC 12228)—62.5 μg/mL. A higher MBC value (250 μg/mL) is observed for clinical isolates of both bacteria. In turn, for the bacteria reference cultures, a lower MBC value (62.5 μg/mL) is observed against *S. epidermidis* than against *S. aureus* (125 μg/mL).

A U-shaped histogram is displayed in the test sections (see Figure 7). This is well observed in the negative control (PRF_CLP_broth), where the absorption capacity gradually decreases with increasing control dilution. The antibacterial data of all prepared PRF_CLP samples showed differences between the donors and the related MIC and MBC values of the samples (Figure 7). For PRF_CLP samples from donor 2 and donor 3 blood, all antibacterial data can be found in an additional file (Figure S3).

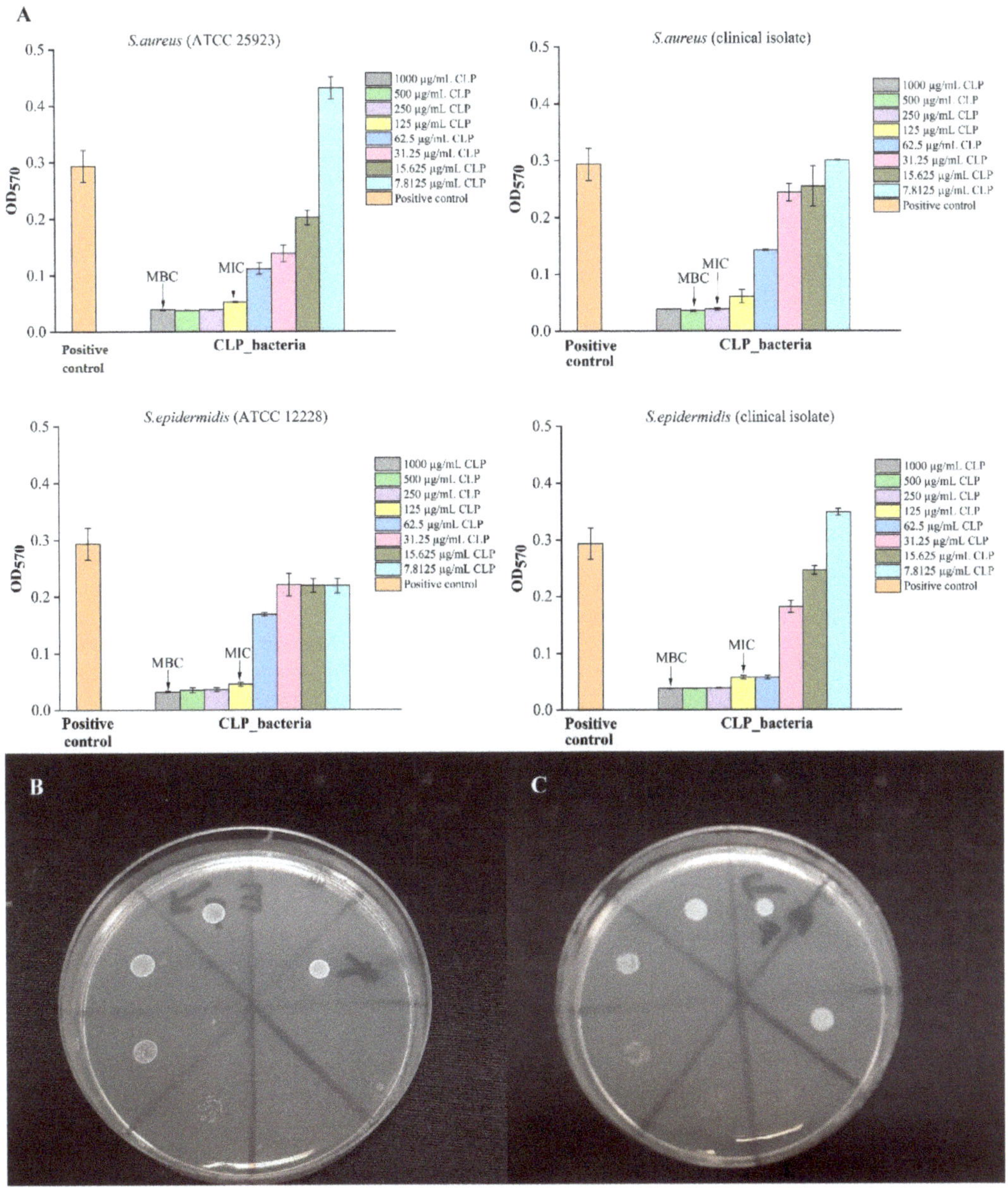

Figure 5. Antibacterial properties of different CLP solutions at various concentrations: (**A**) detected MIC and MBC concentrations for 4 bacteria (*S. aureus* (ATCC 25923), *S. epidermidis* (ATCC 12228), *S. aureus* (clinical isolate), *S. epidermidis* (clinical isolate); (**B**) MBC test for *S. aureus* (clinical isolate); (**C**) MBC test for *S. aureus* (ATCC 25923). The diameter of the Petri dishes is 8.5 cm.

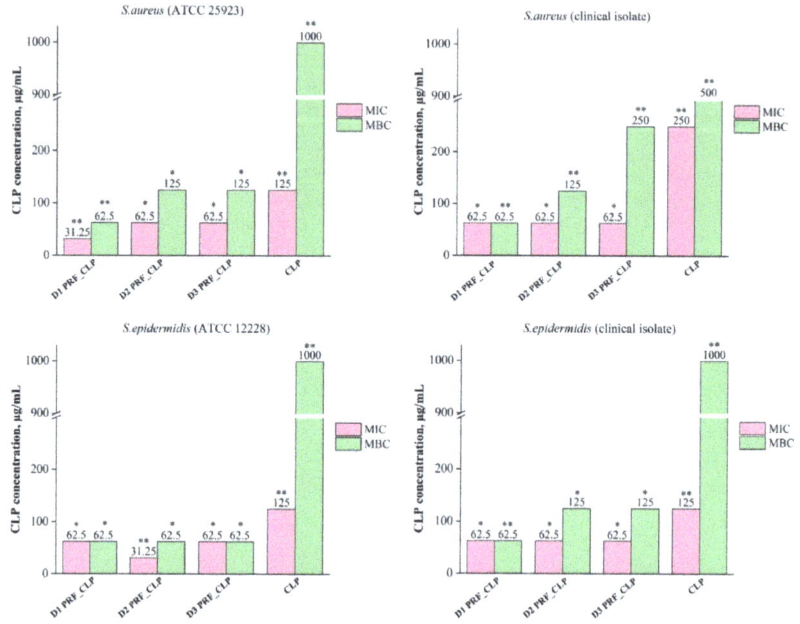

Figure 6. MIC and MBC value differences between CLP and PRF_CLP samples against four bacteria stains (*S. aureus* (ATCC 25923), *S. epidermidis* (ATCC 12228), *S. aureus* (clinical isolate) and *S. epidermidis* (clinical isolate) for all three donors. Samples prepared from donor 1 blood (D1 PRF_CLP); samples prepared from donor 2 (D2 PRF_CLP); samples prepared from donor 3 (D3 PRF_CLP). * $p > 0.05$; ** $p < 0.05$.

Comparing the results of PRF_CLP samples between *S. aureus* reference cultures and clinical isolates, it is observed that only for the donor 3 PRF_CLP samples require a higher CLP concentration (250 µg/mL) against the clinical isolate than against the reference culture (125 µg/mL) (Figure 7). Regarding MIC values, it was observed that only the donor 1 PRF_CLP samples against the clinical isolates required a higher CLP concentration (62.5 µg/mL) than against the reference culture (31.25 µg/mL).

From the results of PRF_CLP samples against the *S. epidermidis* reference culture and clinical isolate (Figure 7), we observed that there is a difference in MIC values for donor 2 PRF_CLP samples, with a higher CLP concentration to the clinical isolate (62.5 µg/mL) than to the reference cultures (31.25 µg/mL) being required to ensure antibacterial activity. MBC values required to provide antibacterial activity against both types of *S. epidermidis* bacteria differ from the *S. aureus* results described above. Looking at the results for donor 2 and donor 3 PRF_CLP samples, it was shown that a higher CLP concentration (125 µg/mL) was required against the *S. epidermidis* clinical isolate and a lower concentration against the *S. epidermidis* reference culture.

Differences in MIC and MBC values against a particular bacterial strain for all three donors are shown in Figure 6. Significantly, a higher MBC value—1000 µg/mL—was observed for CLP samples compared to all donor PRF_CLP samples against each bacterial strain. MBC value against *S. epidermidis* (ATCC 12228) decreased 16-fold for all donor PRF_CLP samples compared to the CLP samples, but decreased 8–16-fold against *S. epidermidis* (clinical isolate) and *S. aureus* (ATCC 25923). The efficacy of PRF_CLP samples against *S. aureus* (clinical isolate) is seen as a 4–16-fold reduction in the MBC value. Thus, indicating that the addition of the required CLP concentration to provide an antibacterial effect against the same bacteria varies greatly depending on the donor PRF. The average

MIC and MBC values of all antibacterial data for all PRF_CLP samples can be found in an additional file (Figures S1 and S2).

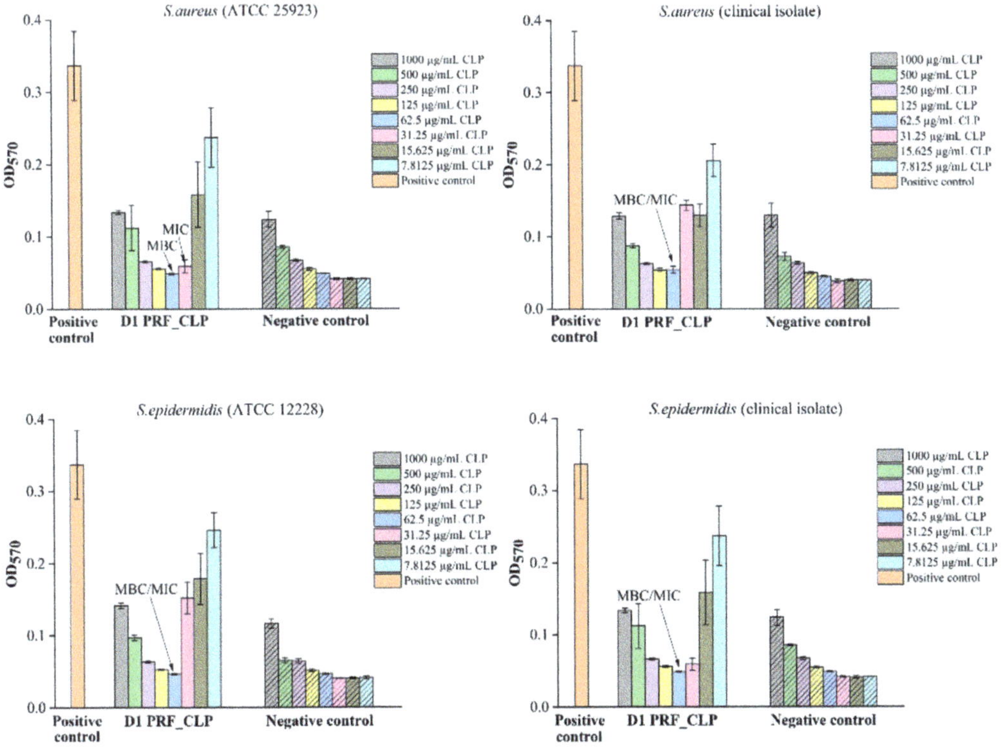

Figure 7. Antibacterial properties of PRF_CLP samples at various concentrations of CLP solution for 4 bacteria strains (*S. aureus* (ATCC 25923), *S. epidermidis* (ATCC 12228), *S. aureus* (clinical isolate) and *S. epidermidis* (clinical isolate) for PRF_CLP samples prepared from donor 1 blood. Pure bacterial suspension (10^6 CFU/mL) as a positive control and pure sterile Mueller–Hinton broth as a negative control were used.

2.4. Cell Viability

The obtained cell cytotoxicity results for PRF and PRF_CLP are shown in Figure 8. Fibroblasts are used for material testing because they have a wide range of functions in the human body, one of them being as part of connective tissue. As PRF has contact with fibroblasts in the body, it is important to test the biomaterial effect on them.

Precise results could be obtained after 24 h and 48 h. The reason for the vague results after 1 h, 2 h and 4 h is that PRF contains many cells, for example, leukocytes, monocytes, red blood cell platelets, neutrophils and lymphocytes [33], which affected cell staining (Figure 9). It should be noted that no difference was observed between PRF samples containing CLP and those not. The experiment had three controls—pure 10 mg/mL CLP solution, untreated cells (positive control) and cells treated with 5% DMSO (negative control).

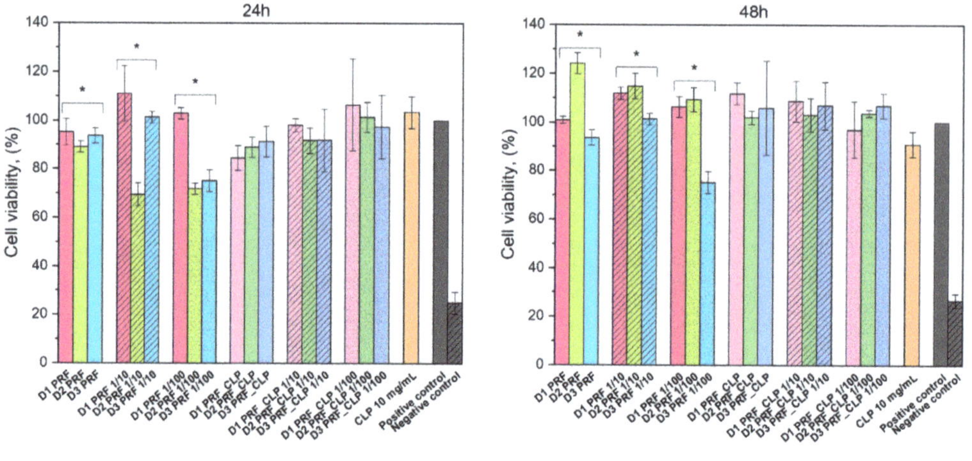

Figure 8. Cytotoxicity of PRF and PRF-CLP extracts and dilutions (significant statistical difference (* $p < 0.05$)).

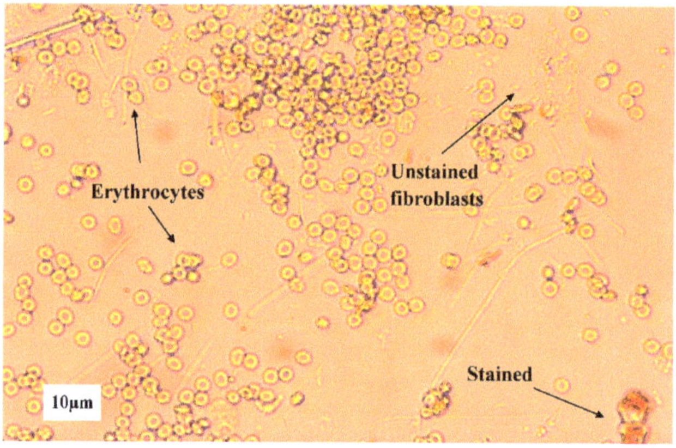

Figure 9. Different blood cells on 3T3 fibroblast cells from D2 PRF sample extract taken after 1 h.

Cell viability was above 70% for both PRF and PRF_CLP extracts and their dilutions were taken after 24 h and 48 h. According to ISO 10993-5:2009, a cytotoxicity effect is considered if the cell viability is decreased by more than 30% [34]. Dilutions did not show significant differences with extracts; however, PRF samples from different donors did have significant statistical differences (* $p < 0.05$). With PRF_CLP samples, there is a small trend of cell viability increasing with dilution, but there is no trend visible with pure PRF samples, which indicates that dilution does not have a significant effect on cell viability.

3. Discussion

This study examined the ability of CLP to convert to clindamycin in the presence of PRF, to provide higher antibacterial activity than PRF and CLP alone. To date, no one has studied the hydrolysis of CLP in the blood without a specific chemical reaction, nor the ability of CLP to enhance the antibacterial properties of PRF. The structure, surface properties, antibacterial properties and drug release kinetics of PRF_CLP were tested.

As observed in the FTIR spectra, CLP interacts with PRF during the incubation for 7 days to provide partial hydrolysis and conversion to clindamycin. After seven days of incubation, a new bond formation and a phosphate group absorption maximum increase over time were observed, indicating structural changes that are likely to be a CLP switch to clindamycin. In addition, other impurities or degradation products than clindamycin can be formed during the degradation of clindamycin phosphate. Brown [19] mentions that in addition to free clindamycin, clindamycin 3-phosphate, clindamycin 4-phosphate and clindamycin 2-phosphate are formed during conversion. In contrast, Wang et al. [30] described the clindamycin phosphate degradation experiment, indicating that in addition to clindamycin, lincomycin-2-phosphate and a small amount of clindamycin B-2-phosphate are formed. Based on the obtained SEM results, we can conclude that the addition of CLP does not significantly affect the structure of PRF. Minor changes are observed during CLP degradation.

Release data suggest that the PRF_CLP sample can be used for one day local therapy, ensuring maximum CLP release within 1 h. Wang et al., 2020, combined clindamycin (2 μg/mL) with PRP, indicating that 90% of the administered dose was excreted within 10 min [35]. As we can see, our material is able to provide longer release kinetics. In the same way, the release time of the drug could be adjusted according to the required therapy by administering drug delivery systems.

The composition of the blood from each of the donors affects the antibacterial properties of the sample, specifically the amount of CLP required to achieve antibacterial activity. Comparing the MIC and MBC values of the PRF_CLP samples with pure CLP samples for all bacteria strains, a decrease in these values is observed with the addition of PRF to the CLP. The widespread increase in staphylococcal resistance to most antimicrobials, especially in resistant strains, points to the need for new effective treatments for staphylococcal infections [36]. Our antibacterial tests showed that the addition of PRF enhances the antibacterial activity of CLP not only against staphylococcal reference cultures but also against clinical isolates. It can be seen that against the clinical isolates of *S. aureus* and *S. epidermidis*, higher CLP concentrations are required in PRF_CLP samples to provide a lower MBC value compared to both bacteria reference cultures. Each donor has different blood properties (such as different white blood cell counts or vitamin D levels) that drastically affect the antibacterial effect and that is why we have such high error limits. All microbiological input data for all three donor PRF_CLP samples are shown in the supplement (Figure S2). The spread of the *S. aureus* strains that are resistant to certain antibiotics has been reported [37]. According to the Daum [38] and Naimi [39] studies, methicillin-resistant *S. aureus* (MRSA) isolates tend to be sensitive to clindamycin and are less likely to be resistant to antibiotics other than the β-lactam class. The same may be for the *S. epidermidis* clinical isolate. Studies from Schilcher et al. [40,41] and Kuriyama et al. [42] showed that the MIC of pure clindamycin in clinical isolates against MRSA can reach > 256 mg/L. Based on the review of the literature, studies have been performed to test the activity of CLP and clindamycin against dermally important microorganisms. The results showed that CLP had antimicrobial activity against the same organisms as clindamycin, with only a 3 to 44 times higher concentration dose [22]. Summarizing all the data, it can be seen that CLP with PRF is a better antibacterial material than pure CLP, and compared to the literature; we have obtained lower MIC values (ranging from 62.5 to 145.8 μg/mL depending on the bacterial strain) than required for clindamycin (>256 μg/mL) [40–42]. Depending on the bacterial strain, the concentration of the drug has to be adjusted.

To ensure that the obtained PRF_CLP matrices can be used for medical applications, in vitro cell viability tests were performed. The highest cell viability can be observed for 48 h extract and dilutions, where it increases above 100% for most of the samples. An increase in viability indicates that PRF increases cell proliferation [43]. PRF is known to be rich in transforming growth factor-β (TGF-β), platelet-derived growth factor (PDGF), vascular endothelial growth factor (VEGF) and epidermal growth factor (EGF) [44], which all have a significant role in new cell formation. Overall, CLP has a favorable effect on cell viability. By adding the antibiotic to PRF, the viability does not go below 80% in the extracts for the prepared time points. Navarro et al. [45] tested periodontal ligament (PDL) cell viability in

PRF and concluded that PRF increases cell viability after PDL is exposed to PRF for 30 min, 1 h and 2 h. In this case, it can be noted that all the PRF ingredients have a favorable effect on PDL cells. The positive effect of PRF was also noticed in a Bucur et al. [46] study on the blood clot effect on fibroblast proliferation and migration. The samples were tested for 24 h and 48 h and in both cases, PRF positively affected cell viability; the same can be observed in our experiment. An interesting difference between the studies is that Bucur et al. filtered the testing solution before applying it to cells to remove blood cells. This should be taken into account for future experiments.

4. Materials and Methods

4.1. Materials

Clindamycin phosphate (CLP, Sigma Aldrich, St. Louis, MO 63103, USA), acetonitrile (≥99.9%, Sigma-Aldrich, St. Louis, MI, USA), phosphoric acid (H_3PO_4; C = 75% *w/w*, Latvijas ķīmija, Riga, Latvia), potassium dihydrogen phosphate (KH_2PO_4, Sigma Aldrich, ≥99%), methanol (≥99.9%, Sigma-Aldrich, St. Louis, MI, USA), Dulbecco's Modified Eagle's Medium (DMEM, Sigma Aldrich, St. Louis, MO, USA), bovine calf serum (CS, Sigma-Aldrich, St. Louis, MO, USA), Penicillin/Streptomycin (P/S, Sigma-Aldrich, St. Louis, MO, USA), dimethylsulfoxide (DMSO, Sigma-Aldrich, St. Louis, MO, USA), neutral red (NR, Sigma Aldrich, St. Louis, MO, USA), Phosphate Buffer Saline (PBS, Sigma-Aldrich, St. Louis, MO, USA), acetic acid (Sigma-Aldrich, St. Louis, MO, USA), ethanol (96%, Latvian Chemistry, Riga, Latvia).

4.2. Blood Collection and Platelet-Rich Fibrin Production

Blood of 3 healthy volunteers with vitamin D levels > 30 ng/mL was collected in 13 mL i-PRF+ tubes (PROCESS FOR PRF, 06000 Nice, France) and immediately placed in a centrifuge ("PRF DUO Quattro"). PRF was obtained by centrifugation at 700 rpm for 5 min (for women) or 6 min (for men). After the centrifugation, the upper layer of liquid PRF (1 mL) from one donor of each tube was transferred into a 50 mL tube, and mixed together for further use.

An amount of 0.5 mL of liquid PRF was used to obtain one PRF sample. To prepare PRF samples with CLP (PRF_CLP), 0.5 mL PRF was added to pre-weighed 0.5 mg CLP with an automatic pipette and mixed well with a spatula. Samples for FTIR and SEM analysis were prepared by incubation (Environmental Shaker-Incubator ES-20, Biosan, Riga, Latvia) at 37 °C for 1, 3 and 7 days and then lyophilized for 72 h. For drug release and cell experiments, coagulated PRF and PRF_CLP samples were used.

Written consent from all of the volunteers for use of their samples in the research studies was obtained. All donors were free of any infectious disease and had no abnormal nicotine or alcohol use. None of the subjects used any anticoagulant drugs. Permission No. 6-2/10/53 of the Research Ethics Committee of Riga Stradins University was obtained for the study.

4.3. Characterization of Prepared Samples

4.3.1. Chemical Structure

The lyophilized PRF and PRF with CLP (PRF_CLP) samples after 1, 3 and 7 days of incubation were investigated with Fourier-transform infrared spectroscopy (FTIR) attenuated total reflection (ATR) method, to identify functional groups in PRF matrix. ATR spectroscopy spectra were taken with Thermo Fisher Scientific Nicolet iS5 with a diamond crystal. Spectra were recorded from 500 to 4000 cm^{-1} with 64 scans and with a resolution of 4 cm^{-1}, optical velocity 0.4747, and aperture 100%.

4.3.2. Morphology

Scanning electron microscope Tescan Mira/LMU (Tescan, Brno, Czech Republic) was used to visualize the microstructure and morphology of obtained PRF and PRF_CLP samples. Prior to examination, samples were fixed to aluminum pin stubs with conductive carbon tape and sputter coated with thin layer of gold at 25 mA for 3 min using Emitech K550X (Quorum Technologies, Ashford, Kent, UK). Secondary electrons created at 5 kV were used.

4.3.3. Evaluation of CLP Kinetics

Evaluation of CLP release kinetics was analyzed using ultra-performance liquid chromatography. The chromatographic method was adapted based on other studies [47,48]. A chromatograph "Waters Acquity UPLC H-class" with a UV/VIS detector "Waters Acquity TUV" at 195 nm and column "Waters Acquity UPLC BEH C18, 1.7 μm, 2.1 × 150 mm" was used for data acquisition. The mobile phase consisted of 0.02M KH_2PO_4 buffer (PH = 2.5 ± 0.02): acetonitrile in ratio 79:21, respectively, and at a flow rate of 0.3 mL/min. The total analysis time for one sample was 7 min. During the analysis, the column temperature was maintained at 40 °C ± 5 °C and the sample temperature at 10 °C ± 5 °C. The limit of quantification and the limit of detection for the developed method were found to be 1.157 μg/mL and 0.382 μg/mL.

Samples for CLP release studies were immersed in 20 mL of DMEM and placed in an incubator at 37 °C ± 5 °C. At the first 2 time points (15 min and 30 min), the solution was completely removed, and at the other time points (1 h, 1.5 h, 2 h, 4 h, 6 h, 17 h, 24 h), 2 mL aliquots of the solution were used. Finally, 2 mL of DMEM was returned after each sample to ensure a constant volume during the release experiment.

4.4. *Preparation of Bacterial Suspension*

Four bacterial strains were used in the study, reference culture of *S. aureus* (ATCC 25923) and *S. epidermidis* (ATCC 12228), and clinical isolates of *S. aureus* and *S. epidermidis*, which previously were isolated from the pure sample and identified with VITEK2 system (bioMérieux, Marcy l'Etoile, France). Before the antibacterial tests, bacterial susceptibility against clindamycin was tested with the disc diffusion method. All bacterial suspensions were prepared according to EUCAST (European Committee on Antimicrobial Susceptibility Testing) standards in optic density of 0.5 according to McFarland standard with optic densitometer (Biosan, Riga, Latvia). All bacterial strains showed sensitivity against clindamycin (2 μg) discs (Liofilchem S.r.l., Roseto degli Abruzzi, Italy).

4.5. *Determination of Antibacterial Properties*

The antibacterial tests were investigated with EUCAST (European Committee on Antimicrobial Susceptibility Testing) standard laboratory antibacterial susceptibility testing method—broth microdilution (Figure 10) [49,50].

4.5.1. Determination of Minimal Inhibitory Concentration

Three different test sample solutions were used: pure PRF, PRF_CLP and pure CLP. Samples with PRF were diluted 1:5, accordingly 2 mL PRF and 8 mL Mueller–Hinton broth (MHB) (Oxoid, UK) to obtain 2 mg/mL stock solution of CLP. A 96-well plate (SARSTEDT, Nümbrecht, Germany) was used in the quantitative assay. Twofold serial dilutions of the pure CLP and PRF_CLP stock solutions (ranging between 2000 and 7.8125 μg/mL) were performed in a 100 μL volume. Each well was seeded with 100 μL of bacterial suspension (10^6 CFU/mL, 0.5 McFarland density), where 200 μL of pure bacterial suspension (10^6 CFU/mL) served as positive control while pure sterile MHB served as negative controls. To detect the MIC and MBC values we used PRF_CLP controls in broth with and without bacteria. After 2-fold dilution, instead of adding bacterial suspension, sterile MHB was added. Then, 96-well plates were incubated in a thermostat (Memmert GmbH, Schwabach, Germany) for 18 h at 37 °C. MIC values were considered as the lowest concentration of the tested solution that inhibits bacterial growth in microdilution wells as visually detected. After incubation, the values of absorbance were measured with microplate reader at 570 nm (Tecan Infinite F50, Männedorf, Switzerland).

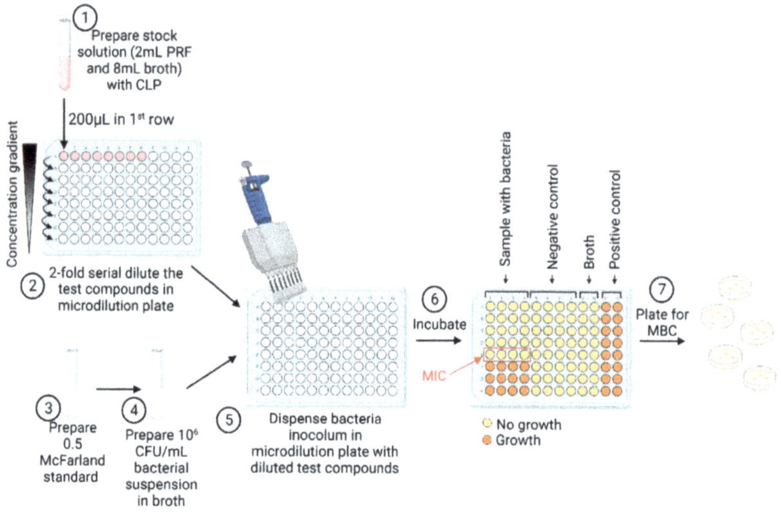

Figure 10. The MIC/MBC assay of CLP, PRF and PRF_CLP samples. Figure created with Biorender.com.

4.5.2. Determination of Minimal Bactericidal Concentration

The lowest concentration at which bacterial growth was completely inhibited by the additional culture method on non-selective media was taken as the MBC value. To determine MBC, extra cultivation of 10 μL samples from the wells (prepared according to the methodology specified in Section 4.5.1) were inoculated on non-selective agar plates (Oxoid, UK); one sample from the well above the MIC value and all remaining below MIC value (MIC values based on data from methodology 4.5.1 were used). Agar plates were incubated in a thermostat (Memmert GmbH, Schwabach, Germany) for 18 h at 37 °C.

4.6. Cell Viability Experiments

PRF with and without CLP was tested on 3T3 mouse fibroblasts. Overall PRFs from 3 different donors were tested.

Prior to cell viability tests, 5000 cells were seeded in a 96-well plate in 200 μL of full cell medium. To prevent the plates from drying out, PBS was added to the outer wells. After seeding the cells, the plates were incubated overnight (37 °C, 5%) (New Brunswick™ S41i CO_2 Incubator Shaker, Eppendorf, Hamburg, Germany).

The following day each PRF sample with and without CLP was submerged in 2 mL of full cell medium. The medium consisted of 89% DMEM, 10% CS and 1% P/S. After 1, 2, 4, 24 and 48 h, all the solution was removed from the testing sample and replaced with a fresh 2 mL cell medium. Extract and 2 types of dilutions—1:10 and 1:100—were directly put onto the cells. Before adding the analyzing solution to the cells, the old medium was removed. The experiment had two types of controls. The positive control consisted of untreated cells with medium; on the other hand, for the negative control, 5% DMSO solution in cell medium was applied to cells to analyze their viability. Each treatment had 6 replicates.

To analyze the PRF extract and its dilutions effect on cell viability, Natural Red (NR) test was used. The tests included PBS, NR and solubility solution (1% acetic acid, 50% ethanol, 49% water).

After 24 h of each time point, the testing solutions were discarded and cells were washed with 200 μL PBS solution. Subsequently, cells were treated with 150 μL NR solution, after which plates were left to incubate for 2 h. Afterward, the solution with dye was taken off, and cells were washed again with 250 μL PBS solution. Finally, cells were solubilized, which was done with a 150 μL solubilization solution. Then, a 540 nm wavelength was used to measure optical density with a microplate reader (Tecan Infinite M Nano, Switzerland). Every plate was analyzed appropriately with the method just described.

4.7. Statistical Evaluation

All results are expressed as the mean ± standard deviation (SD) of at least three independent samples. The reliability of the results was assessed using the unpaired Student's t-test with a significance level of $p < 0.05$. One—and two-way analysis of variance (ANOVA) was performed to assess the differences between the results.

5. Conclusions

The results of the present study show the structure, surface properties, antibacterial properties, drug release kinetics, and cell viability of the PRF_CLP samples. Burst release (80% of CLP after 1 h) was observed for the PRF_CLP samples; thus, the development of more advanced drug delivery systems could be an area for future research. The antibacterial effect of CLP was affected by the addition of PRF, thus providing a reduction in MIC and MBC concentrations compared to pure CLP and pure PRF samples. Cell viability for the PRF_CLP samples increased indicating the ability of PRF to alter cell proliferation. Structural studies have also shown that clindamycin phosphate is converted to clindamycin within the PRF matrix at 37 °C.

This study proves that the presence of PRF in the resulting PRF_CLP samples improves the antibacterial efficacy and may be suitable for medical applications. The results are the first step in finding alternative solutions that can enhance the antibacterial properties of CLP to prevent postoperative infections and could lead to a new method to be developed, which may increase the efficiency of drug delivery and activity. Further clinical trials with larger patient groups are needed to introduce this method for reducing the risk of post-operative infections.

Supplementary Materials: The following supporting information can be downloaded at: https://www.mdpi.com/article/10.3390/ijms23137407/s1.

Author Contributions: Conceptualization, writing—original draft preparation, writing—review and editing, methodology, formal analysis, visualization, K.E.; conceptualization, writing—review and editing, methodology, I.S. (Ingus Skadins); writing, methodology, formal analysis, A.G.; writing, methodology, L.M.; assistance in the development of the UPLC method V.D.; conceptualization, writing—review and editing, methodology, I.S. (Ilze Salma); writing—review and editing, supervision, funding acquisition, project administration, conceptualization, A.D. All authors have read and agreed to the published version of the manuscript.

Funding: This research was funded by the Latvian Council of Science research project No. lzp-2020/1-0054 "Development of antibacterial autologous fibrin matrices in maxillofacial surgery" (MATRI-X).

Institutional Review Board Statement: The study was conducted according to the guidelines of the Declaration of Helsinki, and approved by the Research Ethics Committee at Riga Stradins University, Latvia, Permission No. 6-2/10/53, 28 November 2019.

Informed Consent Statement: Written informed consent has been obtained from the patients to publish this paper.

Data Availability Statement: The data presented in this study are available on request from the corresponding author.

Acknowledgments: The authors acknowledge financial support from the Latvian Council of Science research project "Development of antibacterial autologous fibrin matrices in maxillofacial surgery" (MATRI-X) under agreement No. lzp-2020/1-0054. This work was also supported by the European Union's Horizon 2020 research and innovation programme under the grant agreement No 857287 (BBCE). The authors thank Agnese Brangule for her help with FTIR analysis.

Conflicts of Interest: The authors declare no conflict of interest related to this study.

References

1. Chou, T.; Chang, H.; Wang, J. Autologous platelet concentrates in maxillofacial regenerative therapy. *Kaohsiung J. Med. Sci.* **2020**, *36*, 305–310. [CrossRef] [PubMed]
2. Fan, Y.; Perez, K.; Dym, H. Clinical Uses of Platelet-Rich Fibrin in Oral and Maxillofacial Surgery. *Dent. Clin. N. Am.* **2020**, *64*, 291–303. [CrossRef] [PubMed]
3. Jasmine, S.; Thangavelu, A.; Janarthanan, K.; Krishnamoorthy, R.; Alshatwi, A.A. Antimicrobial and antibiofilm potential of injectable platelet rich fibrin—a second-generation platelet concentrate—against biofilm producing oral *staphylococcus* isolates. *Saudi J. Biol. Sci.* **2020**, *27*, 41–46. [CrossRef] [PubMed]
4. Kour, P.; Pudakalkatti, P.; Vas, A.; Das, S.; Padmanabhan, S. Comparative evaluation of antimicrobial efficacy of platelet-rich plasma, platelet-rich fibrin, and injectable platelet-rich fibrin on the standard strains of *Porphyromonas gingivalis* and *Aggregatibacter actinomycetemcomitans*. *Contemp. Clin. Dent.* **2018**, *9*, S325. [CrossRef]
5. Heal, C.; Buettner, P.; Browning, S. Risk factors for wound infection after minor surgery in general practice. *Med. J. Aust.* **2006**, *185*, 255–258. [CrossRef]
6. Zhang, J.; Xu, Q.; Huang, C.; Mo, A.; Li, J.; Zuo, Y. Biological properties of an anti-bacterial membrane for guided bone regeneration: An experimental study in rats. *Clin. Oral Implant. Res.* **2010**, *21*, 321–327. [CrossRef]
7. Tong, S.Y.C.; Davis, J.S.; Eichenberger, E.; Holland, T.L.; Fowler, V.G. *Staphylococcus aureus* Infections: Epidemiology, Pathophysiology, Clinical Manifestations, and Management. *Clin. Microbiol. Rev.* **2015**, *28*, 603–661. [CrossRef]
8. Pollitt, E.J.G.; Szkuta, P.T.; Burns, N.; Foster, S.J. *Staphylococcus aureus* infection dynamics. *PLoS Pathog.* **2018**, *14*, e1007112. [CrossRef]
9. DeLeo, F.R.; Diep, B.A.; Otto, M. Host Defense and Pathogenesis in *Staphylococcus aureus* Infections. *Infect. Dis. Clin. N. Am.* **2009**, *23*, 17–34. [CrossRef]
10. Martinez-Aguilar, G.; Hammerman, W.A.; Mason, E.O.; Kaplan, S.L. Clindamycin treatment of invasive infections caused by community-acquired, methicillin-resistant and methicillin-susceptible *Staphylococcus aureus* in children. *Pediatr. Infect. Dis. J.* **2003**, *22*, 593–599. [CrossRef]
11. Mohamed, M.A.; Nasr, M.; Elkhatib, W.F.; Eltayeb, W.N.; Elshamy, A.A.; El-Sayyad, G.S. Nanobiotic formulations as promising advances for combating MRSA resistance: Susceptibilities and post-antibiotic effects of clindamycin, doxycycline, and linezolid. *RSC Adv.* **2021**, *11*, 39696–39706. [CrossRef] [PubMed]
12. Foster, T.J.; Geoghegan, J.A.; Ganesh, V.K.; Höök, M. Adhesion, invasion and evasion: The many functions of the surface proteins of *Staphylococcus aureus*. *Nat. Rev. Microbiol.* **2014**, *12*, 49–62. [CrossRef] [PubMed]
13. Fortunato, L.; Bennardo, F.; Buffone, C.; Giudice, A. Is the application of platelet concentrates effective in the prevention and treatment of medication-related osteonecrosis of the jaw? A systematic review. *J. Cranio-Maxillofac. Surg.* **2020**, *48*, 268–285. [CrossRef] [PubMed]
14. Maestre-Vera, J.R. Treatment options in odontogenic infection. *Med. Oral Patol. Oral Cir. Bucal* **2004**, *9* (Suppl. S25–S31), 19–24.
15. Li, H.; Deng, J.; Yue, Z.; Zhang, Y.; Sun, H.; Ren, X. Clindamycin hydrochloride and clindamycin phosphate: Two drugs or one? A retrospective analysis of a spontaneous reporting system. *Eur. J. Clin. Pharmacol.* **2017**, *73*, 251–253. [CrossRef] [PubMed]
16. Yang, Y.; Aloysius, H.; Inoyama, D.; Chen, Y.; Hu, L. Enzyme-mediated hydrolytic activation of prodrugs. *Acta Pharm. Sin. B* **2011**, *1*, 143–159. [CrossRef]
17. Stanković, M.; Savić, V.; Marinković, V. Determination of Clindamycin Phosphate in Different Vaginal Gel Formulations by Reverse Phase High Performance Liquid Chromatography. *Acta Fac. Med. Naissensis* **2013**, *30*, 63–71. [CrossRef]
18. Morozowich, W.; Karnes, H.A. Case Study: Clindamycin 2-Phosphate, A Prodrug of Clindamycin. In *Prodrugs*; Springer: New York, NY, USA, 2007; pp. 1207–1219.
19. Brown, L.W. High-Pressure Liquid Chromatographic Assays for Clindamycin, Clindamycin Phosphate, and Clindamycin Palmitate. *J. Pharm. Sci.* **1978**, *67*, 1254–1257. [CrossRef]
20. Borin, M.T.; Ryan, K.K.; Hopkins, N.K. Systemic Absorption of Clindamycin after Intravaginal Administration of Clindamycin Phosphate Ovule or Cream. *J. Clin. Pharmacol.* **1999**, *39*, 805–810. [CrossRef]
21. Borin, M.T.; Powley, G.W.; Tackwell, K.R.; Batts, D.H. Absorption of clindamycin after intravaginal application of clindamycin phosphate 2% cream. *J. Antimicrob. Chemother.* **1995**, *35*, 833–841. [CrossRef]
22. Amr, S.; Brown, M.B.; Martin, G.P.; Forbes, B. Activation of clindamycin phosphate by human skin. *J. Appl. Microbiol.* **2001**, *90*, 550–554. [CrossRef]
23. Mostafavi, S.; Karkhane, R.; Riazi-Esfahani, M.; Dorkoosh, F.; Rafiee-Tehrani, M.; Tamaddon, L. Thermoanalytical characterization of clindamycin-loaded intravitreal implants prepared by hot melt extrusion. *Adv. Biomed. Res.* **2015**, *4*, 147. [CrossRef] [PubMed]
24. Kilicarslan, M.; Ilhan, M.; Inal, O.; Orhan, K. Preparation and evaluation of clindamycin phosphate loaded chitosan/alginate polyelectrolyte complex film as mucoadhesive drug delivery system for periodontal therapy. *Eur. J. Pharm. Sci.* **2018**, *123*, 441–451. [CrossRef] [PubMed]
25. Usković, V.; Desai, T.A. Simultaneous bactericidal and osteogenic effect of nanoparticulate calcium phosphate powders loaded with clindamycin on osteoblasts infected with *Staphylococcus aureus*. *Mater. Sci. Eng. C* **2014**, *37*, 210–222. [CrossRef] [PubMed]
26. Cai, S.; Singh, B.R. A Distinct Utility of the Amide III Infrared Band for Secondary Structure Estimation of Aqueous Protein Solutions Using Partial Least Squares Methods. *Biochemistry* **2004**, *43*, 2541–2549. [CrossRef]

27. Jackson, M.; Mantsch, H.H. The Use and Misuse of FTIR Spectroscopy in the Determination of Protein Structure. *Crit. Rev. Biochem. Mol. Biol.* **1995**, *30*, 95–120. [CrossRef]
28. Litvinov, R.I.; Faizullin, D.A.; Zuev, Y.F.; Weisel, J.W. The α-Helix to β-Sheet Transition in Stretched and Compressed Hydrated Fibrin Clots. *Biophys. J.* **2012**, *103*, 1020–1027. [CrossRef]
29. Vukomanović, M.; Zavašnik-Bergant, T.; Bračko, I.; Škapin, S.D.; Ignjatović, N.; Radmilović, V.; Uskoković, D. Poly(d,l-lactide-co-glycolide)/hydroxyapatite core–shell nanospheres. Part 3: Properties of hydroxyapatite nano-rods and investigation of a distribution of the drug within the composite. *Colloids Surf. B Biointerfaces* **2011**, *87*, 226–235. [CrossRef]
30. Wang, S.-M.; Bu, S.-S.; Liu, H.-M.; Li, H.-Y.; Liu, W.; Wang, Y.-D. Separation and characterization of clindamycin phosphate and related impurities in injection by liquid chromatography/electrospray ionization mass spectrometry. *Rapid Commun. Mass Spectrom.* **2009**, *23*, 899–906. [CrossRef]
31. Mohamed, A.; Abd-Motagaly, A.; Ahmed, O.; Amin, S.; Mohamed Ali, A. Investigation of Drug–Polymer Compatibility Using Chemometric-Assisted UV-Spectrophotometry. *Pharmaceutics* **2017**, *9*, 7. [CrossRef]
32. Pradid, J.; Keawwatana, W.; Boonyang, U.; Tangbunsuk, S. Biological properties and enzymatic degradation studies of clindamycin-loaded PLA/HAp microspheres prepared from crocodile bones. *Polym. Bull.* **2017**, *74*, 5181–5194. [CrossRef]
33. Miron, R.J.; Chai, J.; Fujioka-Kobayashi, M.; Sculean, A.; Zhang, Y. Evaluation of 24 protocols for the production of platelet-rich fibrin. *BMC Oral Health* **2020**, *20*, 310. [CrossRef] [PubMed]
34. Mardashev, S.R.; Nikolaev Ya, A.; Sokolov, N.N. Isolation and properties of a homogenous L asparaginase preparation from *Pseudomonas fluorescens* AG (Russian). *Biokhimiya* **1975**, *40*, 984–989.
35. Wang, S.; Li, Y.; Li, S.; Yang, J.; Tang, R.; Li, X.; Li, L.; Fei, J. Platelet-rich plasma loaded with antibiotics as an affiliated treatment for infected bone defect by combining wound healing property and antibacterial activity. *Platelets* **2021**, *32*, 479–491. [CrossRef]
36. Aleksandra, A.; Misic, M.; Mira, Z.; Violeta, N.; Dragana, I.; Zoran, B.; Dejan, V.; Milanko, S.; Dejan, B. Prevalence of inducible clindamycin resistance among community-associated *staphylococcal* isolates in central Serbia. *Indian J. Med. Microbiol.* **2014**, *32*, 49–52. [CrossRef]
37. Indrawattana, N.; Sungkhachat, O.; Sookrung, N.; Chongsa-nguan, M.; Tungtrongchitr, A.; Voravuthikunchai, S.P.; Kong-ngoen, T.; Kurazono, H.; Chaicumpa, W. *Staphylococcus aureus* Clinical Isolates: Antibiotic Susceptibility, Molecular Characteristics, and Ability to Form Biofilm. *Biomed Res. Int.* **2013**, *2013*, 1–11. [CrossRef]
38. Daum, R.S. Skin and Soft-Tissue Infections Caused by Methicillin-Resistant *Staphylococcus aureus*. *N. Engl. J. Med.* **2007**, *357*, 380–390. [CrossRef]
39. Naimi, T.S. Comparison of Community- and Health Care–Associated Methicillin-Resistant *Staphylococcus aureus* Infection. *JAMA* **2003**, *290*, 2976–2984. [CrossRef]
40. Schilcher, K.; Andreoni, F.; Dengler Haunreiter, V.; Seidl, K.; Hasse, B.; Zinkernagel, A.S. Modulation of *Staphylococcus aureus* Biofilm Matrix by Subinhibitory Concentrations of Clindamycin. *Antimicrob. Agents Chemother.* **2016**, *60*, 5957–5967. [CrossRef]
41. Schilcher, K.; Andreoni, F.; Uchiyama, S.; Ogawa, T.; Schuepbach, R.A.; Zinkernagel, A.S. Increased Neutrophil Extracellular Trap–Mediated *Staphylococcus aureus* Clearance Through Inhibition of Nuclease Activity by Clindamycin and Immunoglobulin. *J. Infect. Dis.* **2014**, *210*, 473–482. [CrossRef]
42. Kuriyama, T.; Karasawa, T.; Nakagawa, K.; Saiki, Y.; Yamamoto, E.; Nakamura, S. Bacteriologic features and antimicrobial susceptibility in isolates from orofacial odontogenic infections. *Oral Surg. Oral Med. Oral Pathol. Oral Radiol. Endodontology* **2000**, *90*, 600–608. [CrossRef] [PubMed]
43. Strauss, F.-J.; Nasirzade, J.; Kargarpoor, Z.; Stähli, A.; Gruber, R. Effect of platelet-rich fibrin on cell proliferation, migration, differentiation, inflammation, and osteoclastogenesis: A systematic review of in vitro studies. *Clin. Oral Investig.* **2020**, *24*, 569–584. [CrossRef] [PubMed]
44. Pavlovic, V.; Ciric, M.; Jovanovic, V.; Trandafilovic, M.; Stojanovic, P. Platelet-rich fibrin: Basics of biological actions and protocol modifications. *Open Med.* **2021**, *16*, 446–454. [CrossRef]
45. Navarro, L.B.; Barchiki, F.; Navarro Junior, W.; Carneiro, E.; da Silva Neto, U.X.; Westphalen, V.P.D. Assessment of platelet-rich fibrin in the maintenance and recovery of cell viability of the periodontal ligament. *Sci. Rep.* **2019**, *9*, 19476. [CrossRef] [PubMed]
46. Bucur, M.; Constantin, C.; Neagu, M.; Zurac, S.; Dinca, O.; Vladan, C.; Cioplea, M.; Popp, C.; Nichita, L.; Ionescu, E. Alveolar blood clots and platelet-rich fibrin induce in vitro fibroblast proliferation and migration. *Exp. Ther. Med.* **2018**, *17*, 982–989. [CrossRef] [PubMed]
47. Vella, J.; Busuttil, F.; Bartolo, N.S.; Sammut, C.; Ferrito, V.; Serracino-Inglott, A.; Azzopardi, L.M.; LaFerla, G. A simple HPLC-UV method for the determination of ciprofloxacin in human plasma. *J. Chromatogr. B Anal. Technol. Biomed. Life Sci.* **2015**, *989*, 80–85. [CrossRef]
48. Liu, C.; Chen, Y.; Yang, T.; Hsieh, S.; Hung, M.; Lin, E.T. High-performance liquid chromatographic determination of clindamycin in human plasma or serum: Application to the bioequivalency study of clindamycin phosphate injections. *J. Chromatogr. B Biomed. Sci. Appl.* **1997**, *696*, 298–302. [CrossRef] [PubMed]
49. Balouiri, M.; Sadiki, M.; Ibnsouda, S.K. Methods for in vitro evaluating antimicrobial activity: A review. *J. Pharm. Anal.* **2016**, *6*, 71–79. [CrossRef]
50. Gajic, I.; Kabic, J.; Kekic, D.; Jovicevic, M.; Milenkovic, M.; Mitic Culafic, D.; Trudic, A.; Ranin, L.; Opavski, N. Antimicrobial Susceptibility Testing: A Comprehensive Review of Currently Used Methods. *Antibiotics* **2022**, *11*, 427. [CrossRef]

International Journal of
Molecular Sciences

MDPI

Article

Controllable Nitric Oxide Storage and Release in Cu-BTC: Crystallographic Insights and Bioactivity

Do Nam Lee [1], Yeong Rim Kim [2], Sohyeon Yang [3], Ngoc Minh Tran [4,5], Bong Joo Park [6,*], Su Jung Lee [1], Youngmee Kim [3], Hyojong Yoo [4], Sung-Jin Kim [3] and Jae Ho Shin [2,*]

1 Ingenium College of Liberal Arts (Chemistry), Kwangwoon University, Seoul 01897, Korea
2 Department of Chemistry, Kwangwoon University, Seoul 01897, Korea
3 Nanobio-Energy Materials Center, Department of Chemistry and Nano Science, Ewha Womans University, Seoul 03760, Korea
4 Department of Materials Science and Chemical Engineering, Hanyang University, Ansan-si 15588, Korea
5 Department of Chemistry, University of Sciences, Hue University, Hue City 530000, Vietnam
6 Department of Electrical and Biological Physics, Kwangwoon University, Seoul 01897, Korea
* Correspondence: parkbj@kw.ac.kr (B.J.P.); jhshin@kw.ac.kr (J.H.S.);
Tel.: +82-2-940-8629 (B.J.P.); +82-2-940-5627 (J.H.S.)

Abstract: Crystalline metal–organic frameworks (MOFs) are extensively used in areas such as gas storage and small-molecule drug delivery. Although Cu-BTC (**1**, MOF-199, BTC: benzene-1,3,5-tricarboxylate) has versatile applications, its NO storage and release characteristics are not amenable to therapeutic usage. In this work, micro-sized Cu-BTC was prepared solvothermally and then processed by ball-milling to prepare nano-sized Cu-BTC (**2**). The NO storage and release properties of the micro- and nano-sized Cu-BTC MOFs were morphology dependent. Control of the hydration degree and morphology of the NO delivery vehicle improved the NO release characteristics significantly. In particular, the nano-sized NO-loaded Cu-BTC (NO⊂nano-Cu-BTC, **4**) released NO at 1.81 μmol·mg^{-1} in 1.2 h in PBS, which meets the requirements for clinical usage. The solid-state structural formula of NO⊂Cu-BTC was successfully determined to be $[CuC_6H_2O_5]\cdot(NO)_{0.167}$ through single-crystal X-ray diffraction, suggesting no structural changes in Cu-BTC upon the intercalation of 0.167 equivalents of NO within the pores of Cu-BTC after NO loading. The structure of Cu-BTC was also stably maintained after NO release. NO⊂Cu-BTC exhibited significant antibacterial activity against six bacterial strains, including Gram-negative and positive bacteria. NO⊂Cu-BTC could be utilized as a hybrid NO donor to explore the synergistic effects of the known antibacterial properties of Cu-BTC.

Keywords: nitric oxide; drug delivery; MOFs; antibacterial activity

Citation: Lee, D.N.; Kim, Y.R.; Yang, S.; Tran, N.M.; Park, B.J.; Lee, S.J.; Kim, Y.; Yoo, H.; Kim, S.-J.; Shin, J.H. Controllable Nitric Oxide Storage and Release in Cu-BTC: Crystallographic Insights and Bioactivity. *Int. J. Mol. Sci.* **2022**, *23*, 9098. https://doi.org/10.3390/ijms23169098

Academic Editor: Helena Felgueiras

Received: 11 July 2022
Accepted: 4 August 2022
Published: 13 August 2022

1. Introduction

Nitric oxide (NO) in the environment is mainly derived from natural sources and internal combustion engines. It is typically considered an air pollutant and causes smog and strongly acidic rain. However, since Furchgott et al. reported that NO acts as the endothelium-derived relaxation factor, NO has also been identified as an important physiological and pathological signaling material responsible for regulating the cardiovascular and nervous systems as well as the immune response [1–6]. The deficiency of NO produced endogenously from l-arginine by NO synthase (NOS) causes various diseases, which has driven investigations into the exogenous delivery of NO for therapeutic applications. Because NO is a highly reactive radical and gains an electron through covalent bonding, hydrogen bonding, or coordinative bonding [7–10], several types of NO donors have been explored for efficient NO delivery. These include simple nitrosyl metal complexes of organic nitrates/nitrites, macromolecular scaffolds containing nitrosamines, *N*-diazeniumdiolates (NONOates), and *S*-nitrosothiols [11–15].

Metal–organic frameworks (MOFs) have been used as attractive organic–inorganic hybrid materials that have high porosity and crystallinity and enable the facile tuning of structural composition. Consequently, MOFs have been used as sensors, applied to catalysis and gas sorption and separation, and employed in medicinal applications [16–23]. Moreover, MOFs have been considered the best candidates for controlled NO release as they can physically capture NO in their inner pores, bond with NO via their open metal sites (OMSs), or amine functional group of the linkers comprising the frameworks [24–33]. Cu-BTC, formulated as $Cu_3(BTC)_2$ (MOF-199, copper(II)-benzene-1,3,5-tricarboxylate), is one of the most studied MOFs and is commonly used as a sensor or for gas sorption, gas storage, and catalysis [34–39]. For example, Xiao et al. investigated Cu-BTC as an NO donor due to its high crystallinity and varied porosity and reported that this material could store as much as 9 $mmol \cdot mg^{-1}$ of NO at 196 K but released only 1 $nmol \cdot mg^{-1}$—a very small fraction of the loading—upon exposure to a stream of wet nitrogen gas. However, this irreversible release was detrimental to the application of Cu-BTC for therapeutic purposes [28]. This result also suggested that Cu-BTC predominantly physically absorbs NO in its inner pores, with some NO being partially chemically adsorbed onto its OMSs. To address this limitation, other isostructural MOFs incorporating secondary amine functionalities were developed for enhancing NO release up to 0.51 $\mu mol \cdot mg^{-1}$ [11]. Subsequently, Co-CPO-27 and Ni-CPO-27 linked to the 2,5-dihydroxyterephthalic acid ligand were reported as the best MOF donors, which absorbed 6.5 and 7.0 $\mu mol \cdot mg^{-1}$ of NO, respectively. While they successfully released the absorbed NO completely, their poor biocompatibility limited their applications [40]. The bonding of NO to MOFs has been typically characterized using FTIR spectroscopy, NMR spectroscopy, or theoretical simulations, which revealed the formation of nitrosyl complexes between NO and the OMSs or NONOates derived from secondary amines [31,32,40–43]. However, there are no reports on the characterization of the NO loading modes in the solid state by X-ray crystallography, mainly due to the rapid release of NO in the presence of water vapor and the challenges related to low-temperature measurements. To improve the NO storage/release properties of MOFs, we aimed to understand the bonding characteristics of NO loaded on MOFs by single-crystal X-ray crystallography, which is expected to be significantly different from previous studies [28,31].

Herein, for improving the biocompatibility and NO capacity, nano-sized Cu-BTC was fabricated via a convenient and straightforward ball-milling process of micro-sized Cu-BTC. The hydration degree of Cu-BTC was controlled to enable the coordination of sufficient water molecules to the OMSs. However, the morphology of Cu-BTC can be designed to load NO efficiently in the empty pores by the facile removal of the guest water molecules by activation. Highly improved NO storage/release and antibacterial activities against six bacterial strains, including Gram-positive

Gram-negative bacteria, are discussed.

2. Results and Discussion

2.1. Preparation of Cu-BTC and NO⊂Cu-BTCs

To investigate the NO storage/release properties and antibacterial activities of Cu-BTC, micro-sized Cu-BTC (**1**) was prepared. A previously reported solvothermal method, after slight modification, was used for the reaction of copper(II) nitrate and benzene-1,3,5-tricarboxylic acid in a mixture of ethanol, deionized water, and DMF [44]. The resulting compound **1** was further processed by ball-milling to afford nano-sized Cu-BTC (**2**) (Figure S1). The two NO-loaded Cu-BTC systems, NO⊂micro-Cu-BTC (**3**; NO was loaded on **1**) and NO⊂nano-Cu-BTC (**4**; NO was loaded on **2**) were obtained by charging 10 atm of NO onto activated **1** and **2**, respectively, at 25 °C for three days. The obtained Cu-BTC and NO-loaded Cu-BTC were characterized by X-ray crystallography, PXRD, SEM, Brunauer–Emmett–Teller (BET) measurements, FTIR spectroscopy, and TGA.

2.2. X-ray Crystallography and PXRD

The structures of all Cu-BTC MOFs before and after NO gas loading were determined by X-ray crystallography and PXRD. A single crystal with 0.02 × 0.08 × 0.09 mm^3 dimensions was selected for XRD analysis. Upon the capture of NO gas in **1**, its cubic *Fm-3m* space group (Table 1) and the original framework remained unchanged (Figure 1). X-ray crystallography revealed the moiety formula of **3** to be $CuC_6H_2O_5]\cdot(NO)_{0.167}$. While the occupancies of NO were fixed to obtain the best fit with the largest residual peaks, the actual occupancies should be larger than the fixed occupancies. The single-crystal structure of **3** showed that the remaining water molecules were coordinated to the OMSs. NO interacts through weak hydrogen bonding between the hydrogen atom of the coordinated water and the nitrogen atom of NO (Cu–O–H···N–O, 3.308 Å). Weak interactions between the nitrogen atom of NO and the carboxylate oxygen atoms of the BTC linkers (Cu–O–C–O···NO, 3.999 Å) were also observed (Figure 2 and Table S1).

Table 1. Crystallographic data for NO⊂Cu-BTC.

Empirical Formula	$C_6H_2CuO_5$ $(NO)_{0.17}$
Formula weight	222.62
Temp. (K)	223(2)
Wavelength (Å)	0.71073
Space group	*Fm-3m*
a (Å)	26.3068(11)
b (Å)	26.3068(11)
c (Å)	26.3068(11)
α (°)	90.00
β (°)	90.00
γ (°)	90.00
Volume ($Å^3$)	18,206(2)
Z	48
Density (calc.) (Mg m^{-3})	0.975
Absorption coeff. (mm^{-1})	1.429
Crystal size (mm)	0.090 × 0.080 × 0.020
Reflections collected	148,341
Independent reflections	1177 [R(int) = 0.1842]
Data/restraints/parameters	1177/1/40
Goodness-of-fit on F^2	1.291
Final R indices [I>2σ(I)]	R1 = 0.1149, wR2 = 0.2110
R indices (all data)	R1 = 0.1264, wR2 = 0.2170
Largest diff. peak and hole (e.Å-3)	0.697 and −0.564
CCDC	2,073,930

Notably, this is the first report of a single-crystal X-ray structure that clearly shows the NO loading structure, which comprises NO interacting with the coordinated water molecules and the carboxylate groups of the BTC linkers. The NO loading mode of 3 in this study was significantly different from previous results that characterized the adsorption of NO to the OMSs as chemisorption [28,31]. Figure 3 shows the XRD patterns of the simulated and NO-loaded Cu-BTC MOFs of different sizes. All XRD patterns coincided well with the simulated pattern. The main peaks at 6.82°, 9.64°, 11.76°, and 13.57° corresponding (2 0 0), (2 2 0), (2 2 2), and (4 0 0) of the Cu-BTC pattern were maintained in nano-Cu-BTC and micro-Cu-BTC. The (2 0 0) peak was not shown in NO loaded Cu-BTC MOFs. Particularly, the PXRD of **4** obtained after storing NO for 1 month did not show any structural changes, and the original framework of Cu BTC remained unchanged. These results indicate that the robust structure of Cu-BTC was stably maintained after storing NO for a long time, which could enable it to perform the reversible NO release mechanism.

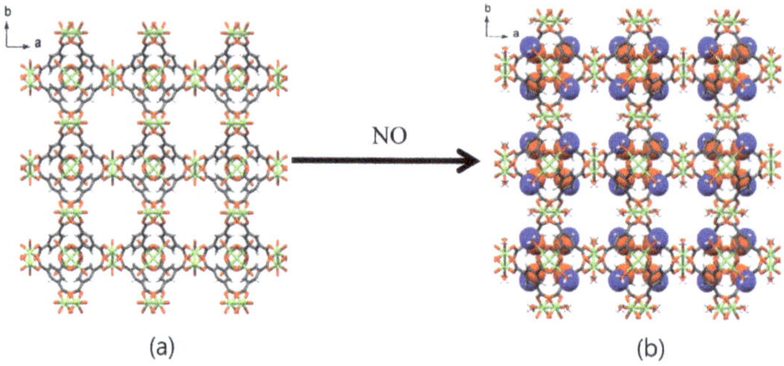

Figure 1. (**a**) Structure of Cu-BTC, *Fm-3m*, a = b = c = 26.3015(4) Å, V = 18194.6(5) Å^3. (**b**) Structure of NO⊂micro-Cu-BTC, *Fm-3m*, a = b = c = 26.3068(11) Å, V = 18205.6(5) Å^3. NO molecules are shown in space filled models. The color codes: green, Cu; grey, carbon; red, oxygen; blue, nitrogen.

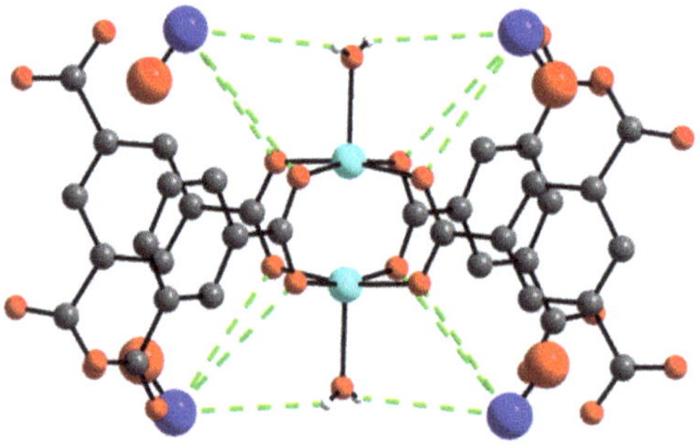

Figure 2. Fragment structure showing weak hydrogen bonding interactions between NO and the coordinated water molecules, and interactions between NO and carboxylate oxygen atoms. Color codes: green, Cu; grey, carbon; red, oxygen; blue, nitrogen. Hydrogen atoms, except those of water, were omitted. The large spheres represent NO for clarity.

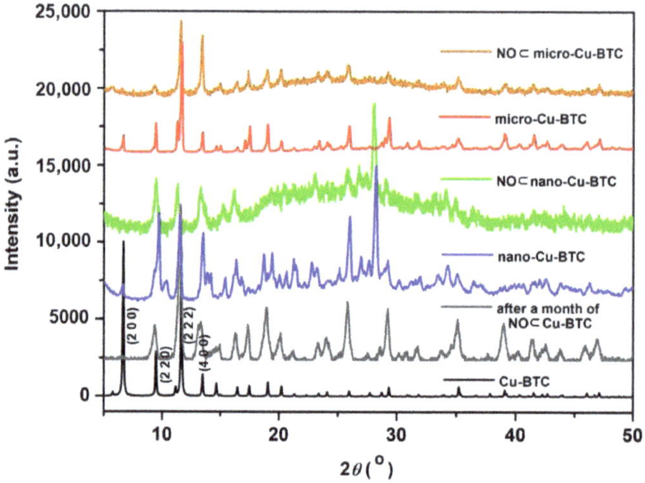

Figure 3. Powder X-ray diffraction (PXRD) of micro-sized Cu-BTC **1** (red), nano-sized Cu-BTC **2** (blue), NO⊂micro-Cu-BTC **3** (yellow), NO⊂nano-Cu-BTC **4** (green), and NO⊂micro-Cu-BTC **3** after loading NO (grey).

2.3. SEM, BET Measurements, FTIR, and TGA

The morphologies of the Cu-BTCs before and after loading NO were imaged using SEM. As shown in Figure 4a, truncated octahedral crystals larger than 10 μm in length were observed, which is in good agreement with the previous reports [45–47]. In contrast to the micro-sized crystal, **2** was seen as an irregular lump comprising an agglomerated powder with sizes in the range of less than 500 nm to greater than 1 μm (Figure 4b). This may be attributed to the loss of crystallinity during the ball-milling process, which could cause the transformation to the agglomerated powder [48]. The morphologies of the Cu-BTCs were well maintained after loading NO (Figure 4c,d).

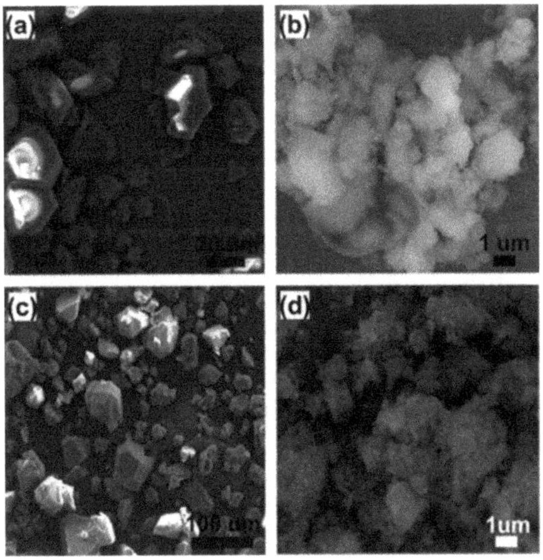

Figure 4. Scanning electron microscopy (SEM) images of (**a**) micro-sized Cu-BTC (**1**), (**b**) nano-sized Cu-BTC (**2**), (**c**) NO⊂micro-Cu-BTC (**3**), and (**d**) NO⊂nano-Cu-BTC (**4**).

In addition, the surface properties of **1** and **2** were analyzed by N_2 sorption measurements at 77 K. A high BET surface area of 799 $m^2 \cdot g^{-1}$ was achieved by **1**, and its nitrogen sorption (Figure 5a) showed a characteristic type-I isotherm [49,50]. The increased adsorption uptakes at low relative pressures ($P/P_0 \leq 0.1$) are due to the presence of micro pores, whereas a hysteresis at high relative pressures ($0.3 \leq P/P_0 \leq 0.9$) indicates the existence of textural meso or macro pores, formed as a result of the specific crystal packing. The large surface area of **1** might have originated from its high crystallinity. In contrast, **2** exhibited a much lower BET surface area (27 $m^2 \cdot g^{-1}$) than **1**. Further, **2** exhibited a characteristic type-II isotherm, proving that it is composed of both mono and multilayers (Figure 5c) with mixed micro pore diameters ranging from 0.4 to 2.0 nm (Figure 5d) [50]. The smaller surface area of the nano-sized crystal of **2** can be attributed to the agglomeration of nano powder and/or the defects of its inner pores formed during the ball-milling process [51]. Furthermore, the vertical nature of the N_2 adsorption isotherms of **1** at low pressures supports the hypothesis that these adsorption/desorption properties are derived from the strong adsorption on the surface and the micro pore filling. The plot of **2** suggests that intra-agglomerate voids arise from the presence of some meso and macro pores formed by multilayers in the samples [52,53]. We have summarized the nitrogen sorption properties of the micro-sized Cu-BTC and the nano-sized Cu-BTC on Table S2. These results match well with the SEM images shown in Figure 4b, showing the lump shape composed of the agglomerated powder.

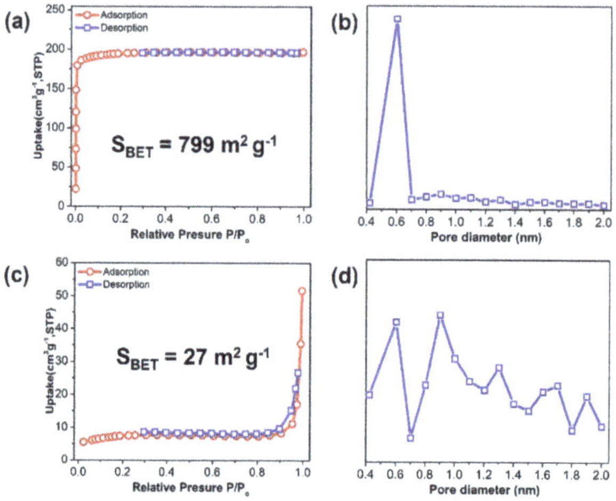

Figure 5. N_2 sorption, measured at 77 K, and pore size of **1** (**a**,**b**) and **2** (**c**,**d**).

Cu-BTC was degassed at 300 °C under 1×10^{-4} mbar of pressure using a vacuum to ensure complete dehydration. The loading of NO onto this MOF was confirmed based on the appearance of stretching peaks in the 1890–1000 cm^{-1} region of its FTIR spectrum, which is attributed to the formation of the nitrosyl complex by the coordination of NO on the reactive OMSs [28]. Further, the FTIR spectra of **3** and **4** were scanned at various times after the NO was released (Figures 6 and 7). The Cu-BTC MOFs before and after loading NO showed weak bands at 488 and 721 cm^{-1}, which are attributed to the bending and stretching modes of Cu–O, respectively. The higher intensity absorption peaks at 1368, 1445, and 1640 cm^{-1} are assigned to the stretching modes of the carboxylate moiety of BTC; specifically, the stretching mode of C–O, and the asymmetric and symmetric stretching modes of C=O, respectively [34,35,54]. However, in this study, a new peak representing the coordination of NO to Cu in the 1890–1900 cm^{-1} range did not appear after NO loading. Rather, a strong, broad O–H stretching band at ~3400 cm^{-1} was observed, which corresponds to the water molecules coordinating with the OMSs. This evidence of water coordinating with Cu agrees with the NO loading mode determined by the crystallographic structure of **3**.

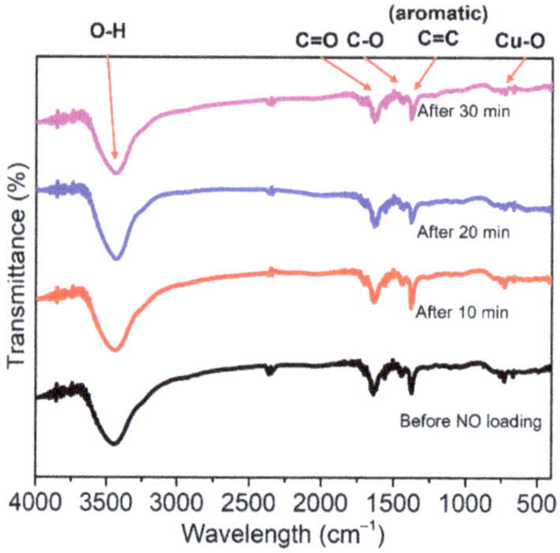

Figure 6. FTIR spectra of **1** (black) and **3** after releasing NO for 10, 20, and 30 min (red, blue, and pink, respectively).

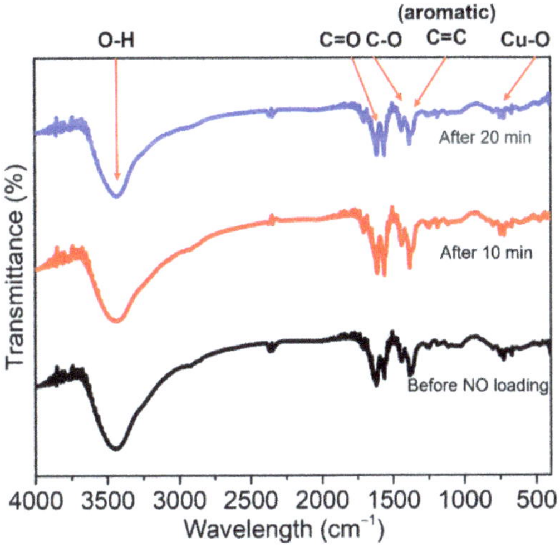

Figure 7. FTIR spectra of **2** (black) and **4** after releasing NO for 10 and 20 min (red and blue, respectively).

TGA was carried out to analyze the amount of water molecules coordinated to the OMSs and the amount of guest water molecules captured in the inner pores or on the surface, depending on the activation. When as-prepared **1** and **2** were heated up to 800 °C under an inert atmosphere, an initial weight loss occurred up to 150 °C, which was due to the desorption of the physically absorbed water (Figure 8). Then, slow weight loss caused by the desorption of the water molecules coordinating with the OMSs continued up to 350 °C. The final prominent weight loss step appeared at 350 °C in both the samples and was attributed to the decomposition of the BTC linker (approximately 38% weight loss). The largest difference in the initial weight loss ratio depending on the morphologies of **1** and **2** was 9%. Furthermore, the hydration of **2** could be reduced from 27% to 20.6% upon activation at 150 °C for 24 h (Figure 8b). The hydration of Cu-BTC was adequately lowered to 20.6% (150 °C) by controlling the morphology and activation. We attempted to investigate the hydration effect on NO storage and release.

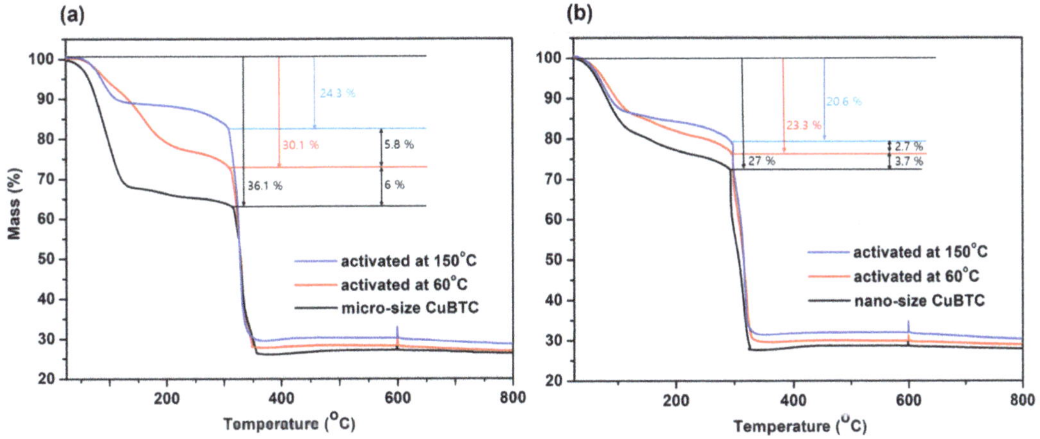

Figure 8. TGA of **1** (**a**) and **2** (**b**). Black line, as-prepared; red line, activated at 60 °C; blue line, activated at 150 °C.

2.4. NO Release from NO⊂Cu-BTC

The amount of NO released from NO⊂Cu-BTC was estimated from the intensity of the chemiluminescence of excited NO_2 that was produced from the reaction of the NO with ozone at the outlet stream of the PBS solution at 37 °C. Cu-BTC is a well-known MOF that adsorbs 3 $\mu mol \cdot mg^{-1}$ of NO at room temperature; however, 2.21 $\mu mol \cdot mg^{-1}$ of NO was strongly chemisorbed onto the OMSs of the MOF, and only a minor fraction of the chemisorbed NO, less than 0.02%, was released upon exposure to water or wet gas [28].

The chemisorption of NO onto the OMSs inhibits its release sufficiently, thus inhibiting the therapeutic applications of our MOFs. Thus, we attempted to control the chemisorption of NO onto the OMSs by adjusting the hydration degree, NO charging pressure, and the morphologies of the sample to enhance the NO release ability of Cu-BTC.

Figure 9 shows the NO release tendency of NO⊂micro-Cu-BTC **3** as a function of the NO charging pressure in a range of 2 to 12 atm. The total amount of NO released (t[NO]) increased up to 0.34 $\mu mol \cdot mg^{-1}$ with increasing charging pressure. Further, to investigate the effect of dehydration on NO release, unactivated (i.e., non-dehydrated) Cu-BTC and Cu-BTC activated (i.e., dehydrated) at 150 °C for 24 h were examined. The t[NO] value of dehydrated **3** increased approximately two-fold, from 0.34 (non-dehydrated) to 0.68 $\mu mol \cdot mg^{-1}$, and the duration of NO release (t_d) was longer than that of the non-dehydrated sample. Furthermore, the t[NO] value of dehydrated **4** increased significantly from 0.25 (non-dehydrated) to 1.81 $\mu mol \cdot mg^{-1}$, and the maximum flux of NO release ($[NO]_m$) increased proportionally from 4.78 (non-dehydrated) to 52.7 $ppm \cdot mg^{-1}$ (Figure 10). The notable difference between dehydrated **3** and **4** was attributable to the different surface areas and porosities, which were derived from their morphologies (Table 2). These results confirm that more regular micro pores exist on **3** than on **4**, as shown on Figure 5. As the guest water molecules trapped in these regular inner pores cannot be easily released, the loading of NO on the micro pores of **3** is more difficult compared to that of **4**. As a result, NO can be adsorbed in more empty pores and on the surface of **4**, and t[NO] reaches to 1.81 $\mu mol \cdot mg^{-1}$ upon exposure to water, which is sufficiently high for therapeutic applications [55].

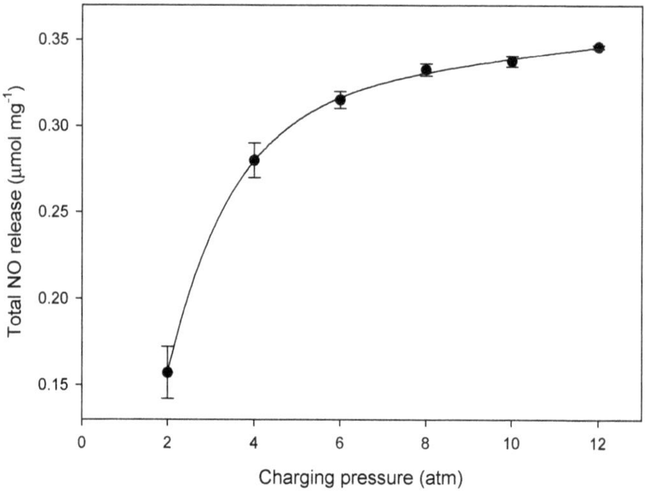

Figure 9. Plot of total NO release of NO⊂micro-Cu-BTC **3** in deoxygenated phosphate-buffered saline (PBS, 0.01 M, pH 7.4) at 37 °C as a function of varying NO charging pressure.

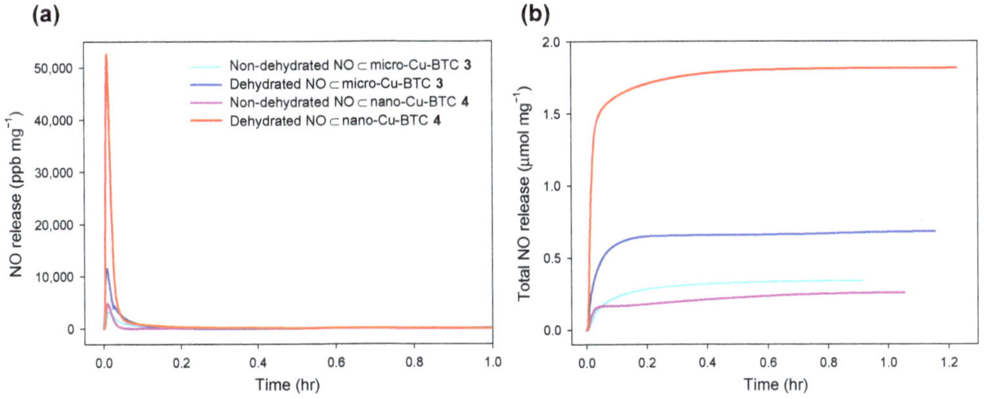

Figure 10. (**a**) Real-time NO release profiles and (**b**) total amount of NO released for NO⊂Cu-BTC in deoxygenated PBS (0.01 M, pH 7.4) at 37 °C: sky-blue line, non-dehydrated NO⊂micro-Cu-BTC **3**; blue line, dehydrated NO⊂micro-Cu-BTC **3**; pink line, non-dehydrated NO⊂nano-Cu-BTC **4**; red line, dehydrated NO⊂nano-Cu-BTC **4**.

Table 2. NO release properties of NO⊂Cu-BTC [a,b].

	t[NO] (μmol·mg^{-1})		t_m (s)		[NO]$_m$ (ppm·mg^{-1})		$t_{1/2}$ (s)		t_d (h)	
	3	4	3	4	3	4	3	4	3	4
Non-dehydrated	0.34	0.25	50	40	3.25	4.78	185	75	0.9	1.1
Dehydrated	0.68	1.81	33	39	11.5	52.7	73	58	1.2	1.2

[a] Values were determined using a Sievers chemiluminescence NO analyzer (NOA 280i) in deoxygenated PBS (0.01 M, pH 7.4) at 37 °C. [b] t[NO], total amount of NO released; [NO]$_m$, maximum flux of NO release; t_m, time necessary to reach [NO]$_m$; $t_{1/2}$, half-life of NO release; t_d, duration time of NO release for sustained fluxes of NO ≥ 1 ppb·mg^{-1}.

2.5. Antibacterial Properties

Therapeutic applications involving NO are popular in various areas, such as immunology, studies on antibacterial and anticancer agents, as well as wound healing. However, NO sometimes exhibits a dual effect depending on its concentration, flux, and duration when used as an antibacterial agent [6,55–57]. To evaluate the antibacterial activity of our NO-releasing Cu-BTC, an inhibition zone assay based on a modified disk diffusion method was carried out using two Gram-negative strains (*Escherichia coli* (*E. coli* ATCC11775) and *Pseudomonas aeruginosa* (*P. aeruginosa* ATCC9027)), two Gram-positive strains (*Staphylococcus aureus* (*S. aureus* ATCC14458) and *Bacillus cereus* (*B. cereus* ATCC11706)), and two methicillin-resistant *Staphylococcus aureus* strains (MRSA KCCM40510 and clinically isolated MRSA) (Figure 11). The inhibition zone of the six bacteria exposed to both Cu-BTC and NO⊂Cu-BTC ranged from 47.858 to 803.39 mm^2, and the zone was relative smaller for *S. aureus*, compared to that for the other five bacteria exposed to NO⊂Cu-BTC. In contrast, the inhibition zone for *S. aureus* exposed to Cu-BTC was 376.84 mm^2, which was larger than that of *S. aureus* exposed to NO⊂Cu-BTC (Table 3). The NO-releasing Cu-BTC was more effective in inhibiting the growth of the five tested bacteria than the growth of *S. aureus*. Furthermore, the data for the *P. aeruginosa* strains, which displayed the least susceptibility, and *E. coli*, which displayed the greatest susceptibility, were consistent with those in previous reports [17,55]. The bacterial species were determined as being susceptible to NO⊂Cu-BTC in the following order: *E. coli* > MRSA (clinically isolated) > *S. aureus* > MRSA (KCCM 40510) > *B. cereus* > *P. aeruginosa*. Thus, NO⊂Cu-BTC exhibited more selective and synergistic antimicrobial activities toward a wide range of bacteria than Cu-BTC.

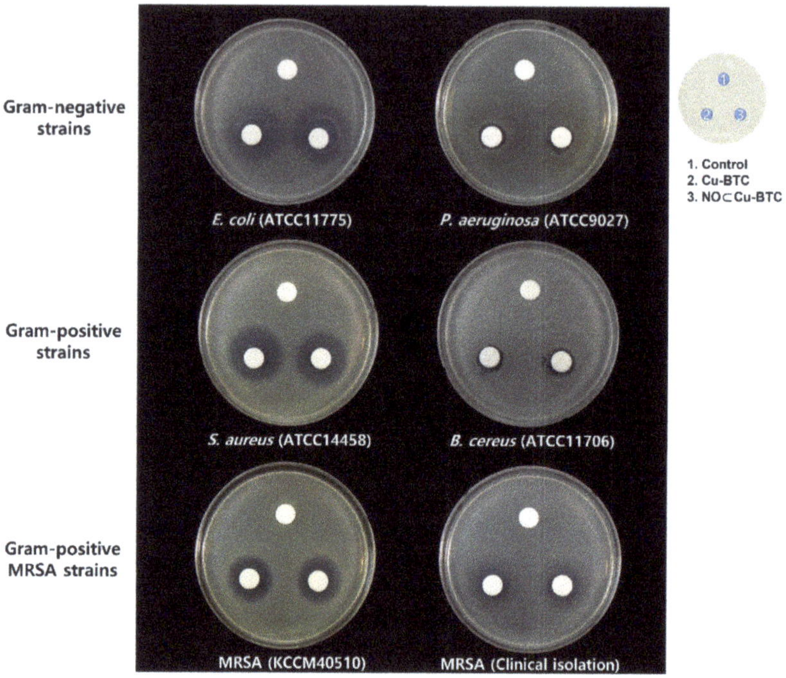

Figure 11. Inhibition zone assay of Cu-BTC (BTC: benzene-1,3,5-tricarboxylate) and NO⊂Cu-BTC (NO: nitric oxide) toward six strains of bacteria tested by disc diffusion method.

Table 3. Inhibition zone of Cu-BTC and NO⊂Cu-BTC toward six strains of bacteria.

Bacterial Strains *		Inhibition Zone (mm^2)		*p* Value
		Cu-BTC	**NO⊂Cu-BTC**	
Gram-negative strains	*E. coli* (ATCC11775)	712.3 ± 38.6	803.4 ± 54.7	<0.024
	P. aeruginosa (ATCC9027)	47.8 ± 22.2	52.3 ± 26.2	<0.21
Gram-positive strains	*S. aureus* (ATCC14458)	414.2 ± 18.4	376.8 ± 21.6	<0.016
	B. cereus (ATCC11706)	51.5 ± 7.3	74 ± 8.8	<0.003
Gram-positive MRSA strains	MRSA (KCCM40510)	271.4 ± 8.1	297.4 ± 8.1	<0.0018
	MRSA (Clinical isolation)	501.1 ± 5.6	573.3 ± 6.9	<0.00057

* Escherichia coli (*E. coli* ATCC11775); Pseudomonas aeruginosa (*P. aeruginosa* ATCC9027)); Staphylococcus aureus (*S. aureus* ATCC14458); Bacillus cereus (*B. cereus* ATCC11706)); methicillin-resistant Staphylococcus aureus strains (MRSA KCCM40510 and clinically isolated MRSA). Data are mean zone inhibition (mm^2) ± standard deviation (S.D.) of three replicates (n = 3, $p < 0.05$).

3. Materials and Methods

3.1. Preparation of Cu-BTC 1 and 2

The Micro-sized Cu-BTC (**1**) was prepared according to a reported protocol with slight modifications [45]. In a typical synthesis, copper(II) nitrate trihydrate ($Cu(NO_3)_2{\cdot}3H_2O$, 99%, Acros, Seoul, Korea) (0.725 g, 3.0 mmol) was dissolved in 10 mL of deionized water. In a separate vial, 1,3,5-benzenetricarboxylic acid (H_3BTC, $C_9H_6O_6$, 98%, Acros, Seoul, Korea) (0.210 g, 1.0 mmol) was dissolved in 10 mL of ethanol. To a solution of H_3BTC stirring at 500 rpm for 10 min at room temperature, the $Cu(NO_3)_2$ solution was quickly added. Then, 0.7 mL of DMF was added to the solution. The reaction mixture was placed in a temperature-controlled oven at 80 °C for 24 h. After cooling to 25 °C, the product was collected by centrifugation, washed several times with solvents (deionized water and ethanol), and dried under vacuum for 24 h before further use.

Nano-sized Cu-BTC (**2**) was prepared from **1** by ball-milling at 350 rpm for 6 h with a balls-to-Cu-BTC weight ratio of 50:1 using the Fritsch™ Planetary Mill Pulverisette 5 (Idar-Oberstein, Germany). Powder X-ray diffraction (PXRD), FTIR, and scanning-electron microscopy (SEM) were used for further characterization of the Cu-BTC MOFs.

3.2. X-ray Crystallography

X-ray diffraction data for NO⊂Cu-BTC were collected on a Bruker APX-II diffractometer (Ames, IA, USA) equipped with a monochromator with a Mo Kα (λ = 0.71073 Å) incident beam at the National Research Facilities and Equipment Center (NanoBio-Energy Materials Center) at Ewha Womans University. A crystal was mounted on a glass fiber. The CCD data were integrated and scaled using the Bruker-SAINT software package (Bruker Nano, Inc., 2019), and the structure was solved and refined using SHEXL-2014 (Sheldrick, 2014) [58]. All hydrogen atoms were placed at the calculated positions. The crystallographic data are listed in Table 1, and the bond lengths and angles are listed in Table S1. The CCDC reference number is 2073930 for NO⊂Cu-BTC.

3.3. NO Storage/Release of Cu-BTC

For the dehydration process, 10 mg of **1** and **2** were dehydrated in a vacuum at 150 °C for 24 h. The activated Cu-BTCs were placed in a 40 mL vial, and the vial was placed in a Parr bottle (200 mL) that was connected to an in-house NO reactor. The reactor was flushed with Ar gas (99.99%) thrice for 10 min each to remove oxygen before charging NO. The reaction bottle was then charged under 10 atm of NO using ultrapure grade (99.5%) NO gas provided by Dong-A Specialty Gases (Seoul, Korea), which was purified over KOH pellets to remove trace NO degradation products. The bottle was then sealed for 72 h at 25 °C. Prior to removing the NO-charged Cu-BTCs, unreacted NO was purged from the chamber with Ar thrice. The NO⊂Cu-BTCs (**3** and **4**) were stored in a sealed container at −20 °C until further use. The NO release profiles of NO⊂Cu-BTC were monitored in deoxygenated phosphate-buffered saline (PBS; 0.01 M, pH 7.4) at 37 °C using a Sievers 280i chemiluminescence NO analyzer (Boulder, CO, USA). NO released from NO⊂Cu-BTC was transported to the analyzer by a stream of Ar gas (70 mL·min^{-1}) passed through the reaction cell. The instrument was calibrated with air passed through a zero filter (0 ppm NO) and 45 ppm of NO standard gas balanced with N_2 purchased from Dong-Woo Gas Tech (Siheung, Korea). The total amount of NO released, t[NO]; maximum flux of NO release, $[NO]_m$; time necessary to reach $[NO]_m$, t_m; half-life of NO release, $t_{1/2}$; and duration time of NO release for sustained fluxes of NO ≥ 1 ppb·mg^{-1}, t_d, were determined for the evaluation of NO⊂Cu-BTC.

3.4. Antibacterial Test

To confirm the antibacterial activity of the two types of Cu-BTC, we used six strains of bacteria, which included two drug-resistant bacteria. Two Gram-negative strains (*Escherichia* coli ATCC 11775 and *Pseudomonas aeruginosa* ATCC 9027) and two Gram-positive strains (*S. aureus* ATCC 14458 and *B. cereus* ATCC11706) were acquired from the American Type Culture Collection (ATCC, Rockville, MD, USA). One methicillin-resistant bacteria, *S. aureus* (MRSA KCCM 40510), was purchased from the Korean Culture Center of Microorganisms (KCCM, Sedaemun-Gu, Seoul, Korea), and clinically isolated MRSA was kindly provided by the Yonsei Medical Center in Seoul. Gram-negative and Gram-positive bacteria were grown on a plate count agar (PCA, Becton, Dickinson and Company, Sparks, MD, USA) at 35 °C for 24 h. MRSA strains were grown on Brain Heart Infusion agar (BHIA, Becton, Dickinson and Company) at 35 °C for 24 h. The antibacterial activities of Cu-BTC and NO⊂Cu-BTC were evaluated using a disk diffusion method from the National Committee for Clinical Laboratory Standards (NCCLS 2003a), protocol M2-A8. A bacterial suspension for each strain was prepared by the resuspension of each bacterial colony in sterilized 0.85% saline solution, and the optical density of the suspension solution was adjusted to 0.5 McFarland turbidity standards (~10^7 CFU/mL). Each bacterial suspension was applied to the entire surface of the PCA and BHIA plates, and the agar plates were incubated for 10 min at room temperature. Next, three 10 mm Whatman filter paper disks were placed on each agar plate, as shown in Figure 1, and each suspension solution (final concentration: 1 mg/mL in 0.85% saline solution) of Cu-BTC and NO⊂Cu-BTC was applied to the paper disk. The agar plates treated with each sample were incubated at 35 °C for 24 to 48 h, and the zone of inhibition of each agar plate was measured by subtracting the diameter of each disk from the diameter of the total inhibition zone using ImageJ software (NIH, Bethesda, MD, USA). All experiments were carried out in triplicate with results expressed as a mean with standard deviations (S.D). Statistical comparisons between Cu-BTC and NO⊂Cu-BTC performed using Stutens's *t*-test and a difference with $p < 0.05$ was considered statistically significant.

3.5. Instrumentation

The PXRD patterns of the Cu-BTCs were recorded using a Rigaku MiniFlex diffractometer (Rigaku Corp., Neu-Isenburg, Germany). FTIR spectra were measured on a Nicolet iS10 FTIR spectrometer with KBr pellets (Thermo Fisher Scientific, Waltham, MA, USA). TGA was performed using a TG 209 F3 Tarsus® instrument (NETZSCH, Burlington, MA, USA). The surface morphology and elemental composition of Cu-BTC were characterized using SEM-EDS (FE-SEM, JEOL JSM-5800F, Peabody, MA, USA). N_2 adsorption isotherms were obtained by using a BELSORP-mini II instrument (BEL Japan, Inc., Tokyo, Japan). High-purity (99.999%) gases were used throughout the adsorption experiments. All samples were activated by rinsing them thoroughly, followed by drying under vacuum for 24 h prior to the gas sorption measurements.

4. Conclusions

Microporous Cu-BTC MOFs with two different morphologies (micro-sized and nano-sized) were prepared, and their NO sorption/release properties were investigated. NO was captured in Cu-BTC by partial hydrogen bonding with water molecules coordinated to Cu and ON$\cdots$O interactions with the oxygen atoms of the BTC linker. The solid-state structural analysis of Cu-BTC revealed a stable structure upon NO loading and releasing. When the nano-sized Cu-BTC MOF was activated, the total amount of NO released was significantly higher than that released from the micro-sized Cu-BTC, owing to the lower hydration and different morphological characteristics of the former. Furthermore, the NO⊂Cu-BTC MOFs showed bactericidal properties against five strains of bacteria that were superior to those of the Cu-BTC MOFs. These results reveal that the NO release of Cu-BTC can be highly enhanced by controlling the hydration degree and morphology of the MOF, and the resultant NO delivery vehicle system exhibits synergistic therapeutic effects. This study paves the way for the development of various MOFs as promising hybrid NO donor materials through simple physical modifications for application as drug delivery systems.

Supplementary Materials: The following supporting information can be downloaded at: https://www.mdpi.com/article/10.3390/ijms23169098/s1.

Author Contributions: Conceptualization, J.H.S. and D.N.L.; methodology, Y.R.K. and N.M.T.; validation, Y.K., S.Y. and S.-J.K.; formal analysis, Y.R.K., Y.K., B.J.P. and N.M.T.; Investigation, Y.K., S.Y. and S.J.L.; data curation, Y.R.K., Y.K., S.-J.K., B.J.P. and N.M.T.; writing—original draft preparation, D.N.L. and H.Y.; writing—review and editing, Y.K., H.Y., J.H.S., B.J.P. and D.N.L.; supervision, D.N.L. and J.H.S.; funding acquisition, Y.K., H.Y. and D.N.L. All authors have read and agreed to the published version of the manuscript.

Funding: This work was supported by the Basic Science Research Program of the National Research Foundation of Korea [grant numbers 2017R1D1A1A02017607, 2018R1D1A1B07045327, 2020R1A2C1004006, 2021R1A2C1004285], by Institute of Information & communications Technology Planning & Evaluation (IITP) grant funded by the Korea government (MSIT) (No.2021-0-00894), and by Kwangwoon University in the year 2022.

Institutional Review Board Statement: Not applicable.

Informed Consent Statement: Not applicable.

Data Availability Statement: Not applicable.

Conflicts of Interest: The authors declare no conflict interest.

References

1. Furchgott, R.F.; Khan, M.T.; Jothianandan, D. Similarities on behavior of nitric oxide and endothelium derived relaxing factor in a perfusion cascade bioassay system. *Fed. Proc.* **1987**, *46*, 385.
2. Ignarro, L.J.; Buga, G.M.; Wood, K.S.; Byrns, R.E.; Chaudhuri, G. Endothelium-derived relaxing factor produced and released from artery and vein is nitric oxide. *Proc. Natl Acad. Sci. USA* **1987**, *84*, 9265–9269. [CrossRef]
3. Arnold, W.P.; Mittal, C.K.; Katsuki, S.; Murad, F. Nitric oxide activates guanylate cyclase and increases guanosine 3′:5′-cyclic monophosphate levels in various tissue preparations. *Proc. Natl Acad. Sci. USA* **1977**, *74*, 3203–3207. [CrossRef] [PubMed]
4. Fang, F.C. Perspectives Series: Host/Pathogen Interactions, Perspectives series: Host/pathogen interactions. Mechanisms of nitric oxide-related antimicrobial activity. *J. Clin. Investig.* **1997**, *99*, 2818–2825. [CrossRef] [PubMed]
5. Luo, J.D.; Chen, A.F. Nitric Oxide: A newly discovered function on wound healing. *Acta Pharmacol. Sin.* **2005**, *26*, 259–264. [CrossRef]
6. Mocellin, S.; Bronte, V.; Nitti, D. Nitric, a double edged sword in cancer biology: Searching for therapeutic opportunities. *Med. Res. Rev.* **2007**, *27*, 317–352. [CrossRef] [PubMed]
7. Cavalieri, F.; Finelli, I.; Tortora, M.; Mozetic, P.; Chiessi, E.; Polizio, F.; Brismar, T.B.; Paradossi, G. Polymer microbubbles as diagnostic and therapeutic gas delivery device. *Chem. Mater.* **2008**, *20*, 3254–3258. [CrossRef]
8. Riccio, D.A.; Schoenfisch, M.H. Nitric oxide release: Part I. Macromolecular scaffolds. *Chem. Soc. Rev.* **2012**, *41*, 3731–3741. [CrossRef]
9. Horcajada, P.; Serre, C.; Maurin, G.; Ramsahye, N.A.; Balas, F.; Vallet-Regí, M.; Sebban, M.; Taulelle, F.; Férey, G. Flexible porous metal-organic frameworks for a controlled drug delivery. *J. Am. Chem. Soc.* **2008**, *130*, 6774–6780. [CrossRef] [PubMed]
10. Huxford, R.C.; Rocca, J.D.D.; Lin, W. Metal-organic frameworks as potential drug carriers. *Curr. Opin. Chem. Biol.* **2010**, *14*, 262–268. [CrossRef] [PubMed]
11. Hrabie, J.A.; Keefer, L.K. Chemistry of the nitric oxide-releasing diazeniumdiolate ("nitrosohydroxylamine") functional group and its oxygen-substituted derivatives. *Chem. Rev.* **2002**, *102*, 1135–1154. [CrossRef] [PubMed]
12. Lyn, D.L.H.; Williams, H. The Chemistry of S-Nitrosothiols. *Acc. Chem. Res.* **1999**, *32*, 869–876. [CrossRef]
13. Parzuchowski, P.G.; Frost, M.C.; Meyerhoff, M.E. Synthesis and characterization of polymethacrylate-based nitric oxide donors. *J. Am. Chem. Soc.* **2002**, *124*, 12182–12191. [CrossRef]
14. Jeong, H.; Park, K.; Yoo, J.C.; Hong, J. Structural heterogeneity in polymeric nitric oxide donor nanoblended coatings for controlled release behaviors. *RSC Adv.* **2018**, *8*, 38792–38800. [CrossRef] [PubMed]
15. de Oliveira, M.G.G. S-Nitrosothiols as platforms for topical nitric oxide delivery. *Basic Clin. Pharmacol. Toxicol.* **2016**, *119* (Suppl. S3), 49–56. [CrossRef] [PubMed]
16. Rosi, N.L.; Eckert, J.; Eddaoudi, M.; Vodak, D.T.; Kim, J.; O'Keeffe, M.; Yaghi, O.M. Hydrogen storage in microporous metal-organic frameworks. *Science* **2003**, *300*, 1127–1129. [CrossRef]
17. Peng, Y.; Krungleviciute, V.; Eryazici, I.; Hupp, J.T.; Farha, O.K.; Yildirim, T. Methane storage in metal–organic frameworks: Current records, surprise findings, and challenges. *J. Am. Chem. Soc.* **2013**, *135*, 11887–11894. [CrossRef] [PubMed]
18. Sumida, K.; Rogow, D.L.; Mason, J.A.; McDonald, T.M.; Bloch, E.D.; Herm, Z.R.; Bae, T.H.; Long, J.R. Carbon Dioxide capture in metal-organic frameworks. *Chem. Rev.* **2012**, *112*, 724–781. [CrossRef]
19. Alavijeh, R.K.K.; Beheshti, S.; Akhbari, K.; Morsali, A. Investigation of reasons for metal–organic framework's antibacterial activities. *Polyhedron* **2018**, *156*, 257–278. [CrossRef]
20. Chowdhury, P.; Bikkina, C.; Meister, D.; Dreisbach, F.; Gumma, S. Comparison of adsorption isotherms on Cu-BTC metal organic frameworks synthesized from different routes. *Micropor. Mesopor. Mater.* **2009**, *117*, 406–413. [CrossRef]
21. Moellmer, J.; Moeller, A.; Dreisbach, F.; Glaeser, R.; Staudt, R. High pressure adsorption of hydrogen, nitrogen, carbon dioxide and methane on the metal–organic framework HKUST-1. *Micropor. Mesopor. Mater.* **2011**, *138*, 140–148. [CrossRef]
22. Martín-Calvo, A.; García-Pérez, E.; García-Sánchez, A.; Bueno-Pérez, R.; Hamad, S.; Calero, S. Effect of air humidity on the removal of carbon tetrachloride from air using Cu-BTC metal-organic framework. *Phys. Chem. Chem. Phys.* **2011**, *13*, 11165–11174. [CrossRef] [PubMed]
23. Chowdhury, P.; Mekala, S.; Dreisbach, F.; Gumma, S. Adsorption of CO, CO_2 and CH_4 on Cu-BTC and MIL-101 metal organic frameworks: Effect of open metal sites and adsorbate polarity. *Micropor. Mesopor. Mater.* **2012**, *152*, 246–252. [CrossRef]
24. Férey, G.; Latroche, M.; Serre, C.; Millange, F.; Loiseau, T.; Percheron-Guégan, A. Hydrogen adsorption in the nanoporous metal-benzenedicarboxylate $M(OH)(O_2C\text{-}C_6H_4\text{-}CO_2)$ ($M = Al^{3+}, Cr^{3+}$), MIL-53. *Chem. Commun. (Camb)* **2003**, *2976*, 2976–2977. [CrossRef] [PubMed]

25. Ferey, G.; Mellot-Draznieks, C.; Serre, C.; Millange, F.J.; Dutour, S. Surble and I. Margiolaki, A. chromiumterephthalate-based solid with unusually large pore volumes and surface area. *Science* **2005**, *309*, 2040–2042. [CrossRef]
26. Horcajada, P.; Serre, C.; Vallet-Regí, M.; Sebban, M.; Taulelle, F.; Férey, G. Metal-organic frameworks as efficient materials for drug delivery. *Angew. Chem. Int. Ed. Engl.* **2006**, *45*, 5974–5978. [CrossRef]
27. Bauer, S.; Serre, C.; Devic, T.; Horcajada, P.; Marrot, J.; Férey, G.; Stock, N. High-throughput assisted rationalization of the formation of metal organic frameworks in the iron(III) aminoterephthalate solvothermal system. *Inorg. Chem.* **2008**, *47*, 7568–7576. [CrossRef]
28. Xiao, B.; Wheatley, P.S.; Zhao, X.; Fletcher, A.J.; Fox, S.; Rossi, A.G.; Megson, I.L.; Bordiga, S.; Regli, L.; Thomas, K.M.; et al. High-capacity hydrogen and nitric oxide adsorption and storage in a metal-organic framework. *J. Am. Chem. Soc.* **2007**, *129*, 1203–1209. [CrossRef]
29. McKinlay, A.C.; Xiao, B.; Wragg, D.S.; Wheatley, P.S.; Megson, I.L.; Morris, R.E. Exceptional behavior over the whole adsorption-storage-delivery cycle for no in porous metal organic frameworks. *J. Am. Chem. Soc.* **2008**, *130*, 10440–10444. [CrossRef] [PubMed]
30. Peikert, K.; McCormick, L.J.; Cattaneo, D.; Duncan, M.J.; Hoffmann, F.; Khan, A.H.; Bertmer, M.; Morris, R.E.; Fröba, M. Tuning the nitric oxide release behavior of amino functionalized HKUST-1. *Micropor. Mesopor. Mater.* **2015**, *216*, 118–126. [CrossRef]
31. Khan, A.H.; Peikert, K.; Hoffmann, F.; Fröba, M.; Bertmer, M. Nitric oxide adsorption in Cu3btc2-type MOFs-physisorption and chemisorption as NONOates. *J. Phys. Chem. C* **2019**, *123*, 4299–4307. [CrossRef]
32. Pinto, R.V.; Antunes, F.; Pires, J.; Graça, V.; Brandão, P.; Pinto, M.L. Vitamin B3 metal-organic frameworks as potential delivery vehicles for therapeutic nitric oxide. *Acta Biomater.* **2017**, *51*, 66–74. [CrossRef] [PubMed]
33. Tanabe, K.K.; Cohen, S.M. Post synthetic modification of metal-organic frameworks-a progress report. *Chem. Soc. Rev.* **2011**, *40*, 498–519. [CrossRef]
34. DeCoste, J.B.; Peterson, G.W.; Schindler, B.J.; Killops, K.L.; Browe, M.A.; Mahle, J.J. The effect of water adsorption on the structure of the carboxylate containing metal–organic frameworks Cu-BTC, Mg-MOF-74, and UiO-66. *J. Mater. Chem. A* **2013**, *1*, 11922. [CrossRef]
35. Chen, M.; Ye, Q.; Jiang, S.; Shao, M.; Jin, C.; Huang, Z. Two-step elution recovery of cyanide platinum using functional metal organic resin. *Molecules* **2019**, *24*, 2779. [CrossRef]
36. Kaur, R.; Kaur, A.; Umar, A.; Anderson, W.A.; Kansal, S.K. Metal organic framework (MOF) porous octahedral nanocrystals of Cu-BTC: Synthesis, properties and enhanced adsorption properties. *Mater. Res. Bull.* **2019**, *109*, 124–133. [CrossRef]
37. Davydovskaya, P.; Pohle, R.; Tawil, A.; Fleischer, M. Work function based gas sensing with Cu-BTC metal-organic framework for selective aldehyde detection. *Sens. Actuators B* **2013**, *187*, 142–146. [CrossRef]
38. Hosseini, M.S.; Zeinali, S.; Sheikhi, M.H. Fabrication of capacitive sensor based on Cu-BTC (MOF-199) nanoporous film for detection of ethanol and methanol vapors. *Sens. Actuators B* **2016**, *230*, 9–16. [CrossRef]
39. Kidanemariam, A.; Lee, J.; Park, J. Recent innovation of metal-organic frameworks for carbon dioxide photocatalytic reduction. *Polymers* **2019**, *11*, 2090. [CrossRef]
40. Eubank, J.F.; Wheatley, P.S.; Lebars, G.; McKinlay, A.C.; Leclerc, H.; Horcajada, P.; Daturi, M.; Vimont, A.; Morris, R.E.; Serre, C. Porous, rigid metal (III). *APL Mater.* **2014**, *2*, 124112. [CrossRef]
41. Nguyen, J.G.; Tanabe, K.K.; Cohen, S.M. Postsynthetic diazeniumdiolate formation and NO release from MOFs. *CrystEngComm* **2010**, *12*, 2335. [CrossRef]
42. Gallis, D.F.S.S.; Vogel, D.J.; Vincent, G.A.; Rimsza, J.M.; Nenoff, T.M. NOx Adsorption and optical detection in rare earth metal−organic frameworks. *ACS Appl. Mater. Interfaces* **2019**, *11*, 43270–43277. [CrossRef] [PubMed]
43. Pirillo, J.; Hijikata, Y. Trans Influence across a Metal−Metal Bond of a Paddle-Wheel Unit on Interaction with Gases in a Metal−Organic Framework. *Inorg. Chem.* **2020**, *59*, 1193–1203. [CrossRef] [PubMed]
44. Jeong, N.C.; Samanta, B.; Lee, C.Y.; Farha, O.K.; Hupp, J.T. Coordination-chemistry control of proton conductivity in the iconic metal−organic framework material HKUST-1. *J. Am. Chem. Soc.* **2012**, *134*, 51–54. [CrossRef] [PubMed]
45. Majano, G.; Pérez-Ramírez, J. Room temperature synthesis and size control of HKUST-1. *Helv. Chim. Acta* **2012**, *95*, 2278–2286. [CrossRef]
46. Umemura, A.; Diring, S.; Furukawa, S.; Uehara, H.; Tsuruoka, T.; Kitagawa, S. Morphology design of porous coordination polymer crystals by coordination modulation. *J. Am. Chem. Soc.* **2011**, *133*, 15506–15513. [CrossRef]
47. Emam, H.E.; Darwesh, O.M.; Abdelhameed, R.M. In-growth metal organic framework/synthetic hybrids as antimicrobial fabrics and its toxicity. *Colloids Surf. B Biointerfaces* **2018**, *165*, 219–228. [CrossRef]
48. Song, F.; Zhong, Q.; Zhao, Y. A protophilic solvent-assisted solvothermal approach to Cu-BTC for enhanced CO_2 capture. *Appl. Organomet. Chem.* **2015**, *29*, 612–617. [CrossRef]
49. Schlesinger, M.; Schulze, S.; Hietschold, M.; Mehring, M. Evaluation of synthetic methods for microporous metal-organic frameworks exemplified by the competitive formation of $[Cu_2(btc)_3(H_2O)_3]$ and $[Cu_2(btc)(OH)(H_2O)]$. *Micropor. Mesopor. Mater.* **2010**, *132*, 121–127. [CrossRef]
50. Brunauer, S.; Deming, L.S.; Deming, W.E.; Teller, E. On a Theory of the van der Waals Adsorption of Gases. *J. Am. Chem. Soc.* **1940**, *62*, 1723–1732. [CrossRef]
51. Wei, X.; Wang, X.; Gao, B.; Zou, W.; Dong, L. Facile ball-milling synthesis of CuO/biochar nanocomposites for efficient removal of reactive Red 120. *ACS Omega* **2020**, *5*, 5748–5755. [CrossRef] [PubMed]

52. Kitagawa, S.; Kitaura, R.; Noro, S. Functional porous coordination polymers. *Angew. Chem. Int. Ed. Engl.* **2004**, *43*, 2334–2375. [CrossRef] [PubMed]
53. Kumar, R.S.; Kumar, S.S.; Kulandainathan, M.A. Microporous and mesoporous materials efficient electrosynthesis of highly active Cu3(BTC)2-MOF and its catalytic application to chemical reduction. *Micropor. Mesopor. Mater.* **2013**, *63*, 57. [CrossRef]
54. Kim, K.J.; Li, Y.J.; Kreider, P.B.; Chang, C.H.; Wannenmacher, N.; Thallapally, P.K.; Ahn, H.G. High-rate synthesis of Cu–BTC metal–organic frameworks. *Chem. Commun. (Camb)* **2013**, *49*, 11518–11520. [CrossRef] [PubMed]
55. Friedman, A.; Blecher, K.; Sanchez, D.; Tuckman-Vernon, C.; Gialanella, P.; Friedman, J.M.; Martinez, L.R.; Nosanchuk, J.D. Susceptibility of Gram-positive and -negative bacteria to novel nitric oxide-releasing nanoparticle technology. *Virulence* **2011**, *2*, 217–221. [CrossRef]
56. Lis, M.J.; Caruzi, B.B.; Gil, G.A.; Samulewski, R.B.; Bail, A.; Scacchetti, F.A.P.; Moisés, M.P.; Bezerra, F.M.M. In-Situ Direct synthesis of HKUST-1 in wool fabric for the improvement of antibacterial properties. *Polymers* **2019**, *11*, 713. [CrossRef]
57. Duncan, M.J.; Wheatley, P.S.; Coghill, E.M.; Vornholt, S.M.; Warrender, S.J.; Megson, I.L.; Morris, R.E. Antibacterial efficacy from NO-releasing MOF–polymer films. *Mater. Adv.* **2020**, *1*, 2509. [CrossRef]
58. Sheldrick, G.M. Crystal structure refinement with SHELXL. *Acta Crystallogr. Sect. C Struct. Chem.* **2015**, *71*, 3–8. [CrossRef]

MDPI
St. Alban-Anlage 66
4052 Basel
Switzerland
Tel. +41 61 683 77 34
Fax +41 61 302 89 18
www.mdpi.com

International Journal of Molecular Sciences Editorial Office
E-mail: ijms@mdpi.com
www.mdpi.com/journal/ijms

www.ingramcontent.com/pod-product-compliance
Lightning Source LLC
LaVergne TN
LVHW070400100526
838202LV00014B/1354